Pharmacy Workforce Support Personnel

Pharmacy Workforce Support Personnel

Special Issue Editors

Shane P. Desselle
Kenneth C. Hohmeier

MDPI • Basel • Beijing • Wuhan • Barcelona • Belgrade

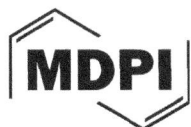

Special Issue Editors
Shane P. Desselle
Touro University California
College of Pharmacy
USA

Kenneth C. Hohmeier
University of Tennessee Health
Sciences Center
USA

Editorial Office
MDPI
St. Alban-Anlage 66
4052 Basel, Switzerland

This is a reprint of articles from the Special Issue published online in the open access journal *Pharmacy* (ISSN 2226-4787) from 2019 to 2020 (available at: https://www.mdpi.com/journal/pharmacy/special_issues/Pharmacy_Workforce_Support).

For citation purposes, cite each article independently as indicated on the article page online and as indicated below:

LastName, A.A.; LastName, B.B.; LastName, C.C. Article Title. *Journal Name* **Year**, *Article Number*, Page Range.

ISBN 978-3-03936-543-2 (Hbk)
ISBN 978-3-03936-544-9 (PDF)

© 2020 by the authors. Articles in this book are Open Access and distributed under the Creative Commons Attribution (CC BY) license, which allows users to download, copy and build upon published articles, as long as the author and publisher are properly credited, which ensures maximum dissemination and a wider impact of our publications.

The book as a whole is distributed by MDPI under the terms and conditions of the Creative Commons license CC BY-NC-ND.

Contents

About the Special Issue Editors vii

Preface to "Pharmacy Workforce Support Personnel" ix

Shane P. Desselle and Kenneth C. Hohmeier
Pharmacy Technicians Help to Push Boundaries in Delivering Quality Care
Reprinted from: *Pharmacy* 2020, *8*, 98, doi:10.3390/pharmacy8020098 1

Bjarke Abrahamsen, Rikke Nørgaard Hansen, Marianne Bjørn-Christensen, Tina Druskeit and Charlotte Rossing
Using Real-Life Data to Strengthen the Education of Pharmacy Technician Students: From Student to Research Assistant
Reprinted from: *Pharmacy* 2020, *8*, 62, doi:10.3390/pharmacy8020062 5

Maryam Jetha, Ali Walji, Paul Gregory, Dalya Abdulla and Zubin Austin
Pharmacist—Pharmacy Technician Intraprofessional Collaboration and Workplace Integration: Implications for Educators
Reprinted from: *Pharmacy* 2020, *8*, 95, doi:10.3390/pharmacy8020095 12

Jon Schommer, William Doucette, Matthew Witry, Vibhuti Arya, Brianne Bakken, Caroline Gaither, David Kreling and David Mott
Pharmacist Segments Identified from 2009, 2014, and 2019 National Pharmacist Workforce Surveys: Implications for Pharmacy Organizations and Personnel
Reprinted from: *Pharmacy* 2020, *8*, 49, doi:10.3390/pharmacy8020049 25

Taylor G. Bertsch and Kimberly C. McKeirnan
Perceived Benefit of Immunization-Trained Technicians in the Pharmacy Workflow
Reprinted from: *Pharmacy* 2020, *8*, 71, doi:10.3390/pharmacy8020071 47

Tamera D. Hughes, Lana M. Minshew, Stacey Cutrell and Stefanie P. Ferreri
T.E.A.M.S.Work: Leveraging Technicians to Enhance ABM Med Sync in
Community Pharmacies
Reprinted from: *Pharmacy* 2020, *8*, 51, doi:10.3390/pharmacy8020051 57

Chelsea Renfro, Davis Coulter, Lan Ly, Cindy Fisher, Lindsay Cardosi, Mike Wasson and Kenneth C. Hohmeier
Exploring Pharmacy Technician Roles in the Implementation of an Appointment-Based Medication Synchronization Program
Reprinted from: *Pharmacy* 2020, *8*, 28, doi:10.3390/pharmacy8010028 64

Deeb Eid, Joseph Osborne and Brian Borowicz
Moving the Needle: A 50-State and District of Columbia Landscape Review of Laws Regarding Pharmacy Technician Vaccine Administration
Reprinted from: *Pharmacy* 2019, *7*, 168, doi:10.3390/pharmacy7040168 73

Shane P. Desselle, Kenneth C. Hohmeier and Kimberly C. McKeirnan
The Value and Potential Integration of Pharmacy Technician National Certification into Processes That Help Assure a Competent Workforce
Reprinted from: *Pharmacy* 2019, *7*, 147, doi:10.3390/pharmacy7040147 94

Juanita A. Draime, Emily C. Wicker, Zachary J. Krauss, Joel L. Sweeney and Douglas C. Anderson
Description of Position Ads for Pharmacy Technicians
Reprinted from: *Pharmacy* **2020**, *8*, 88, doi:10.3390/pharmacy8020088 107

David P. Zgarrick, Tatiana Bujnoch and Shane P. Desselle
Wage Premiums as a Means to Evaluate the Labor Market for Pharmacy Technicians in the United States: 1997–2018
Reprinted from: *Pharmacy* **2020**, *8*, 42, doi:10.3390/pharmacy8010042 120

Ryan Burke
Embracing the Evolution of Pharmacy Practice by Empowering Pharmacy Technicians
Reprinted from: *Pharmacy* **2020**, *8*, 66, doi:10.3390/pharmacy8020066 129

Melanie Boughen and Tess Fenn
Practice, Skill Mix, and Education: The Evolving Role of Pharmacy Technicians in Great Britain
Reprinted from: *Pharmacy* **2020**, *8*, 50, doi:10.3390/pharmacy8020050 133

Kristenbella AYR Lee, Joanna E. Harnett, Carolina Oi Lam Ung and Betty Chaar
Impact of Up-Scheduling Medicines on Pharmacy Personnel, Using Codeine as an Example, with Possible Adaption to Complementary Medicines: A Scoping Review
Reprinted from: *Pharmacy* **2020**, *8*, 65, doi:10.3390/pharmacy8020065 142

Mira El-Souri, Rikke Nørgaard Hansen, Ann Moon Raagaard, Birthe Søndergaard and Charlotte Rossing
Pharmacy Technicians' Contribution to Counselling at Community Pharmacies in Denmark
Reprinted from: *Pharmacy* **2020**, *8*, 48, doi:10.3390/pharmacy8010048 153

Rebecca Chamberlain, Jan Huyton and Delyth James
Pharmacy Technicians' Roles and Responsibilities in the Community Pharmacy Sector: A Welsh Perspective
Reprinted from: *Pharmacy* **2020**, *8*, 97, doi:10.3390/pharmacy8020097 164

About the Special Issue Editors

Shane P. Desselle, RPh, Ph.D., FAPhA is Professor of Social and Behavioral Pharmacy at Touro University California. He received in B.S. in Pharmacy from University of Louisiana Monroe (ULM) in 1990 and his PhD from ULM in 1995. He has served on the faculty at Long Island University Brooklyn, as Director of Assessment at Duquesne University, Associate Dean and Chair at University of Oklahoma, and Dean at California Northstate University. He is founding Editor-in-Chief of Research in Social and Administrative Pharmacy and Co-editor of Pharmacy Management, Essentials for All Settings, 5th ed, one of the most widely used pharmacy texts in the world. Professor Desselle won the American Association of Colleges of Pharmacy (AACP) Sustained Contribution in Social Sciences Award in 2019 in recognition of his research, teaching, and service in pharmacy education. He conducts research in advancement of pharmacist roles for patient safety, creation of standards for pharmacist care of patients using complementary medicines, and professionalization of pharmacy technicians to advance the delegatory authority of pharmacists. Dr. Desselle has over 100 full-text original research articles in peer-reviewed journals.

Kenneth C. Hohmeier, PharmD is an Associate Professor & Director of Community Affairs in the Department of Clinical Pharmacy and Translational Science at the University of Tennessee Health Science Center. Dr. Hohmeier has an extensive background in pharmacy practice and practice-based and implementation science research, including post-graduate residency training in community pharmacy, credentials in lean six sigma and change leadership, and attending the University of Pennsylvania's Implementation Science Institute. He has successfully established and provided clinical pharmacist services within several community pharmacy settings in a wide variety of rural, suburban, and urban locations. His background also includes extensive leadership experience both in practice and within professional organizations, with past and current positions held at local, regional, and national levels including the American Pharmacists Association, Ohio Pharmacists Association, and Tennessee Public Health Association. His specific areas of research focus are in clinical service implementation in community pharmacy settings, medication therapy management, and innovative clinical pharmacy practice models. He has served as PI or Co-PI on 15 grant-funded projects, most of which explore expanded roles of pharmacy technicians and pharmacists in the community pharmacy to increase patient care activities, such as vaccinations, medication therapy management (MTM), and other clinical services.

Preface to "Pharmacy Workforce Support Personnel"

Pharmacy care has evolved considerably in recent decades. This evolution has quickened in recent years owing to the realization that pharmacy workforce support personnel, namely pharmacy technicians, had to become more widely recognized as integral to this transition. Much of the research on pharmacy technicians has occurred within the past 5–10 years. The research has centered on evolving scopes of practice, pharmacist delegation, quality of work life, and patient safety. This special themed issue of the journal, Pharmacy, is comprised of the most recent research and scholarly commentary on pharmacy technicians, addressing even more advanced roles, their certification and education, skills mix, desired characteristics by employers, and their job earnings, which still are lacking, given their new roles. The papers in this themed issue highlight the progress that has been made but also the challenges that still remain in the transitioning of pharmacy technician jobs into more stable, rewarding, and life-long careers.

Shane P. Desselle, Kenneth C. Hohmeier
Special Issue Editors

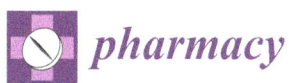

Editorial

Pharmacy Technicians Help to Push Boundaries in Delivering Quality Care

Shane P. Desselle [1,*] and Kenneth C. Hohmeier [2]

1. California College of Pharmacy, Touro University, Vallejo, CA 94592, USA
2. College of Pharmacy, University of Tennessee Health Sciences Center, Nashville, TN 37211, USA; khohmeie@uthsc.edu
* Correspondence: shane.desselle@tu.edu or sdesselle68@gmail.com

Received: 30 May 2020; Accepted: 1 June 2020; Published: 7 June 2020

We are so pleased that *Pharmacy* dedicated a themed Special Issue to pharmacy workforce supportpersonnel, namely technicians. Pharmacy technicians are increasingly recognized for their roles in supporting the delivery of pharmacy care services. The literature of pharmacy technicians has swelledin the past few years, with too many instances of their involvement to entirely enumerate here. We will point out a recently published systematic review that illuminates pharmacy technicians' evolving role in medication therapy management (MTM) [1]. That review underscored the importance of pharmacy technicians in assisting with medication reconciliation and the documentation of services provided. Another study has proffered a new paradigm of practice, the Optimizing Care Model, which leveragesthe concept of tech-check-tech into an organizational culture and workflow redesign concept that helps maximize technicians' effectiveness and allows pharmacists to expand their autonomy [2]. In fact, this study has served as the basis for practice change in one U.S. state to facilitate delegation to pharmacy technicians and has the support of the National Association of Chain Drug Stores, which might drive yet further change more rapidly [3].

It is anticipated that the articles published in this Special Issue will help further advance pharmacy care both in the U.S. and globally. Two of the articles in this themed issue demonstrate the effectivenessof integrating pharmacy technicians into medication synchronization (med sync) programs. Med sync programs have the potential to greatly improve medication adherence, and their success will be aided by further standardization of operational processes [4].Among those processes include a redefinition of technician roles and the use of appointment-based models (ABM) to facilitate patient interaction and prospective drug utilization review. The first of the two articles on med sync ABM employedqualitativeresearch to describe technicians' job descriptions for this type of service [5]. The tasks in which techniciansmight assume greatest responsibility include identifying patients for marketing and enrollment, reviewing patients' medication lists, choosing alignment dates based on patient preference, contacting patients in preparation for dispensing, and engaging in pickup or delivery of medications. A second study employed the Consolidated Framework for Implementation Research (CFIR) to examine not only initial design, but the sustainability of med sync ABM services [6]. The study found that among pharmacy technicians engaged in helping coordinate and deliver these services, in an absence of proper planning for workflow and job redesign, that other tasks might sometimes get short shrift; however, they expressed confidence that minor system flaws can be adjudicated and expressed considerable enthusiasm for their role in helping patients.

Another study in this issue took a holistic approach in examining the evolving roles of pharmacists, technicians and other support personnel, concurrently [7].The study authors demonstrated an increase in the amount of time spent by pharmacists in direct patient care through a segmentation analysis that also bore witness to these pharmacists better integrating those direct patient care activities with distributive functions as well as use of remote locations to provide services. They emphasized the need for training, continuing education, monitoring, regulations, and process designs to keep up with these changes, and hopefully even get ahead of the curve. Boughen and Fenn provided similar optimism and words of advice in moving forward for technician practice in the United Kingdom (U.K.) [8]. The authors described a model of technician education that employed pyramidal structures of technician activities, beginning with assembling medications, up to advanced communication, coupled with education standards that begin with basic customer service and lead up to assistance with medication optimization. They also call for additional research that aims to optimize evolving technician roles in the context of improving patient safety.

In regard to education, Denmark has always been a beacon for its training of their pharmaconomists, who study for three years and require an in-residence component in a national program. Among other rather advanced education paradigms, pharmaconomists receive extensive training in patient communication. El-Souri et al. document how the advanced communication skills of pharmaconomists result in their ability to have identify large numbers of potential and actual drug-related problems during patient consultation, along with the ability to actually resolve many of those problems themselves [9]. The authors suggest that future studies be geared toward affecting policies that might advance patient safety that much further. The training that pharmaconomists receive in Denmark is even further enhanced by strategies often being employed in other health professions programs. In one study noted here, pharmaconomists in training tackled research problems with the requirement that they perform and make formal presentations on their findings, thus sharpening their reasoning, literature review, and communication skills, all while using the opportunity to remain abreast of key pharmacy issues ongoing regionally and throughout the world [10].

The issue of technician education and training has indeed received considerable attention around the world. In the U.S., more states are requiring certification, particularly in light of what has been regarded as uneven quality in technician vocational programs [11]. In this Special Issue, Desselle et al. ascribed value to a national certification process adjudicated by either of two vendors [12]. Pharmacists witness first-hand the value of certification, but especially when it is combined with other education and better linked with formal on-the-job training programs. Pharmacists in the study recognize the contribution of certification for imparting greater professionalism and more advanced knowledge in basic pharmacology and math skills, but recognize the need for certification processes to include more "soft skills" such as advanced communication, leadership, and ethical decision-making. It is hoped that technicians being better prepared and deploying such skills will inspire greater confidence among pharmacists and delegating emerging responsibilities to them. The findings of Jetha et al. further corroborate this notion, suggesting that further integration of such skills into technician education and training is necessary to maximize the benefit of future technician deployment and regulation [13]. An official from one of the certifying organizations in the U.S. speaks to this, and also indicates that they are working with various stakeholders, such as large employers and regulators to improve technician mobility across various settings in considering these basic skills, but also within organizations, such as with career laddering mechanisms [14]. Career ladders provide hope and aspirations to employees that they might make increasingly substantial contributions to the organization and fulfill personal self-actualization goals. The move toward career laddering for technicians has been called for in other research [15,16]. It might very well be demonstration of advanced skills, such as communication, upon which employers decide to use as a basis for job mobility and career laddering, rather than more technical tasks.

Being on the proverbial "front line", technicians are the persons most likely to come into contact with patients with questions around use of opioids, complementary medicine, and a growing array of products transitioning to over-the counter status [17]. Technicians must have the judgment and temperament to field those sensitive questions and know which ones to triage to pharmacists. These are all part of the move toward professional socialization and enhancement of more global competencies among technicians, and are concurrent with the expanding role of the pharmacist in patient care. In this themed issue, Draime et al. analyzed 14 days' worth of job advertisement listings for pharmacy technicians [18]. Among the more common sought-after job qualifications were communication, office etiquette, and professionalism. This comports with other recent studies demonstrating a desire by both technicians and their employers for enhanced professionalization and socialization into the field, so as to make it more endearing as a life-long career [19,20].

Policymakers and regulators must be more nimble and proactive in anticipating needed practice change. A study in Wales saw increases in technicians assuming leadership roles [21]. The study authors recommend not only that technicians seek development opportunities in this area but also that pharmacists become more adept at the art of delegation and work with profession leaders to optimize appropriate staffing levels and skills mix of support personnel to advance practice. Eid et al. pointed out that U.S. state board of pharmacy regulations were often overly prescriptive and favored the term "not expressly prohibited" in regard to many pharmacy technician roles [22]. This might be an improvement over them being previously being prohibited. However, some states like Idaho have taken a different tact, where instead of listing functions that a technician can do, it lists a very succinct list of those that they cannot perform, and instead simply leave it up to the pharmacist to determine the scope of technician practice activities under their supervision [23]. As regulations must keep pace with practice change, so must salary and other economic levers. Zgarrick et al. point out that while technicians are being asked to do more, their salary is not keeping up with these extra responsibilities and additional stressors on the job [24]. They analyzed data from the Bureau of Labor and Statistics to find that technicians have not enjoyed any wage premiums; in fact, those wage premiums (expectations for pay above the rate of inflation) have been flat or even negative in the past decade, and express concern that technicians can sometimes find better-paying jobs among unskilled labor positions. It will be especially important that improvements be made in earning potential and career mobility, as we have likely seen only the beginning in a wave of changes for pharmacy technician practice. Technicians have been involved in coordinating immunization activities, but now are gaining approval as immunizers and are thus side-by-side with pharmacists in helping them to take center stage in public health initiatives [25]. Properly trained technicians can help prevent pharmacists from being overwhelmed during certain seasonal events such as influenza upticks and inspire confidence among patients that pharmacies are an appropriate place to seek health solutions.

The articles in this themed SpecialIssue help to underscore the importance of pharmacy technicians. They also show how far we have come in better integrating technicians into the support of pharmacist-led, patient-centered services. At the same time, we still have much room for improvement, and those issues and gaps are identified. The profession of pharmacy will advance only as far as its constituent workforce personnel advances as well.

Author Contributions: S.P.D. reviewed the literature and conceptualized the paper. K.C.H. assisted with evaluation of articles comprising the special issue and in writing this manuscript. All authors have read and agreed to the published version of the manuscript.

Funding: This research received no external funding.

Conflicts of Interest: The authors declare no conflict of interest.

References

1. Gernant, S.A.; Nguyen, M.O.; Siddiqui, S.; Schneller, M. Use of pharmacy technicians in elements of medication therapy management delivery: A systematic review. *Res. Social. Pharm. Adm.* **2018**, *14*, 883–890. [CrossRef] [PubMed]
2. Hohmeier, K.C.; Desselle, S.P. Exploring the implementation of a novel optimizing care model in the community pharmacy setting. *J. Am. Pharm. Assoc.* **2019**, *59*, 310–318. [CrossRef] [PubMed]
3. *Optimizing Patient Care in Pharmacies is Focus of New Rule Backed by PSW*; NACDS. Available online: https://www.nacds.org/news/optimizing-patient-care-in-pharmacies-is-focus-of-new-rule-backed-by-psw-nacds/?MessageRunDetailID=1454377707&PostID=12364229&utm_medium=email&utm_source=rasa_io. (accessed on 26 March 2020).
4. Patti, M.; Renfro, C.P.; Posey, R. Systematic review of medication synchronization in community pharmacy practice. *Res. Social. Adm. Pharm.* **2019**, *15*, 1281–1288. [CrossRef] [PubMed]

5. Hughes, T.D.; Minshew, L.M.; Cutrell, S.; Ferreri, S.P. TEAMS work: Leveraging technicians to enhance ABM med sync in community pharmacies. *Pharmacy* **2020**, *8*, 51. [CrossRef] [PubMed]
6. Renfro, C.; Coulter, D.; Ly, L. Exploring pharmacy technician roles in the implementation of an appointment-based medication synchronization program. *Pharmacy* **2020**, *8*, 28. [CrossRef]
7. Schommer, J.; Doucette, W.; Witry, M. Pharmacist segments identified from 2009–2014, and 2019 national pharmacist workforce surveys: Implications for pharmacy organizations and personnel. *Pharmacy* **2002**, *8*, 49. [CrossRef]
8. Boughen, M.; Fenn, T. Practice skill mix, and education: The evolving role of pharmacy technicians in Great Britain. *Pharmacy* **2020**, *8*, 50. [CrossRef]
9. El-Souri, M.; Hansen, R.N.; Raagaard, A.M. Pharmacy technicians' contribution to counselling in community pharmacies in Denmark. *Pharmacy* **2020**, *8*, 48. [CrossRef]
10. Abrahamsen, B.; Hansen, R.N.; Bjorn-Christensen, M.; Druskeit, T.; Rossing, C. Using real-life data to strengthen the education of pharmacy technician students: From student to research assistant. *Pharmacy* **2020**, *8*, 62. [CrossRef]
11. Anderson, D.C.; Draime, J.A.; Anderson, T.S. Description and comparison of pharmacy technician training programs in the United States. *J. Am. Pharm. Assoc.* **2016**, *56*, 231–236. [CrossRef]
12. Desselle, S.P.; Hohmeier, K.C.; McKeirnan, K.C. The value of potential integration of pharmacy technician national certification into processes that help assure a competent workforce. *Pharmacy* **2019**, *7*, 147. [CrossRef] [PubMed]
13. Jetha, M.; Walji, A.; Gregory, P.; Abdulla, D.; Austin, Z. Pharmacist-pharmacy technician intraprofessional collaboration and workplace integration: Implications for educators. *Pharmacy* **2020**, *8*, 95. [CrossRef] [PubMed]
14. Burke, R. Embracing the evolution of pharmacy practice by empowering pharmacy technicians. *Pharmacy* **2020**, *8*, 66. [CrossRef] [PubMed]
15. Mattingly, A.N.; Mattingly, T.J. Advancing the role of the pharmacy technician: A systematic review. *J. Am. Pharm. Assoc.* **2018**, *58*, 94–108. [CrossRef]
16. Desselle, S.P. An in-depth examination of into pharmacy technician worklife though an organizational behavior framework. *Res. Social. Adm. Pharm.* **2016**, *12*, 722–732. [CrossRef]
17. Lee, K.A.Y.R.; Harnett, J.; Lam, C.O.L.; Chaar, B. Impact of up-scheduling medicines on pharmacy practice, using codeine as an example with possible adaption to complementary medicines: A systematic scoping review. *Pharmacy* **2020**, *8*, 65. [CrossRef]
18. Draime, J.A.; Wicker, E.C.; Krauss, J. Description of position ads for pharmacy technicians. *Pharmacy* **2020**, *8*, 88. [CrossRef]
19. Wheeler, J.S.; Renfro, C.P.; Wang, J. Assessing pharmacy technician certification: A national survey comparing certified and noncertified pharmacy technicians. *J. Am. Pharm. Assoc.* **2019**, *59*, 369–374.e2. [CrossRef]
20. Desselle, S.P.; Hoh, R.; Rossing, C. Work preferences and general abilities among US pharmacy technicians and Danish pharmaconomists. *J. Pharm. Pract.* **2020**, *33*, 142–152. [CrossRef]
21. Chamberlain Huyton, I.; James, D. Pharmacy techniciansroles and responsibilities in the community pharmacy sector. A Wales perspective. *Pharmacy* **2020**, *8*, 97. [CrossRef]
22. Eid, D.; Osborne, J.; Borowicz, B. Moving the needle: A 50-state and District of Columbia landscape review of laws regarding pharmacy technician vaccine administration. *Pharmacy* **2019**, *7*, 168. [CrossRef] [PubMed]
23. Adams, A.J. Advancing technician practice: Deliberations of a regulatory board. *Res. Social. Adm. Pharm.* **2018**, *14*, 1–5. [CrossRef] [PubMed]
24. Zgarrick, D.P.; Bujnoch, T.; Desselle, S.P. Wage premiums as a means to evaluate the labor market for pharmacy technicians in the United States: 1997–2018. *Pharmacy* **2020**, *8*, 42. [CrossRef] [PubMed]
25. Bertsch, T.; McKeirnan, K.C. Perceived benefit of immunization trained technicians in the pharmacy workflow. *Pharmacy* **2020**, *8*, 71. [CrossRef]

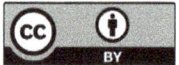

© 2020 by the authors. Licensee MDPI, Basel, Switzerland. This article is an open access article distributed under the terms and conditions of the Creative Commons Attribution (CC BY) license (http://creativecommons.org/licenses/by/4.0/).

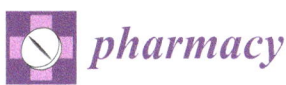

Commentary

Using Real-Life Data to Strengthen the Education of Pharmacy Technician Students: From Student to Research Assistant

Bjarke Abrahamsen [1,*], Rikke Nørgaard Hansen [1], Marianne Bjørn-Christensen [2], Tina Druskeit [2] and Charlotte Rossing [1]

[1] Department of Research and Development, Danish College of Pharmacy Practice, Milnersvej 42, Hillerød 3400, Denmark; RNH@pharmakon.dk (R.N.H.); cr@pharmakon.dk (C.R.)
[2] Department of Education, Danish College of Pharmacy Practice, Milnersvej 42, Hillerød 3400, Denmark; mb@pharmakon.dk (M.B.-C.); tdo@pharmakon.dk (T.D.)
* Correspondence: bja@pharmakon.dk

Received: 5 March 2020; Accepted: 5 April 2020; Published: 8 April 2020

Abstract: This commentary is based on the experience of teaching and observations of how pharmacy technician students can expand their perspective on patient safety by using real-life student-gathered patient data collected from community pharmacies. Pharmacy technicians in Denmark work extensively with counselling on the safe and efficient use of medications. Final-year pharmacy technician students can take the elective course in Clinical Pharmacy in Community Pharmacy, which targets the students who wish to work in depth with patient communication and quality assurance in counselling. One assignment that forms part of the course is for students to collect data about patients' beliefs about medications. Teachers' observations suggest that when students gather and work with their own data, they change their perspective on patients' beliefs about medications. It also strengthens the students' awareness of their responsibility for ensuring patient safety and contributes valid data to research in pharmacy practice.

Keywords: social pharmacy; pharmacy technician student; education; pharmaceutical care; patient safety; pharmacy practice research; medication beliefs

---

1. Pharmacy Technicians Contributing to Patient Safety and Efficient Use of Medications through Education and Practice

Community pharmacies in Denmark contribute to the healthcare system by offering a variety of pharmacy services to support the patients' optimal use of medications [1]. In Denmark, the number of community pharmacies is lower than the European average, with 8.6 community pharmacies per 100,000 citizens compared to the European average of 32 community pharmacies per 100,000 citizens [2]. In Denmark, community pharmacies must be owned by a pharmacist holding a five-year MSc university degree in Pharmacy. Throughout the opening hours of a community pharmacy, a pharmacist must be available in person at the main pharmacy and in close contact for pharmacy branches related to the main pharmacy. The largest group of personnel at Danish community pharmacies is pharmacy technicians who hold a three-year degree, as outlined below. The allocation of responsibilities between pharmacists and pharmacy technicians is decided at each pharmacy according to the Danish Healthcare Quality Program [3] with the owner having the overall responsibility. However, some pharmacy services, such as the new medicine service and medication review, must be undertaken by a pharmacist. Pharmacy technicians have direct patient contact; they counsel patients at community pharmacies and deliver some pharmacy services, e.g., the inhaler technique assessment service. Representative mapping of pharmacy technicians counselling activities in Danish community pharmacies shows that 58.9% of all patients served by a pharmacy technician received counselling [4]. Counselling was provided to all groups of patients; patients getting prescription drugs, over-the-counter drugs, presenting with a symptom, or requesting a non-medical product. Furthermore, pharmacy technicians identified drug-related problems (DRP) for 17.8% of all pharmacy customers and counselled them accordingly, solving or partly solving 70.4% of all identified DRP. The study investigated 17,682 customers served by 76 pharmacy technicians from 38 community pharmacies over a duration of five days [4]. According to the survey on the scope of practice for pharmacy technicians from 2017, pharmacy technicians from other European countries have similar work activities, such as receiving prescriptions, investigating the dose and type of drug, and counselling patients about their medicines. The survey shows that British and Portuguese pharmacy technicians are most comparable with Danish pharmacy technicians [5].

Another study based on answers to a questionnaire from 313 Danish community pharmacy technicians showed that they rank the task of providing customers with information as one of their top three task preferences [6]. Around 68% of pharmacy technician students, as well as qualified pharmacy technicians, hold a position within a community pharmacy [7]. Because most pharmacy technicians working in community pharmacies in Denmark have close communication with patients, they require strong communication competences. This commentary reports experiences with strengthening patient communication skills through an assignment for final-year pharmacy technician students complementing existing courses on safe and efficient use of medications. It reports how the students were prepared for the assignment, how they worked with real patient data, and how the teachers observed changes in the pharmacy technician students' perspective of patients' use of medications.

2. Preparing Pharmacy Technicians in Terms of Patient Safety

The Danish Pharmacy Technician program is a three-year education program equivalent to 180 ECTS (European Credit Transfer System) points. The academic part, which takes place at the Danish College of Pharmacy Practice, corresponds to 85 ECTS points. Students spend a total of 23 weeks taking eight courses at college. Each course lasts two or three weeks, and there are three courses in year one, two in year two, and three in the final year of the program. The practical part of the education program corresponds to 95 ECTS points and takes place at a community pharmacy, where students are employed full-time and are part of the pharmacy schedule except when taking courses at college.

The overall objective of the Danish Pharmacy Technician program is to educate and provide students with the tools and knowledge that enable them to assess and provide professional information and improve patient safety while working in a systematic, methodical, and quality-conscious way to meet needs of the society. The competences that Danish pharmacy technicians gain are professional knowledge, an ethical approach, and a sense of accountability, where consideration of medication user conditions is essential for their practice.

Pharmacy technician students in their final year can choose the elective course in Clinical Pharmacy in Community Pharmacy equivalent to 13 ECTS points. The course focuses on patient safety, patient counselling, rational pharmacotherapy, and awareness of the role of community pharmacies in the healthcare sector. The course particularly targets the pharmacy technician students who wish to work extensively with patient communication and quality assurance of the counselling related to medication safety and rational pharmacotherapy.

The course comprises a total of 16 learning objectives, with four learning objectives associated with the pharmacy technician students' responsibility for providing patient safety and supporting safe and efficient use of medications. The learning objectives relevant to the focus of this commentary are to:

- Become aware of the responsibility of community pharmacies to ensure patient safety;
- Be able to discuss patient safety in the context of community pharmacy practice;
- Acquire the relevant theory and methods for practicing pharmaceutical care and patient safety;
- Be able to counsel using the patient's perspective on health and disease.

The teaching approach is to establish a link between students' own practical experience and the acquired theory. This is achieved through students working alone, in groups, and at plenary sessions discussing the subjects based on their experience.

3. Educational Intervention—Using Real-Life Data

Part of the course on clinical pharmacy in community pharmacy is a specific assignment using student-gathered data. This is to target the teaching and augment students' perspectives on issues such as awareness of how different behaviors can affect adherence to medications and how pharmacy staff can support the patient's adherence. The assignment has the following learning objectives:

- To become aware of how patients' concerns and requirements influence initiation and continuation of their use of medications (student level);
- To collect data on concerns and necessity for patients' use of medications (course level).

The assignment is centered around students' collection of data based on patient interviews uncovering patients' beliefs about their medications. In the assignment discussed in this commentary, the students were introduced to the theory of the Beliefs about Medicines Questionnaire [8]. The students discussed how a patients' view on necessity and concerns about their medicines could affect their initiation, continuation, and overall adherence to their treatment. The students were prepared for the task through an introduction to the questionnaire before their community pharmacy placement. The students were requested to collect and register data from patients, one questionnaire per patient, during their seventh community pharmacy placement. All data were initially recorded by the students on paper before being electronically registered, also by the students, using a web-based survey tool. In 2018, SelectSurvey was used, and in 2019, Microsoft Forms were used. During their community pharmacy placement, the students received e-mail reminders about data collection and could contact a teacher if they had any questions.

3.1. Outline for the 2018 Approach

- Registered students for the course: 99
- Number of e-mail reminders: 1
- Number of students to contact a teacher: 0
- Students were asked to collect data from 10 patients
- Returned questionnaires: 231 (equaling 2.3 datasets per student)

3.2. Outline for the 2019 Approach

- Registered students for the course: 70
- Number of e-mail reminders: 3
- Number of students to contact a teacher: 0
- Students were asked to collect data from 6 patients
- Returned questionnaires: 311 (equaling 4.4 datasets per student)

4. Qualified Teaching Using Patient Data

Following the data gathering, the results were discussed once students were back at college. Starting with a plenary session, a researcher presented the results and an analysis of the data. The students were encouraged to ask questions about the results and to share their immediate reflections. This session was followed by group discussions where students worked with the results and discussed how to use their new knowledge to generate questions which could be used in a counselling situation to identify patients' perspectives on their use of medications. In the final plenary session, the groups presented their work and received feedback from the teachers and other students.

During the students' subsequent eighth community pharmacy placements, they presented the results of the study to their pharmacy mentor together with suggestions of how to use the results in counselling situations to identify the patients' perspectives on their use of medications. The future use of the results and suggestions was left to the community pharmacy to decide as part of their ongoing quality improvement.

Listed in Table 1 is the summary of what the teachers observed during the teaching in relation to both learning objectives for the course and for the assignment.

Table 1. Summary of the teachers' observations regarding learning objectives.

Learning Objectives for the Course	Summary of Teachers' Observations
Become aware of the responsibility of a community pharmacy to ensure patient safety.	The students became aware that different patients have different needs to discuss and learn how to use medications.
Be able to discuss patient safety in the context of community pharmacy practice.	The students worked extensively with data in groups as well as in plenary sessions. Furthermore, the students presented and discussed the results as part of their subsequent community pharmacy placement.
To acquire the relevant theory and methods to practice pharmaceutical care and patient safety.	Through the work with data, subjects like pharmaceutical care and patient safety were put into the context of the students' work at a community pharmacy.
Be able to counsel using the patient's perspective on health and disease.	By generating questions and interventions, the students demonstrated how to counsel and acknowledge patients' different beliefs about medications.
Learning objectives of the assignment	
Become aware of how patients' concerns and requirements influence initiation and continuation of their use of medications (student level).	The students became aware of patients' concerns and requirements for their medications by comparing their data with pooled data. The students learned first-hand how patients sometimes think differently from pharmacy technicians. Most patients had different views on medication than the students. For example, the students experienced that patients often expressed more concern and less necessity about using medications compared to what the students would expect when they looked at the collected data. The students learned that by using appropriate counselling they can uncover patients' concerns and requirements for medications. This can be done by showing an interest in the patient, listening to the patient, and using questions to target the patients' beliefs about medications, thus facilitating patient safety. Examples of the questions generated include: • "Some patients don't consider this medication necessary, how do you feel about having to take the medication?" • "What thoughts do you have about this medication?" • "Do you know why your doctor has found it necessary for you to use this medication?" • "Some patients are concerned about the side effects. Do you have concerns?" • "Are you managing to take a tablet every morning?" • "How important is it for you to take your medication every day?" • "Do you know the consequences of not taking your medicine every day?" Finally, the students also saw the benefits of a follow-up to support the patient. Through the follow-up, a community pharmacy can uncover patients' concerns and support their use of medications.
Collect patient data on concerns and necessity during community pharmacy placement (course level).	The students registered data during their community pharmacy placement according to the instructions in the questionnaire. These data proved to be of high quality and valid for use in research projects.

5. Discussion

Data collection by students was introduced in 2015 to strengthen the students' perspective on the patients' use of medications and to complement the teaching of the subject already established. By having a questionnaire, students get the experience of asking questions that they may not have the time or courage to ask during a busy working day at the pharmacy. Since 2018, patients have been asked to give their consent for the use of data for research purposes. Both the questionnaire and the introduction were improved to facilitate and support data collection. All students collected and registered data, but not all students registered the intended number of completed questionnaires. From 2018 to 2019, the questionnaire was further improved, and the requested number of questionnaires (one per patient) was reduced from 10 to 6. The changes in the questionnaire, introduction and the possibility for support may be some of the reasons for the increase in the number of completed questionnaires per student from 2.3 to 4.4.

Obtaining student-gathered data from patients representing several community pharmacies and discussing the data in groups as well as during plenary sessions has, according to the teachers' observations, facilitated a change in the students' perspective of patients' beliefs about medications. The teachers' observations highlighted the fact that students' perspectives went from being limited to demonstrating a more empathic understanding of patients' different views, which can have a direct effect on the patients' use of medication. By generating questions and listening to the patients' answers, students demonstrated how to use the knowledge they gained to meet the learning objectives for both student and course levels. During the students' seventh community pharmacy placement, e-mails were sent to remind students to collect and register data. From 2018 to 2019, the total number of returned questionnaires increased from 2.3 to 4.4, possibly due to the increase in reminders from one to three. Students could also contact a teacher with questions about the assignment, but no students used this option. The course is the students' first experience with collecting data for both teaching and research in community pharmacy practice. This adds an increased focus on preparing students to collect valid data. Discussing data collection and introducing students to the theory before the community pharmacy placement is one way to prepare students.

Over the past 20 years, involving MSc in Pharmacy students in pharmacy practice research has proven fruitful for both students and researchers [9]. During a six-month community pharmacy internship, MSc in Pharmacy students contributed to several published studies through data collection using questionnaires and interviews with patients, pharmacy staff, and general practitioners [9].

In 2016, the International Pharmaceutical Federation (FIP) developed a set of Workforce Development Goals (WDG) at the Global Conference on Pharmacy and Pharmaceutical Education, where milestones were established for impactful global development of pharmacy and pharmaceutical science education [10]. Thirteen goals were set under three clusters: academy (focus on schools, universities, and education providers); professional development (focus on the pharmaceutical workforce); and systems (focus on policy development, governmental strategy and planning, and monitoring systems) [10].

This commentary demonstrates that the Danish Pharmacy Technician program supports the three WDG set for the academia. Under the academic capacity, the Danish education of pharmacy technicians is regulated at the governmental level, including pharmaceutical sciences and clinical practice to support the skills required of qualified pharmacy technicians. The education supports a quality-assured needs-based education and training system. Finally, the training in community pharmacy practice and early career development are supported by offering postgraduate training on the core skills needed to work as a pharmacy technician in a Danish community pharmacy [10].

6. Limitations

The students were introduced to collection and registration of data, but no actual control of possible selection bias, errors in data registration, or how the students interacted with patients took place. The evaluation of the teaching and the effect of the students gathering patient data are based on the teachers' observations, leading to a possible bias where the teachers favor a more positive outcome. A formal evaluation of the students' outcome by researchers would have been of great value and is a possibility in the courses in the coming years.

7. Conclusion

Involving pharmacy technician students in data collection at the patient level, according to the teachers' observations, has strengthened the students' awareness of their responsibility to ensure patient safety. The students collected the data that can be used for teaching as well as research and, when discussing the data, the teachers observed an advanced level of understanding from students of how optimal counselling can uncover and accommodate patients' concerns and beliefs about the necessity of using medications. Furthermore, the teachers' observations showed that by generating questions and interventions, the pharmacy technician students demonstrated how to counsel and acknowledge patients' different beliefs about medications. Overall, this commentary reports the experiences from an assignment where students, in addition to their formal academic training, have to relate to real-life data about the patients' perspective of using medications. The teachers' reflections indicate that students working with the data they have collected themselves could be a method to strengthen the students' perspective on optimal patient counselling.

Author Contributions: The following statements should be used: conceptualization, B.A., R.N.H., and C.R.; investigation, B.A. and C.R.; resources, M.B.-C. and T.D.; writing—original draft preparation, B.A.; writing—review and editing, R.N.H. and C.R.; project administration, B.A. and R.N.H. All authors have read and agreed to the published version of the manuscript.

Funding: This research received no external funding.

Conflicts of Interest: The authors declare no conflict of interest.

References

1. Abrahamsen, B.; Burghle, A.H.; Rossing, C. Pharmaceutical Care Services Available in Danish Community Pharmacies. *Int. J. Clin. Pharm.* **2020**. [CrossRef] [PubMed]
2. Pharmaceutical Group of the European Union (PGEU) Annual Report 2018. Available online: https://pgeu-annual-report.eu/accessibility-of-healthcare-services.html (accessed on 19 February 2020).
3. The Danish Institute for Quality and Accreditation in Healthcare. Introduction to DDKM. Available online: https://www.ikas.dk/den-danske-kvalitetsmodel/ddkm-in-english/introduction-to-ddkm/ (accessed on 25 March 2020).
4. El-Souri, M.; Hansen, R.N.; Raagaard, A.M.; Søndergaard, B.; Rossing, C. Pharmacy technicians' contribution to counselling at community pharmacies in Denmark. *Pharmacy* **2020**, *8*, 48. [CrossRef] [PubMed]
5. European Association of Pharmacy Technicians. Community Pharmacy Technicians—European Survey. 2017. Available online: https://www.eapt.info/app/download/28926841/EAPT+European+Survey+%282017%29+Community+Pharmacy+Technicians.pdf (accessed on 19 February 2020).
6. Desselle, S.P.; Hoh, R.; Rossing, C.; Holmes, E.R.; Gill, A.; Zamora, L. Work Preferences and General Abilities Among US Pharmacy Technicians and Danish Pharmaconomists. *J. Pharm. Pract.* **2018**. [CrossRef] [PubMed]
7. Bjarke, A. (Ed.) *Pharmacy Technicians Employed in Community Pharmacy*; Danish Association of Pharmaconomists: Copenhagen, Denmark, 2020.
8. Horne, R.; Weinman, J.; Hankins, M. The beliefs about medicines questionnaire: The development and evaluation of a new method for assessing the cognitive representation of medication. *Psychol. Health* **1999**, *14*, 1–24. [CrossRef]

9. Sørensen, E.W.; Haugbølle, L.S.; Herborg, H.; Tomsen, D.V. Improving situated learning in pharmacy internship. *Pharm. Educ.* **2018**, *5*, 223–233. [CrossRef]
10. International Pharmaceutical Federation. *Pharmaceutical Workforce Development Goals*; International Pharmaceutical Federation: Hague, The Netherlands, 2016.

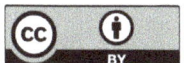

© 2020 by the authors. Licensee MDPI, Basel, Switzerland. This article is an open access article distributed under the terms and conditions of the Creative Commons Attribution (CC BY) license (http://creativecommons.org/licenses/by/4.0/).

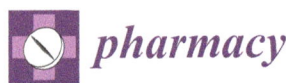

Article

Pharmacist—Pharmacy Technician Intraprofessional Collaboration and Workplace Integration: Implications for Educators

Maryam Jetha [1], Ali Walji [1], Paul Gregory [1], Dalya Abdulla [2] and Zubin Austin [3,*]

1. Leslie Dan Faculty of Pharmacy, University of Toronto, Toronto, ON M5S 3M2, Canada; maryam.jetha.16@ucl.ac.uk (M.J.); ali.walji16@ucl.ac.uk (A.W.); streetsoccercanada@mac.com (P.G.)
2. Faculty of Applied Health and Community Studies, Sheridan College Institute of Technology and Advanced Learning, Brampton, ON L6Y 5H9, Canada; dalya.abdulla@sheridancollege.ca
3. Leslie Dan Faculty of Pharmacy and the Institute for Health Policy, Management, and Evaluation—Faculty of Medicine, University of Toronto, Toronto, ON M5S 3M2, Canada
* Correspondence: zubin.austin@utoronto.ca; Tel.: +1-(416)-978-0186

Received: 14 May 2020; Accepted: 30 May 2020; Published: 1 June 2020

Abstract: Globally, concerns have been expressed regarding the impact of regulation of pharmacy technicians. After more than a decade of experience with technician regulation in Ontario, Canada, uptake of the full scope of practice for technicians has been sporadic at best. The objective of this study was to examine barriers and facilitators to intraprofessional collaboration between pharmacists and pharmacy technicians for the purpose of identifying possible curricular or educational interventions to enhance workplace integration. A qualitative, interview-based study of 24 pharmacists, technicians, educators, pharmacy managers, and owners was undertaken using a semi-structured interview guide. Key findings of this research include: (i) Confirmation of suboptimal utilization of regulated technicians in practice; (ii) identification of crucial knowledge and skills gaps for both pharmacists and technicians; and (iii) proposals for undergraduate education and training, and continuing professional development learning opportunities to address these gaps. In order to achieve the promise and potential of regulation of pharmacy technicians, system-wide change management—beginning with education—will be required and will benefit from multiple stakeholder engagement and involvement.

Keywords: pharmacy technician; collaboration; community pharmacy practice; pharmacy technician education; continuing professional development

1. Introduction

Historically, the role of the pharmacy technician in Ontario, Canada, has grown out of the work of those who assisted pharmacists in day-to-day dispensary related duties [1]. As an unregulated workforce under direct supervision and control of pharmacists, pharmacy assistants performed a wide variety of activities, including dispensing, compounding, inventory control, and in some cases, provision of education, support, or information to patients. In this role, assistants had little or no formal legal liability, no professional responsibilities, and unstandardized education, training, and practice-readiness assessment [2,3]. It is difficult to pinpoint when and the reasons why the assistant role evolved into the (unregulated) pharmacy technician role, and why the change in title occurred. Formal education, assessment, and clinical training programs for pharmacy technicians began to proliferate in the 1980s and 1990s, usually in second-order post-secondary educational institutions (e.g., community colleges rather than universities) [1,3,4]. Over time, standardized curricula and assessment models evolved, as did a growing professional ethos that viewed the pharmacy technician role as complementary to, rather than completely subsumed under, the role of the pharmacist [2]. As the technical complexity of pharmacy work evolved, thus too has the job description, expectations, and academic requirements for pharmacy technicians. In many jurisdictions—including Ontario—pharmacy technicians and pharmacy assistants work side by side, potentially leading to confusion for both the public and pharmacists who may not understand the distinction between the two roles and titles [3–5].

The regulation of pharmacy technicians was initially proposed and enacted as part of a broader strategy to support pharmacists in providing an expanded scope of practice and more impactful patient care services to the public [5,6]. A recent study suggested that regulated pharmacy technicians could yield time savings of close to 20%, allowing pharmacists greater opportunities for patient care [6]. Other studies suggest that the quality of pharmacy technician-led dispensing was higher, with lower error rates and greater operational efficiency [7]. Regulators viewed regulation as an important step in enhancing standardization of education and training, ensuring minimal competency, and providing a formal vehicle for defining responsibility and legal liability for the work undertaken by pharmacy technicians [8]. In regulating pharmacy technicians, there was also an implicit understanding that a professional ethos would grow, and standards of practice, competency expectations, and continuing professional development requirements would evolve [9,10]. Many jurisdictions in Europe, the UK, the US, and Canada began to develop formal frameworks for the regulation of pharmacy technicians while still maintaining an informal and unregulated pharmacy assistant role [11,12].

Ontario is the largest province in Canada; at present, there are 4861 registered pharmacy technicians [1]. The Ontario College of Pharmacists (the regulatory body for the profession) has implemented a regulatory scheme for pharmacy technicians that provides opportunities for pharmacists to focus on cognitive services while providing a high degree of independence for technicians to perform a variety of other important dispensary-related activities (see Table A1) [1,10]. It was hoped that this scheme would promote greater intraprofessional collaboration, facilitating expanded opportunities for pharmacists to engage in cognitive services aimed at enhancing patient care outcomes. Anecdotally, this hope has not been fully realized, particularly in the community pharmacy sector [10]. Regulated technicians continue to be underutilized with respect to their knowledge and skills, and pharmacists are unclear as to how best to leverage this workforce to open up additional opportunities for non-technical patient care services [13]. Worse, regulated technicians have noted that, despite additional educational requirements and regulatory obligations (both of which are costly and time-consuming), they have not enjoyed enhanced professional, employment, or remuneration opportunities commensurate with their increasingly professionalized role [13]. While regulated pharmacy technicians in the hospital sector appear somewhat better integrated with the intraprofessional workflow, community-based regulated pharmacy technicians appear to be less impactful—and satisfied—than was initially hoped [10,14,15].

Recently, there has been increased interest in exploring barriers and enablers to the integration of regulated technicians in the workforce. Renfro et al. examined employer perceptions of pharmacy technicians in community settings and highlighted knowledge and skills gaps related to interpersonal competencies that may limit fuller integration [16]. Banks et al. have examined the economic benefits of pharmacy technicians practicing at advanced scope; they similarly note that further development of the technician curriculum may be required in order to truly unleash the potential of the role, though they do not provide specific recommendations for curricular content reform [17]. Desselle has used an organizational behavior framework to describe pharmacy technician work life. This work highlighted the need for self-actualization and the quest to provide value to the organization as important issues and signpost ways in which current education and training programs serve as barriers and facilitators to fuller integration [11]. Across much of this literature, there is little explicit focus on pharmacy technician curriculum and training as an object of research interest.

The objective of this research was to understand and describe barriers and facilitators to intraprofessional collaboration and integration between community-based regulated pharmacy technicians and pharmacists, with a particular emphasis on educational and curricular gaps in knowledge and skills.

2. Materials and Methods

As there has been little formal research exploring the issue of integration and collaboration between pharmacists and regulated pharmacy technicians, exploratory research was used in order to explore the boundaries of this research while providing opportunities to define future areas for focused research. A qualitative research method was selected in order to support the integration of diverse opinions and experiences and to ensure multiple stakeholders were involved and engaged in the research process. Semi-structured interviews were identified as the main data-gathering tool for this research; one-on-one interviews with multiple stakeholders would allow for the fullest exploration of different experiences and beliefs in a manner that would encourage individual participants to be honest and forthright in their disclosures. Since the emphasis in this project was on implications for educators, 3 major cohorts were identified for inclusion as participants: Regulated pharmacy technicians (both senior-level students and recently qualified individuals), community pharmacists (both practitioners and managers/owners), and educators (in both pharmacy technician and pharmacy programs). While each cohort would bring different perspectives, there would also be significant overlap between categories; for example, some participants would be both pharmacy owners and pharmacy educators. The term "educator" in this study was applied broadly and included those who delivered formal planned lectures within a post-secondary education program, as well as those who served as clinical mentors/preceptors to trainees (either pharmacy technician or pharmacy students) within their community practices, and for whom teaching was not a primary professional identity. Given the exploratory nature of this research, we felt it was important to support a broad array of different participants with diverse experiences and backgrounds, all focused on the same topic of interest; to that end, the same semi-structured interview guide (see Table A2) was used for all participants—regardless of background—though latitude was built into this protocol to support the participant's emphasizing areas or topics of specific personal interest.

A combination of convenience, snowballing, and purposive sampling was used to recruit participants. Convenience sampling involved research team members approaching known informants with specific expertise or interest in this research area with an invitation to participate. Snowball sampling involved asking these participants to recommend other colleagues who they felt might be interested in participating and who may be valuable in helping the research team address our objectives. Purposive sampling involved a deliberate attempt to ensure that convenience and snowball sampling methods did not inadvertently result in excess of certain categories of participants (e.g., too many regulated technicians or too few pharmacy educators). Importantly, no attempt was made to ensure the demographic representativeness of participants. Initial recruitment for this study was undertaken through a general announcement placed on social media (Facebook and Instagram), indicating the purpose of the study and inviting individuals who were interested in participating to self-identify. Participants were then informally approached by members of the research team to consider involvement in a 30–45-min audiotaped interview to discuss issues related to pharmacist-pharmacy technician integration and collaboration. If agreeable, participants completed informed consent pursuant to a research protocol approved by the University of Toronto. Participants were informed that no compensation was available for involvement in this study. A research team member would then arrange to interview the participant at a mutually convenient time in person, by phone, or through a mutually agreed-upon technology platform (such as skype, GoogleHangouts, Facebook Messenger, etc.). In addition to audio and/or video recording of interviews, researchers maintained field notes to help confirm understanding of content.

Verbatim transcripts of all interviews were produced and analyzed using an inductive coding method described by Yin [18]. The trustworthiness of data interpretation was established through triangulation principles described by Lincoln and Guba [19]: Each transcript was reviewed by a minimum of 2 independent researchers who developed, then reconciled coding structures to categorize data and develop themes. Field notes were used to confirm thematic understanding, and the coding structure evolved iteratively with subsequent analyses. According to the research protocol, interviews were to progress to data saturation, the point at which no additional new information or themes were identified. In practice (given the inevitable lag time between interview, transcription, individual coding, and team reconciliation of themes), more interviews than were necessary were undertaken beyond the point of saturation, and these additional interviews were then available for use for confirmatory and triangulation purposes. All data for this study were managed and maintained using a combination of nVivo 11.1, Microsoft Excel, and Microsoft Word.

3. Findings and Discussion

A total of 24 individuals from different backgrounds participated in this research; see Table A3 for the demographic profile of participants. As noted, there were 9 recent pharmacy technician graduates, 9 students currently enrolled in pharmacy technician education programs, and 6 were community pharmacists who also participated (to varying degrees and intensity) as pharmacy technician or pharmacy educators (either as formal lecturers in academic programs or as clinical mentors/preceptors for experiential training).

Based on this research, three key themes were identified: (a) Integration of regulated pharmacy technicians in community pharmacy is neither consistent nor is it widespread; (b) fuller integration is limited due to identified knowledge and skills gaps that potentially could be addressed through educational programs for pharmacists and pharmacy technicians; and (c) lack of a clear business model to ensure the sustainability of an integrated workforce is a major obstacle to fuller integration.

(a) Integration of regulated pharmacy technicians in community pharmacy is neither consistent nor is it widespread

Across all interviews and participants, a clear and common perspective was the "disappointing" way in which the integration of regulated pharmacy technicians has progressed in community practice in Ontario.

> "Well you can't help but feel a bit depressed by it. I mean in school they tell us that we are going to be regulated and professionals and this will open up so many opportunities and jobs and like we are really needed and everything. But then when you start working—well, it was exactly the same as before I went to school, I got a little bit of a raise but really nothing, and the job was still the same."

Most participants in this research suggested that a career pathway for regulated technicians was clearer and better established within hospital pharmacies rather than in community practice, in part because the work of pharmacists and technicians is more clearly delineated.

> "Of course it works better in hospital because everyone—well, there is a specific job for the [regulated] technician and the pharmacist doesn't do that anymore."

Similar to findings by Alkhateeb et al [20], most of the pharmacy technicians (students, recent graduates, and teachers) also noted that larger organizations, some of which are unionized, create better working conditions for a fuller expression of the regulated pharmacy technician roles and responsibilities.

> "I guess it makes sense. I mean a typical drug store, they don't have the resources so of course there are limits. I think it's also that in hospital some of the [regulated technicians] are unionized, right, so the unions, well they fight for the rights of the technicians to make sure they are respected and all that."

A key finding of this study was confirmation that, despite over a decade of legislation and support, integration of regulated pharmacy technicians in community practice has been sporadic at best, and most regulated technicians are not practicing to their fullest potential or scope.

(b) Fuller integration is limited due to identified knowledge and skills gaps that could potentially be addressed through educational programs for pharmacists and pharmacy technicians.

Participants in this study described the integration of regulated technicians into community practice as a process that appears to have become stalled or incomplete. When asked to reflect upon causes, all participants highlighted gaps in knowledge and skill that limited capacity for integration. Key gaps included: (i) Communication/interpersonal skills; (ii) conflict management and negotiation skills; (iii) professionalism and professional ethics; and (iv) practice management/practice readiness. Importantly, these gaps were almost entirely and consistently framed around so-called "soft-skills" deficits, rather than foundational knowledge (e.g., pharmacology, jurisprudence), or technical/procedural skills (e.g., dispensing, compounding, bulk manufacturing, etc.). Though describing the same or substantially similar gaps, pharmacists in this study framed the issue as one of "trusting" regulated technicians with certain tasks, while technicians framed the same issue as one of "self-confidence" in performing tasks.

> "I say this as someone who is both a manager of a pharmacy and who teaches in [a technician education program]. Even some of my best students … well, you have to have faith, you have to trust them to do certain things on their own, without you there and I'm not sure most of them … well, the program just doesn't provide them with that level of preparation to deal with real world issues and patients."

(i) Key communication/interpersonal gaps related to the basic understanding of patient psychology, motivational interviewing, and human behavior, as opposed to basic customer service skills. Understanding of issues such as the psychology of health and illness, complex family dynamics, managing cultural diversity, and cultural competency, and dealing with diverse sexualities and orientations were all identified as crucial for success in community practice but frequently absent in the formal education, training, and assessment of regulated technicians. Most participants described the need for nuanced and sophisticated interpersonal skills in community pharmacy practice as an essential factor for success; pharmacists, technicians, students and educators all agreed that pharmacy technician education programs do not adequately prepare students for this reality and that in most cases students selecting these programs do not have significant natural strengths in these areas:

> "Working with patients—it's really hard. And I think most pharmacy technicians, I mean the kind of person that studies this—well, they likely are more on the technical side not the personal side so this won't be something that comes naturally or easily to them, working with difficult situations and patients. That's why the programs—the teachers—really need to step up and make sure this is part of the program itself, to teach people to get them ready for reality. Otherwise no, integration will never happen, it can't happen".

(ii) Conflict Management and Negotiation Skills One particular sub-type of communication skills was strongly emphasized as a knowledge and skill gap by all participants in this research—the ability to manage conflict and successfully negotiate outcomes with diverse patients and colleagues. Conflict management consistently emerged as one of the most important skills deficits that limited fuller integration of pharmacy technicians into community practice, and again was framed as a "Trust" issue by pharmacists and a "self-confidence" issue by technicians. As noted by Pervanas et al. [21]. This is particularly important in the context of communication across dispensing errors or near misses. Most participants expressed the belief that conflict management and negotiation are skills that can be taught and assessed, and strongly endorsed the idea that this should be integral to the technician education program and curriculum, on part with basic courses such as pharmacology or pharmacy math:

> "It's the most common thing in [community pharmacy] right? You're always getting into disagreements or arguments – about insurance, drug shortages, whatever. And I know for myself, my nature—I'm just not the kind of person that knows how to argue properly or to stand up for myself or just stay calm when things get heated. It's really frustrating—I mean, I don't think I actually SHOULD be

trusted with some of the jobs regulated technicians are eligible to do ... I know I don't have the skills you need so I'm glad the pharmacist is there to do it instead. I just wish though they had taught me more about this in school."

(iii) Professionalism and Professional Ethics The question of whether pharmacy technicians are "professionals" is one that has parallels for pharmacists; the technical focus of the field itself may suggest they are not professionals, while the responsibilities and unique skills associated with the role are highly suggestive of profession-hood. Participants in this study noted challenges they experienced in articulating what professional status means in the context of pharmacy technicians and tended to revert to a series of behavioral characteristics (e.g., punctuality, reliability, honesty) rather than character traits or occupational characteristics associated with specific and unique knowledge and skills. Further to this point, most participants in this study noted that the current structure of community pharmacy practice limited the formation of a professional identity as pharmacists maintained significant control over most activities. This inhibition of professional identity formation was seen as significantly detrimental to fuller integration in practice.

"You know, I find it ironic I guess. For years I've heard pharmacists complain about doctors holding them back, putting them down, not letting them do their best or their jobs to the fullest, and how this wastes [the pharmacist's] talent and potential as a professional. That's exactly what pharmacists are doing to [pharmacy technicians]. They don't let us flourish, and then they complain we're not professional enough or integrating well enough!"

For many technicians in this study, a large part of this problem relates to the lack of a truly independent scope of practice unique from pharmacists; so long as pharmacists can (legally) do everything regulated technicians can do, there would be no need for a separate profession. In the absence of a unique skill set and body of knowledge that does not duplicate what pharmacists already do, no unique professional ethics can—or needs to—evolve, and this further stunts the development of the field into a profession and limits true integration.

"Let's be real ... at the end of the day it still all comes down to what the pharmacist wants and does and as long as that's the case, we'll always only be helpers, not actual professionals. If there were actually real decisions I had to make on my own, and take responsibility—then yeah I'd be a professional. But I'm not. What frustrates me though is that a lot of times I know these pharmacists—well besides a degree there's nothing special about them that is different from most [regulated pharmacy technicians] but still, that's the way it is."

Most participants in this study identified the need for and value of focused education and training in the area of professionalism and professional ethics as a way of enhancing both self-confidence and trustworthiness in pharmacy technicians to assume more complex layers of responsibility and thereby integrate more fully into practice. The notion that professionalism and professional ethics are things that can be taught, learned, and assessed—and should be within the pharmacy technician education program—was widely endorsed by all participants in this study and highlighted as a specific strategy to enhance better uptake of technicians in community practice.

(iv) Practice Management/Practice Readiness A final category of knowledge and skills gaps identified by participants in this study that limited full integration in community practice were practice management and practice readiness capabilities. These capabilities were broadly framed as a series of attributes related to self-motivation, ability to balance risks and benefits, capacity to make and carry out decisions in information-imperfect environments, and ability to take on and assume responsibility rather than simply defer to another authority. Such attributes are essential to smooth day to day management and functioning of a community pharmacy, but are rarely explicitly addressed, taught, or assessed in pharmacy technician education programs.

"I guess the biggest issue I have with trusting [regulated pharmacy technicians] to do more is the sense that most of them—well that I know at least—well, they are a bit passive. They don't seem to want to take on responsibility to manage their own problems but instead are always asking for permission, instead of showing initiative. I get that of course—but if they don't have confidence in their own ability, why should I have confidence in their abilities? So it ends up that they end up being stuck in low level positions, and then complain that we aren't letting them live up to their potential."

The circularity in the logic of the comment above highlights a dilemma that was described by many participants, a push-pull between pharmacists and technicians with respect to how much independent responsibility is expected, allowed, or tolerated. Without opportunities to test-drive independent responsibility, these skills cannot develop or flourish—but without self-motivation and initiative to drive the process forward, such opportunities are rarely freely given. The extent to which these are issues of personality and character vs. issues of skills training and curriculum development are unclear; nonetheless, many participants noted how important these capabilities are for successful workplace integration and endorsed the notion that these need to be explicitly included within pharmacy technician education programs. Desselle et al. [22] highlighted similar issues in their examination of future trends in pharmacy technician education. Participants in this study confirmed this perspective and signposted future opportunities for greater partnerships between pharmacy technician and pharmacist education programs, as well as greater alignment within workplaces and with professional associations to take a more coordinated approach to workforce integration.

(c) Lack of a clear business model to ensure the sustainability of an integrated workforce is a major obstacle to fuller integration.

The final common theme through this research was related to the lack of a viable, sustainable business model for integrating higher-paid regulated pharmacy technicians into practice. Commensurate with their knowledge, skills, training, qualifications, and advanced credential, there is a general expectation that regulated pharmacy technicians should be remunerated at a higher level than regulated pharmacy assistants. As this research highlighted, the lack of a clear role for technicians in practice connects to a lack of a viable business plan related to higher rates of remuneration:

"It's a chicken and egg thing ... the [regulated technicians] think they deserve to be paid more—higher—than the pharmacy assistants. That's fair, makes sense. But where does that money come from? What are they doing to add sufficient value and generate additional revenue to make this possible? That's not clear yet. It's not up to [regulated pharmacy technicians] to figure this out ... it's up to pharmacy owners and businesses to create the business plan that makes this possible, and so far – we haven't. So that means integration doesn't happen as well as it could because no one can figure out how to pay for it. Maybe this is something that pharmacy researchers should be working on to help the profession deal with this."

A business plan that simultaneously appropriately compensates regulated pharmacy technicians, creates additional value in the business to warrant and support this increased compensation, and is both viable and sustainable appears difficult to develop given the current financial climate in community pharmacy. While the initial premise of regulation of technicians focused on the notion that regulated technicians would take over technical dispensary duties, freeing up time for pharmacists to undertake more remunerative cognitive service activities such as medication reviews or immunization consultations, the economics of this business case has not been sustainable or viable given significant reductions in income sources from cognitive services for community pharmacy. As a result, no participant in this study was able to identify a best-practice model for sustainable, viable, economically feasible integration of regulated pharmacy technicians in the workplace. Further research into this theme is required to better understand economic barriers and facilitators that were described as important by participants.

4. Strengths and Limitations

This study is unique in attempting to explore the issue of pharmacy technician workplace integration from the perspective of curriculum and training, using the qualitative method focused on multiple-stakeholder perspectives. The research method used triangulatory processes designed to confirm themes across multiple stakeholders; all transcripts were read and assessed independently by two coders who achieved consensus on code definitions and theme descriptions, further enhancing the trustworthiness of analysis/interpretation.

There are, however, limitations to this research. The qualitative method used and the narrow geographical focus of this study limit generalizability outside of the specific context of Ontario, Canada. While the study method involved interviews until thematic saturation, it is difficult to know if a different cohort of participants would have identified other factors not identified in this research. Findings were based on a participant pool of 24—while this is a reasonably robust number in terms of qualitative studies [9], these participants were not demographically representative, and were identified through purposive, convenience, and snowball sampling methods, which further limits the generalizability of findings. The inclusion of more community pharmacists and community pharmacists with no connection to formal education or clinical training of pharmacy or pharmacy technician students may have also yielded additional or different data for analysis and could be considered in the future. However, as a first step to address a complex issue of topical importance across different jurisdictions, this research has signposted some valuable areas for future exploration and research and has been valuable in highlighting opportunities for evidence-based quality improvement in education and practice.

5. Conclusions

The integration of regulated pharmacy technicians in community pharmacy practice continues to be a vexing issue in many different jurisdictions. This study has helped identify potential areas for curricular quality improvement in pharmacy technician education programs that may enhance the quality and extent of integration. Most of these areas fall into a broad category of "soft-skills" training needs; further work is required to verify the results of this study and determine the feasibility of teaching, learning, and assessment of these soft skills as a method for enhancing the impact that regulated pharmacy technicians may have on community practice and their patients. Particular areas for curricular attention include interpersonal communication skills appropriate for clinical/care workplaces, conflict management and negotiation, intraprofessional collaboration skills, and practice management competencies. There may also be opportunities to consider joint pharmacy/pharmacy technician student education workshops or events in order to start to build a more intraprofessionally collaborative culture at the student level. Another important insight from this study is the need for further work to identify financially viable and sustainable practice models that integrate regulated technicians into the workforce. In recognition of their advanced education, qualifications, and scope of practice, it is reasonable that regulated pharmacy technicians expect and deserve a wage premium compared to unregulated technicians: Understanding how to accommodate this wage premium within an existing business and financial structure, and leveraging the advanced education, qualifications, and scope of practice to generate additional revenue to support payment of higher wages has not been clearly determined within most practices in this study, and this further limits workplace integration. Educators and researchers have an important potential role in working with individual practices and the profession as a whole to provide business plan templates that can support employers in making decisions to hire and retain regulated technicians in a fiscally responsible and sustainable manner.

In a recent study by Anderson et al. [23], the lack of standardization in pharmacy technician education and training programs was identified as a potential barrier to fuller utilization of technicians and integration in practice. Similarly, Wheeler et al. have noted that "(w)ith ongoing pharmacist practice transformation, an approach that ensures uniform technician education ... is vital to support a practice model designed to transform medication management across the continuum of care [24]".

This research has potentially contributed valuable information regarding specific areas for focus in enhancing the quality, rigor, and impact of the educational programs, which form the foundation of regulated pharmacy technician practice.

Author Contributions: Conceptualization, D.A. and Z.A. methodology: A.W., M.J., and P.G.; software P.G.; validation, A.W., M.J., P.G., and Z.A.; formal analysis, P.G.; investigation, A.W., M.J., and P.G.; writing—original draft preparation, A.W. and M.J.; writing—review and editing, P.G. and Z.A.; supervision, D.A. and Z.A.; project administration, D.A. and Z.A.; funding acquisition, Z.A. All authors have read and agreed to the published version of the manuscript.

Funding: This research was funded by an unrestricted grant from the Ontario College of Pharmacists, the regulatory body for pharmacy practice in Ontario Canada Grant Number 21374.

Conflicts of Interest: The authors declare no conflict of interest.

Appendix A

Table A1. Allocation of task responsibilities in community pharmacy.

Pharmacy Task	Who Can Perform
Input a Prescription	Pharmacy Assistant, Pharmacy Technician, Pharmacist
Prepare a Prescription	Pharmacy Assistant, Pharmacy Technician, Pharmacist
Final Check of Product Preparation	Pharmacy Technician, Pharmacist
Check of Clinical Appropriateness	Pharmacist
Patient Consultation	Pharmacist

Table A2. Semi-structured interview protocol.

Opening Questions
1. Tell me a little about your background, i.e.,
• What steps did you take/currently taking to become a Pharmacist/Technician/Assistant (location, education, college/school)?
• Why did you decide to pursue this path?
• How long have you been practicing?
2. What employment experience have you had?
• Name of Pharmacy? Urban, suburban or rural area?
• What was the daily prescription volume of the store?
• Who does the pharmacy team in your store consist of on a typical shift? (i.e., ratio of pharmacists, pharmacy technicians, students, pharmacy assistants)
NB: If no pharmacy technician hired—ask why this is the case
Theme 1: Work environment
1. Would you mind explaining to me the pharmacy workflow and staff roles every time a new prescription arrives? How do you work as a team?
Educators only: What do you understand are areas where your students struggle with the most in the workplace? How do you feel these can be addressed?
2. On the first day, how are you provided information about your own role and those of other staff?

Table A2. *Cont.*

Opening Questions
3. In your experience, what worked well to optimise your role in the pharmacy?
a. Probe: Any workplace practices, policies, training, physical design of pharmacy, i.e., designated workstations, workflow?
4. In your experience, what areas could be improved to better facilitate team work?
a. Probe: Any workplace practices, policies, training, physical design of pharmacy, i.e., designated workstations, workflow?
Theme 2: Scope of practice
1. How do you feel you/pharmacy technician makes a difference to the pharmacy?
2. What do you know about your scope/ the scope of practice of pharmacy technicians? Where did you learn about it?
Educators only: Do you feel the students have a complete understanding of your scope of practice as a pharmacy technician student? How do they learn this?
3. What do you feel differentiates a pharmacist from a regulated pharmacy technician?
4. What do you feel differentiates a pharmacy technician from a pharmacy assistant?
Theme 3: Education
1. How effectively did your school curriculum prepare you for real world work and what specifically was in that curriculum?
2. What do you learn at school about workplace integration and delegating or communicating effectively as part of a team? What could be improved?
Educators only: What do students learn at college about workplace integration, delegating or communicating effectively as part of a team?
3. How would you like this information to be provided if at all and what would be the ideal package to help you successfully integrate?
Theme 4: Professional Identity & Confidence in the workplace
1. How confident (if you were to rate out of ten) are you in interacting with the following groups?
a. Interacting with patients
b. Interacting with licensed Pharmacy Technicians
c. Interacting with Pharmacy Assistants
d. Interacting with Student Pharmacists
e. Interacting with registered Pharmacists
f. Answering phone calls from other health care practitioners
Educators only: In the workplace, how confident do your graduate pharmacy technicians feel interacting with their community pharmacy team and patients following the course? What has been successful and what may be improved?
2. If you were to speak with your pharmacy team, what would you like to tell them about how you would like to be worked with?
3. In the workplace, do you feel that pharmacy technicians are utilised to their full extent?
4. In your experience, do you feel that enough trust is placed on a pharmacy technician to carry out delegated roles?
Closing questions
1. How do you feel about the future of your career?
2. How do you see your role changing in the next 5 years?
3. You may have alluded to this already, but finally what advice would you give to pharmacists and employers to optimise the role of the regulated pharmacy technician?
4. Any other thoughts or opinions?

Table A3. Demographic Profile of Research Participants (n = 24).

Code	Sex	Age *	Roles	Background
RPT1F30	F	30	Recent Pharm Tech Graduate, employed	Worked as assistant × 5 years prior to enrolling in program
RPT2F28	F	28	Recent Pharm Tech Graduate, employed	Supervises bulk packaging and compounding
RPT3F35	F	35	Pharm Tech Graduate, employed	Works in 3 different community practices
RPT4F48	F	48	Recent Pharm Tech Graduate, employed	Former pharmacist from another country, requalified as technician
RPT5M29	M	29	Recent Pharm Tech Graduate, employed	Worked as assistant × 2 years prior to enrolling in program
RPT6M44	M	44	Recent Pharm Tech Graduate, unemployed	Former pharmacist from another country, requalified as technician, currently attempting licensure as pharmacist
RPT7F49	F	49	Recent Pharm Tech Graduate, employed	Worked as assistant × 22 years prior to enrolling in program
RPT8F22	F	22	Recent Pharm Tech Graduate, employed	Worked as student assistant × 4 years prior to enrolling in program
RPT9F29	F	29	Recent Pharm Tech Graduate, unemployed	Parental leave
PTS1F40	F	40	Pharm Tech Student	Worked as assistant × 20 years prior to enrolling in program
PTS2F57	F	57	Pharm Tech Student	Former pharmacist from another country, attempting to qualify
PTS3F22	F	22	Pharm Tech Student	No previous experience
PTS4F28	F	28	Pharm Tech Student	No previous experience
PTS5F33	F	33	Pharm Tech Student	Worked as assistant × 9 years prior to enrolling in program
PTS6M48	M	48	Pharm Tech Student	Former pharmacist from another country, attempting to qualify
PTS7M42	M	42	Pharm Tech Student	Former pharmacist from another country attempting to qualify
PTS8M30	M	30	Pharm Tech Student	No previous experience
PTS9M22	M	22	Pharm Tech Student	No previous experience
RPH1F52	F	52	Pharmacist, pharmacy owner, and educator	Pharmacist × 30 years, educator × 22 years
RPH2F49	F	49	Pharmacist and educator	Pharmacist × 27 years, educator × 11 years
RPH3M50	M	50	Pharmacist, pharmacy owner, and educator	Pharmacist × 25 years, educator × 12 years
RPH4M46	M	46	Pharmacist, pharmacy owner, and educator	Pharmacist × 20 years, educator × 6 years
PTE1F59	F	59	Pharmacist and pharmacy technician educator	Pharmacist × 32 years, educator × 18 years
PTE2M48	M	48	Pharmacist, pharmacy technician educator, pharmacy manager	Pharmacist × 26 years, educator × 12 years

*: if disclosed by participant.

References

1. Grootendorst, P.; Shim, M.; Tieu, J. Uptake and impact of regulated pharmacy technicians in Ontario community pharmacies. *Can. Pharm. J.* **2018**, *151*, 197–202. [CrossRef] [PubMed]
2. Dolovich, L.; Austin, Z.; Waite, N.; Chang, F.; Farrell, B.; Grindrod, K.; Houle, S.; McCarthy, L.; MacCallum, L.; Sproule, B. Pharmacy in the 21st century: Enhancing the impact of the profession of pharmacy on people's lives in the context of healthcare trends, evidence, and policies. *Can. Pharm. J.* **2019**, *152*, 45–53. [CrossRef] [PubMed]
3. Boughen, M.; Sutton, J.; Fenn, T.; Wright, D. Defining the role of the pharmacy technician and identifying their future role in medicines optimization. *Pharmacy* **2017**, *5*, 40. [CrossRef] [PubMed]
4. Borchert, J.S.; Phillips, J.; Thompson Bastin, M.L.; Livingood, A.; Andersen, R.; Brasher, C.; Bright, D.; Fahmi-Armanious, B.; Leary, M.H.; Lee, J.C. Best practices: Incorporating pharmacy technicians and other support personnel into the clinical pharmacist's process of care. *Am. Coll. Clin. Pharm. White Pap.* **2020**, *2*, 74–81. [CrossRef]
5. Newby, B. Expanding the role of pharmacy technicians to facilitate a proactive pharmacist practice. *Am. J. Health-Syst. Pharm.* **2019**, *76*, 398–402. [CrossRef] [PubMed]
6. Desselle, S.P.; Mckeirnan, K.C.; Hohmeier, K.C. Pharmacists ascribing value of technician certification using an organization behaviour framework. *Am. J. Health-Syst. Pharm.* **2020**, *77*, 457–465. [CrossRef]
7. Adams, A.J.; Martin, S.J.; Stolpe, S.F. "Tech check tech": A review of the evidence of safety and benefits. *Am. J. Health Syst. Pharm.* **2011**, *68*, 1824–1833. [CrossRef]
8. Horon, K.; Hennessy, T. Should pharmacy technicians provide clinical services or perform patient care activities in areas without a pharmacist? *Can. J. Hosp. Pharm.* **2010**, *63*, 391–394. [CrossRef]
9. Mattingly, A.N.; Mattingly, T.J. Advancing the role of the pharmacy technician: A systematic review. *J. Am. Pharm. Assoc.* **2018**, *58*, 94–108. [CrossRef]
10. Gregory, P.; Austin, Z. Professional identity formation: The experience of regulated pharmacy technicians in Ontario. *Can. Pharm. J.* **2020**, *153*, 46–51. [CrossRef]
11. Desselle, S.P. An in-depth examination into pharmacy technician worklife through an organizational behaviour framework. *Res. Soc. Adm. Pharm.* **2016**, *12*, 722–732. [CrossRef] [PubMed]
12. Schafheutle, E.I.; Jee, S.D.; Willis, S.C. Fitness for purpose of pharmacy technician education and training: The case of Great Britain. *Res. Soc. Adm. Pharm.* **2017**, *13*, 88–97. [CrossRef] [PubMed]
13. Koehler, T.; Brown, A. A global picture of pharmacy technician and other pharmacy support workforce cadres. *Res. Soc. Adm. Pharm.* **2017**, *13*, 271–279. [CrossRef] [PubMed]
14. Koehler, T.; Brown, A. Documenting the evolution of the relationship between the pharmacy support workforce and pharmacists to support patient care. *Res. Soc. Adm. Pharm.* **2017**, *13*, 280–285. [CrossRef]
15. Friesner, D.L.; Scott, D.M. Identifying characteristics that allow pharmacy technicians to assume unconventional roles in the pharmacy. *J. Am. Pharm. Assoc.* **2010**, *50*, 686–697. [CrossRef]
16. Renfro, C.; Wheeler, J.S.; McDonough, L.K.; Wang, J.; Hohmeier, K.C. Exploring employer perceptions of pharmacy technician certification in the community pharmacy setting. *Res. Soc. Adm. Pharm.* **2019**. [CrossRef]
17. Banks, V.L.; Barras, M.; Snoswell, C.L. Economic benefits of pharmacy technicians practicing at advanced scope: A systematic review. *Res. Soc. Adm. Pharm.* **2020**. [CrossRef]
18. Yin, R. *Qualitative Research from Start to Finish*; Guildford Press: New York, NY, USA, 2011; pp. 44–86.
19. Lincoln, Y.; Guba, E. *Naturalistic Inquiry*; Sage Publications: Newbury Park, CA, USA, 1985; pp. 88–99.
20. Alkhateeb, F.M.; Shields, K.M.; Broedel-Zaugg, K.; Bryan, A.; Snell, J. Credentialing of pharmacy technicians in the USA. *Int. J. Pharm. Pract.* **2011**, *19*, 219–227. [CrossRef]
21. Pervanas, H.C.; Revell, N.; Alotaibi, A.F. Evaluation of medication errors in community pharmacy settings. *J. Pharm. Technol.* **2016**, *32*, 71–74. [CrossRef]
22. Desselle, S.P.; Hoh, R.; Holmes, E.R.; Gill, A.; Zomora, L. Pharmacy technician self-efficacies: Insight to aid future education, staff development, and workforce planning. *Res. Soc. Adm. Pharm.* **2018**, *14*, 581–588. [CrossRef]

23. Anderson, D.C.; Draime, J.A.; Anderson, T.S. Description and comparison of pharmacy technician training programs in the United States. *J. Am. Pharm. Assoc.* **2016**, *56*, 231–236. [CrossRef] [PubMed]
24. Wheeler, J.S.; Gray, J.A.; Gentry, C.K.; Farr, G.E. Advancing pharmacy technician training and practice models in the United States: Historical perspectives, workforce development needs, and future opportunities. *Res. Soc. Adm. Pharm.* **2020**, *16*, 587–590. [CrossRef] [PubMed]

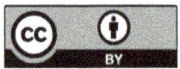 © 2020 by the authors. Licensee MDPI, Basel, Switzerland. This article is an open access article distributed under the terms and conditions of the Creative Commons Attribution (CC BY) license (http://creativecommons.org/licenses/by/4.0/).

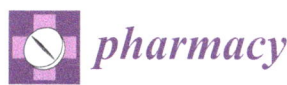

Article

Pharmacist Segments Identified from 2009, 2014, and 2019 National Pharmacist Workforce Surveys: Implications for Pharmacy Organizations and Personnel

Jon Schommer [1,*], William Doucette [2], Matthew Witry [2], Vibhuti Arya [3], Brianne Bakken [4], Caroline Gaither [1], David Kreling [5] and David Mott [5]

1. College of Pharmacy, University of Minnesota, 308 Harvard Street, S.E., Minneapolis, MN 55455, USA; cgaither@umn.edu
2. College of Pharmacy, University of Iowa, S518 PHAR, Iowa City, IA 52242, USA; william-doucette@uiowa.edu (W.D.); matthew-witry@uiowa.edu (M.W.)
3. College of Pharmacy and Health Sciences, St. John's University, St. Augustine Hall, B48, Queens, NY 11439, USA; aryav@stjohns.edu
4. School of Pharmacy, Medical College of Wisconsin, Health Research Center, 8701 Watertown Plank Rd, Milwaukee, WI 53226, USA; bbakken@mcw.edu
5. School of Pharmacy, University of Wisconsin – Madison, 777 Highland Avenue, Madison, WI 53705, USA; david.kreling@wisc.edu (D.K.); david.mott@wisc.edu (D.M.)
* Correspondence: schom010@umn.edu; Tel.: 612-626-9915; Fax: 612-625-9931

Received: 12 February 2020; Accepted: 24 March 2020; Published: 26 March 2020

Abstract: Background/Objective: Findings from the 2009 and 2014 National Pharmacist Workforce Surveys showed that approximately 40% of U.S. pharmacists devoted their time primarily to medication providing, 40% contributed a significant portion of their time to patient care service provision, and the remaining 20% contributed most of their time to other health-system improvement activities. The objective of this study was to characterize the U.S. pharmacist workforce into segments based on the proportion of time they spend in medication providing and patient care services and compare changes in these segments between 2009, 2014, and 2019. **Methods:** Data from 2009, 2014, and 2019 National Pharmacist Workforce Surveys were analyzed. Responses from 1200 pharmacists in 2009, 1382 in 2014, and 4766 in 2019 were used for analysis. Respondents working in the pharmacy or pharmacy-related fields reported both their percent time devoted to medication providing and to patient care services. Medication providing included preparing, distributing, and administering medication products, including associated professional services. Patient care services were professional services designed for assessing and evaluating medication-related needs, monitoring and adjusting patient's treatments, and other services designed for patient care. For each year of data, pharmacist segments were identified using a two-step cluster analysis. Descriptive statistics were used for describing the characteristics of the segments. **Results:** For each year, five segments of pharmacists were identified. The proportions of pharmacists in each segment for the three surveys (2009, 2014, 2019) were: (1) medication providers (41%, 40%, 34%), (2) medication providers who also provide patient care (25%, 22%, 25%), (3) other activity pharmacists (16%, 18%, 14%), (4) patient care providers who also provide medication (12%, 13%, 15%), and (5) patient care providers (6%, 7%, 12%). In 2019, other activity pharmacists worked over 45 hours per week, on average, with 12 of these hours worked remotely. Patient care providers worked 41 hours per week, on average, with six of these hours worked remotely. Medication providers worked less than 40 hours per week, on average, with just one of these hours worked remotely. Regarding the number of patients with whom a respondent interacted on a typical day, medication providers reported 18 per day, patient care providers reported 11 per day, and other activity pharmacists reported 6 per day. In 2009, 8% of patient care providers worked in a setting that was not licensed as a pharmacy.

In 2019, this grew to 17%. **Implications/Conclusions**: The 2019 findings showed that 34% of U.S. pharmacists devoted their time primarily to medication providing (compared to 40% in 2009 and 2014), 52% contributed a significant portion of their time to patient care service provision (compared to 40% in 2009 and 2014), and the remaining 14% contributed most of their time to other health-system improvement activities. Distinguishing characteristics of the segments suggested that recent growth in the pharmacist workforce has been in the patient care services, with more being provided through remote means in organizations that are not licensed as pharmacies. The findings have implications for pharmacist training, continuing education, labor monitoring, regulations, work systems, and process designs. These changes will create new roles and tasks for pharmacy organizations and personnel that will be needed to support emerging patient care services provided by pharmacists.

Keywords: pharmacist; workforce; dispensing; patient care; trends; support personnel

1. Introduction

Findings from the 2009 and 2014 National Pharmacist Workforce Surveys in the United States revealed five segments of pharmacists: (1) medication providers, (2) medication providers who also provide patient care, (3) other activity pharmacists, (4) patient care providers who also provide medication, and (5) patient care providers [1,2]. The findings from 2009 and 2014 showed similar patterns with approximately 40% of U.S. pharmacists devoted primarily to medication providing, 40% contributing a significant portion of their time (typically, 20% or more) to patient care service provision, and the remaining 20% contributing most of their time to business/organization management, research, education, and other health-system improvement activities.

The findings from 2009 and 2014 suggested that there remained a need for, and segment of, pharmacists devoted to specialty practices, dispensing, and patient care services, which are delivered at the point-of-care [2]. At that time, increases in the number of pharmacy graduates per year helped the pharmacy profession meet medication provision needs while, at the same time, expand capacity for new roles in patient care [2]. However, the relatively large cohort of pharmacists trained in the 1970s (capitation years) was retiring at this same time [3], and their contributions needed to be replaced (see Figure 1). Consequently, there still was not a substantial surplus of pharmacists that could have been engaged in more intense advancement of pharmacists' patient care service provision [4]. A recent commentary by Lebovitz and Eddington [5] pointed out that, although pharmacist training focused on clinical knowledge and increased student enrollment during those years, employment in more patient-focused jobs had been minimal.

Since the time the 2009 and 2014 workforce surveys were conducted, considerable shifts in health services and pharmacist roles in the United States have occurred. For example, the pharmacy profession now performs two distinct types of activities: (1) medicine access and supply, and (2) pharmaceutical care [6]. Work system and process designs for medicine access and supply respond to formal requests from prescribers to supply products and associated services as instructed. In contrast, pharmaceutical care involves work systems and processes that focus on decision-making about medicines therapy and planned consultations between pharmacists, prescribers, and patients that facilitate the aim of improving health outcomes [6]. Baines and colleagues described a "blended pharmacy practice" work system and process design that currently is being used as the pharmacy profession attempts to fulfill both types of activities, often in the same location.

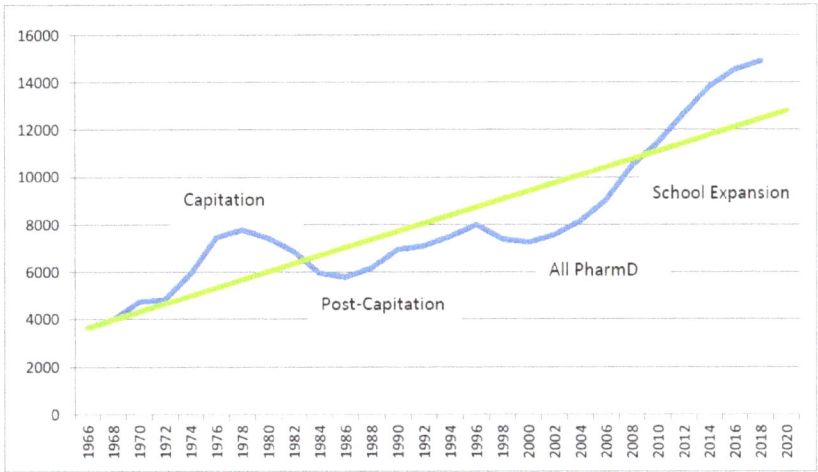

Figure 1. Number of Pharmacist First Professional Degrees by Year of Graduation (1965–2018) with Trend Line. Source: 2017-2018 Profile of Pharmacy Students – American Association of Colleges of Pharmacy, AACP.

Furthermore, the pharmacy profession in the United States is close to gaining provider status, which would provide Medicare coverage for certain pharmacist services in health professional shortage areas or medically underserved areas [5]. Also, changes in laws allowing immunizations, medication therapy management, and collaborative practice agreements are opening up patient-focused jobs for pharmacists. Frogner and colleagues [7] proposed that health care delivery overall is being reorganized to achieve greater value, improve access, integrate care among settings, advance population health, and address social determinants of health. To accomplish this, there is a need for telehealth, the application of digital technology, team-based care, and community-based delivery models [7]. In their commentary, Frogner and colleagues specifically mentioned pharmacists as playing integral roles and the need for changes in their scope-of-practice regulations [7].

Recent market-driven shifts have moved community pharmacy practice from the traditional "locational convenience" strategy to one in which pharmacies are "being organized by their capacity to operate as health care access points that provide and are reimbursed for patient care and public health services" [8–12]. Also, health-system pharmacy practice has been changing from largely acute care models to more comprehensive integrated care models [13] through horizontal integration with clinics and medical centers so that medication and medical costs can be combined in risk portfolios and meet pay-for-performance goals [14].

Vertical integration is affecting pharmacy practice, as well. Insurance companies, wholesalers, manufacturers, integrated delivery networks, pharmacy benefit management companies, pharmacies, clinics, and medical centers are integrating in order to (1) provide coordinated services at a lower cost, (2) improve access to services, (3) leverage data, and (4) bear financial risk for the health outcomes of patient populations [9,14–17].

A special issue in the journal *Pharmacy* focused on pharmacist services and provides further evidence of recent changes in health services and pharmacist roles. In that special issue, Urick and Meggs described the post-pharmaceutical care era and the shift in focus from product to the patient [18]. Ascione proposed the need for pharmacists to be better team members in newly emerging collaborative care and integrated health systems [19]. Goode and colleagues provided a comprehensive categorization of community pharmacy-based patient care services within medication optimization, wellness and prevention screenings, risk assessments, chronic care management, acute care management, patient education, care transitions, and public health domains [20]. Other articles in the special issue further described innovative organizational collaboration [21,22], comprehensive medication management [23,24], transitions of care [25,26], public health initiatives [27–29], and tailored patient-centered care and assessment [30–33]. These are just some examples of the changes in health services and pharmacist roles.

To help make these transitions, significant changes in work systems and processes are being developed, including (1) tech-check-tech processes [34–36], (2) patient-tailored packaging and delivery [37], and (3) technological advances [37]. It appears that the "blended pharmacy practice" work system and the process design described by Baines and colleagues [6] continue to evolve. New ways of delivering products, managing inventory, and reimbursing for product costs are being developed. At the same time, new ways for recruiting and connecting patients with practitioners, achieving patient outcomes, organizing space for patients to receive services, and being reimbursed for value-based outcomes are being developed. These significant changes are likely to influence the types of work activities performed by pharmacists and the time they devote to these activities [2]. This, in turn, will necessitate changes for pharmacy workforce support personnel as they augment the roles that pharmacists and pharmacies will serve in health care.

In light of the expansion of pharmacist roles and congruent changes in systems of care provision, our goal was to repeat the segment analyses conducted in 2009 [1] and 2014 [2] using data from the 2019 National Pharmacist Workforce Survey [38]. As was done in 2009 and 2014, the segmentation analysis was based upon pharmacists' time devoted to medication providing (their traditional role) and to patient care services (their emergent role). A segmentation approach identified key clusters (segments) of the pharmacist workforce and provided a description of their characteristics so that projections could be made regarding future pharmacy profession capacity as cohorts of pharmacists exit the workforce and newly trained pharmacists join the workforce. In addition, the findings were interpreted within the context of the future scope of practice changes that could affect roles filled by pharmacists and pharmacy workforce support personnel.

2. Study Objectives

The overall goal for this study was to repeat the segment analysis of the pharmacist workforce conducted in 2009 [1] and 2014 [2] using data from the 2019 National Pharmacist Workforce Survey. The objectives were to:

1. Identify segments of pharmacists based upon time spent in medication providing and patient care services.
2. Describe segments according to demographic characteristics.
3. Describe segments according to work contributions.
4. Describe segments by work setting.
5. Describe segments according to work activities.
6. Describe year of licensure cohorts to identify trends that might impact future pharmacist capacity for contributing to the U.S. health care system.
7. Compare the findings from the 2019 data with findings from the 2009 and 2014 data.
8. Interpret the findings within the context of future scope of practice changes that could affect roles filled by pharmacists and pharmacy workforce support personnel.

3. Methods

Data from 2009, 2014, and 2019 National Pharmacist Workforce Surveys were analyzed [38–40]. Data in 2009 and 2014 were collected using a mailed questionnaire to a random sample of licensed pharmacists (3000 in 2009 and 5200 in 2014) obtained from a national data warehouse. In 2019, an electronic survey of 96,100 licensed pharmacists obtained from the National Association of Boards of Pharmacy Foundation was used. Responses from 1200 pharmacists in 2009, 1382 in 2014, and 4766 in 2019 were used for analysis. Two continuous variables were the primary focus of this study: (1) percent time spent in medication providing and (2) percent time spent in the patient care services at each respondent's primary place of employment. Respondents reported the proportion of time they spent in each of the activities. These were two of the six work activities included in each survey, which were defined as:

Medication providing: professional services associated with preparing, distributing, and administering medication products, including associated consultation, interacting with patients about the selection and use of over-the-counter products, and interactions with other professionals during the medication dispensing process.

Patient care services: professional services not associated with medication dispensing for assessing and evaluating patient medication-related needs, monitoring and adjusting patients' treatments to attain desired outcomes, and other services designed for patient care.

Business/organization management: managing personnel, finances, and operations.

Research/scholarship: discovery, development, and evaluation of products, services, and/or ideas.

Education: teaching, precepting, and mentoring of students/trainees/technicians.

Other: any activities not described in the above categories.

Data were extracted from each database and analyzed for this report. Two variables (percent time in medication providing and percent time in the patient care services) were utilized for conducting a two-step cluster analysis, with IBM SPSS version 24.0 statistical software (IBM Corp., Armonk, NY, USA). The two-step cluster analysis uses a scalable cluster algorithm. The first step of the analysis is to 'pre-cluster' each case (a record) into many small sub-clusters through a sequential clustering approach. The second step of the analysis is to 'cluster the sub-clusters' resulting from step one into the final cluster solution using an agglomerative hierarchical clustering method. The log-likelihood distance measure (a probability-based distance) is applied for each step of the analysis so that both continuous and categorical variables can be used if so desired [41].

For inclusion in cluster analysis, respondents needed to report both their percent time devoted to medication providing and to patient care services. Respondents who reported that they were: (1) retired, do not practice pharmacy at all, (2) employed in a career not related to pharmacy, or (3) unemployed were not asked the work activity questions and, thus, not included for analysis. Respondents who were included for analysis were those who reported that they were: (1) practicing as a pharmacist, (2) employed in a pharmacy-related field or position, or (3) retired, but still working in a pharmacy or employed part-time as a pharmacist.

Our primary goal was to identify pharmacist segments and describe them using descriptive statistics within the context of the new roles for pharmacists and new work systems that were mentioned in the introduction of this paper. Thus, after pharmacist segments were identified, they were compared across several demographic variables using Chi-Square and Analysis of Variance statistics.

4. Results

Responses from 1200 pharmacists in 2009, 1382 in 2014, and 4766 in 2019 were used for analysis. Cluster analysis identified five segments of pharmacists that we labeled as (1) medication provider, (2) medication provider who also provides patient care, (3) other activity pharmacists, (4) patient care provider who also provides medication, and (5) patient care provider. Figure 2 shows the proportion of pharmacists in each of the five segments, and Table 1 provides a description of each segment in terms of time devoted to medication providing and patient care services.

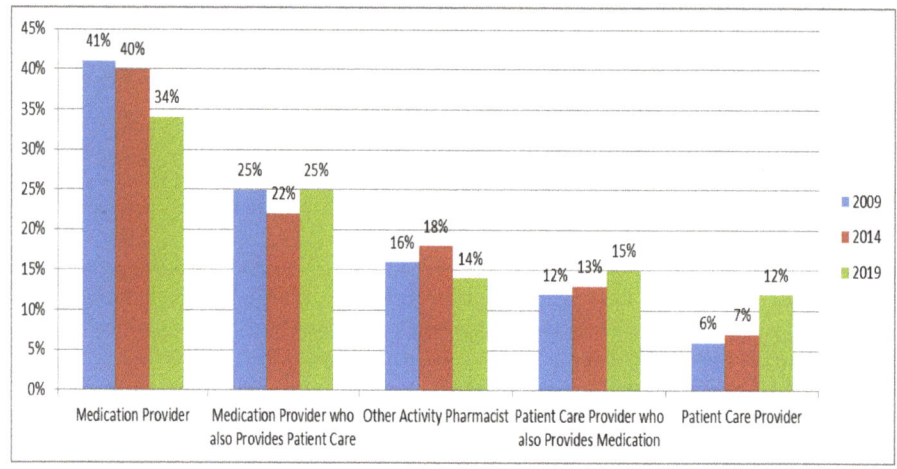

Figure 2. The proportion of U.S. Pharmacists by Segment 2009, 2014, 2019.

Table 1. Description of Pharmacist Segments.

Pharmacist Segment	Segment Size (% of total)			Mean Time Devoted to Medication Providing			Mean Time Devoted to Patient Care Services		
	2009	2014	2019	2009	2014	2019	2009	2014	2019
1: Medication Provider	n = 496 (41%)	n = 555 (40%)	n = 1627 (34%)	88%	83%	88%	5%	6%	4%
2: Medication Provider who also Provides Patient Care	n = 303 (25%)	n = 301 (22%)	n = 1194 (25%)	65%	60%	63%	19%	22%	16%
3: Other Activity Pharmacists	n = 193 (16%)	n = 247 (18%)	n = 680 (14%)	5%	6%	3%	3%	5%	4%
4: Patient Care Provider who also Provides Medication	n = 142 (12%)	n = 184 (13%)	n = 689 (15%)	33%	29%	30%	43%	49%	43%
5: Patient Care Provider	n = 66 (6%)	n = 99 (7%)	n = 576 (12%)	5%	5%	5%	82%	84%	81%
Total	N = 1200	N = 1382	N = 4766	58%	52%	51%	17%	20%	22%

Table 2 provides summary comparisons among the five segments in terms of (1) demographic characteristics, (2) work contributions, (3) work settings by column %, (4) work settings by row %, and (5) time currently spent in work activities.

Table 2. Comparison of U.S. Pharmacist Segments.

	Medication Provider	Medication Provider who also Provides Patient Care	Other Activity Pharmacists	Patient Care Provider who also Provides Medication	Patient Care Provider	Overall
Demographic Characteristics						
Mean Age (years)						
2009	52.0	50.2	49.2	45.6	47.4	50.1
2014	49.5	47.3	49.5	44.5	45.8	48.1
2019	45.1	44.1	48.2	41.9	41.3	44.4
Gender (% female)						
2009	41%	48%	40%	64%	59%	47%
2014	52%	59%	54%	66%	68%	57%
2019	67%	62%	60%	65%	74%	65%
Mean Year of First Licensure						
2009	1982	1983	1984	1988	1988	1983
2014	1989	1992	1989	1994	1993	1991
2019	2000	2001	1996	2003	2004	2001
Hold PharmD (%)						
2009	17%	17%	42%	40%	53%	26%
2014	43%	48%	58%	59%	61%	50%
2019	57%	59%	60%	75%	81%	63%
Residency Training (%)						
2009	3%	4%	19%	25%	26%	9%
2014	6%	5%	27%	30%	34%	15%
2019	4%	6%	26%	28%	40%	15%

Table 2. Cont.

	Medication Provider	Medication Provider who also Provides Patient Care	Other Activity Pharmacists	Patient Care Provider who also Provides Medication	Patient Care Provider	Overall
Both PharmD and Residency (%)						
2009	2%	3%	17%	21%	24%	8%
2014	4%	3%	22%	26%	33%	12%
2019	3%	5%	23%	27%	39%	14%
Work Contributions						
Practicing as a Pharmacist (%)						
2009	89%	93%	45%	94%	97%	84%
2014	90%	95%	59%	94%	93%	86%
2019	99%	99%	62%	99%	99%	94%
Mean Hours Worked/Week						
2009	35.6	38.0	44.7	37.2	39.8	38.1
2014	37.2	39.5	46.4	40.3	40.8	40.0
2019	37.9	40.6	45.8	41.9	41.3	40.7
Mean Hours per Week Worked from Home or Remotely						
2009	-	-	-	-	-	-
2014	-	-	-	-	-	-
2019	1.0	1.5	11.9	2.7	6.0	3.5

Table 2. Cont.

	Medication Provider	Medication Provider who also Provides Patient Care	Other Activity Pharmacists	Patient Care Provider who also Provides Medication	Patient Care Provider	Overall
For Primary Employment, Mean Number of Locations Worked at in a Typical Month						
2009	-	-	-	-	-	-
2014	-	-	-	-	-	-
2019	2.0	1.8	2.2	1.6	1.8	1.9
Mean Number of Patients with whom you Interact as a Pharmacy Care Provider on a Typical Day						
2009	-	-	-	-	-	-
2014	-	-	-	-	-	-
2019	17.6	16.9	5.5	10.4	10.9	11.9
Current Work Setting (Column %)						
2009 Community Pharmacy [a]	78%	67%	10%	23%	1%	-
2014 Community Pharmacy [a]	68%	58%	15%	13%	1%	-
2019 Community Pharmacy [a]	76%	64%	9%	15%	3%	-
2009 Hospital Setting	15%	25%	30%	54%	64%	-
2014 Hospital Setting	17%	28%	23%	70%	49%	-
2019 Hospital Setting	10%	21%	27%	57%	47%	-
2009 Other, Pharmacy Setting [b]	7%	7%	15%	16%	27%	-
2014 Other Pharmacy Setting [b]	14%	14%	16%	14%	36%	-

Table 2. Cont.

	Medication Provider	Medication Provider who also Provides Patient Care	Other Activity Pharmacists	Patient Care Provider who also Provides Medication	Patient Care Provider	Overall
2019 Other Pharmacy Setting [b]	11%	13%	14%	20%	34%	-
2009 Other, Setting Non-Pharmacy [c]	<1%	1%	45%	7%	8%	-
2014 Other, Setting Non-Pharmacy [c]	1%	<1%	46%	3%	14%	
2019 Other Setting Non-Pharmacy [c]	2%	2%	50%	8%	17%	
Current Work Setting (Row %)						
2009 Community Pharmacy [a]	60%	32%	3%	5%	<1%	-
2014 Community Pharmacy [a]	61%	29%	6%	4%	<1%	
2019 Community Pharmacy [a]	57%	35%	3%	5%	<1%	
2009 Hospital Setting	23%	24%	17%	23%	13%	-
2014 Hospital Setting	23%	20%	14%	31%	12%	
2019 Hospital Setting	13%	20%	15%	31%	21%	
2009 Other Pharmacy Setting [b]	29%	16%	23%	18%	14%	-
2014 Other, Pharmacy Setting [b]	36%	18%	18%	12%	16%	
2019 Other, Pharmacy Setting [b]	24%	20%	13%	18%	25%	

Table 2. *Cont.*

	Medication Provider	Medication Provider who also Provides Patient Care	Other Activity Pharmacists	Patient Care Provider who also Provides Medication	Patient Care Provider	Overall
2009 Other, Setting Non-Pharmacy [c]	1%	2%	83%	10%	5%	-
2014 Other, Setting Non-Pharmacy [c]	4%	1%	81%	4%	10%	
2019 Other, Setting Non-Pharmacy [c]	7%	4%	61%	11%	17%	
Mean % of Time Currently Spent in Work Activities						
2009 Medication Providing	88%	65%	5%	33%	5%	58%
2014 Medication Providing	83%	60%	6%	29%	5%	52%
2019 Medication Providing	88%	63%	3%	30%	5%	51%
2009 Patient Care Services	5%	19%	3%	43%	82%	17%
2014 Patient Care Services	6%	22%	5%	49%	84%	20%
2019 Patient Care Services	4%	16%	4%	43%	81%	22%
2009 Business/Org. Management	5%	10%	41%	9%	3%	12%
2014 Business/Org. Management	5%	8%	39%	7%	2%	12%
2019 Business/Org. Management	4%	10%	39%	8%	3%	11%
2009 Research	<1%	1%	18%	4%	3%	4%
2014 Research	<1%	1%	15%	3%	2%	4%
2019 Research	<1%	1%	12%	4%	2%	3%
2009 Education	2%	4%	8%	8%	6%	4%
2014 Education	4%	7%	10%	9%	6%	7%

Table 2. *Cont.*

	Medication Provider	Medication Provider who also Provides Patient Care	Other Activity Pharmacists	Patient Care Provider who also Provides Medication	Patient Care Provider	Overall
2019 Education	3%	7%	12%	11%	7%	7%
2009 Other [d]	1%	1%	25%	5%	2%	5%
2014 Other [d]	1%	2%	24%	3%	2%	6%
2019 Other [d]	1%	2%	29%	3%	1%	6%

Note: All statistical comparisons (ANOVA, Chi-Square) significant at $p < 0.002$. [a] "Community Pharmacy Practice" included independent, chain, mass merchandiser, and supermarket pharmacies. [b] "Other, Pharmacy Setting" included nursing home, long term care, health maintenance organization, nuclear, clinic-based, mail service, central fill, and home health/infusion pharmacies. [c] "Other, Setting Non-Pharmacy" included pharmacy benefit administration, academic, government administration, pharmaceutical industry, consulting companies, professional associations, and other organizations that were not licensed as a pharmacy. [d] Other include activities, such as computer analysis, audit control, continuing education, grants, committee work, communications, consultation, data analysis, drug information services, formulary management, systems implementation, inspections, investigations, information technology work, manufacturing, marketing, medication safety, meetings, policy work, problem resolution, quality assurance, regulatory issues, and writing.

Medication providing: professional services associated with preparing, distributing, and administering medication products, including associated consultation, interacting with patients about the selection and use of over-the-counter products, and interactions with other professionals during the medication dispensing process.

Patient care services: professional services not associated with medication dispensing for assessing and evaluating patient medication-related needs, monitoring and adjusting patients' treatments to attain desired outcomes, and other services designed for patient care.

4.1. Medication Providers

In our study, 41% of pharmacists in 2009, 40% of pharmacists in 2014, and 34% of pharmacists in 2019 who were employed in pharmacy or in a pharmacy-related field were in the medication provider segment. In 2009/2014/2019, these pharmacists devoted an average of 88%/83%/88% of their time to medication providing and only 5%/6%/4% to patient care services, as defined in this study. Table 2 shows that they were the oldest of the five segments in 2009 and 2014, but not in 2019. Also, in 2009 and 2014, they were less likely to be female and hold a PharmD degree compared to other segments. In 2019, this was no longer the case. In all three study years (2009, 2014, and 2019), this segment contributed the fewest hours worked per week of any segment, and relatively few had residency training (see Table 2). This segment of pharmacists primarily worked in community pharmacy practice settings (78% in 2009, 68% in 2014, and 76% in 2019). In 2019, 57% of respondents who worked in community practice settings were identified as being in the "medication provider" segment of pharmacists, which is similar to 61% of the respondents in 2014 and 60% of respondents in 2009. For 2019, three questions were added to the survey and showed that this segment of pharmacists worked an average of 1.0 hour per week from home or remotely, worked at an average of 2.0 locations for their primary employment, and interacted with an average of 17.6 patients per day as a pharmacy care provider (highest among the five segments).

4.2. Medication Providers Who also Provide Patient Care

In our study, 25% of pharmacists in 2009, 22% of pharmacists in 2014, and 25% of pharmacists in 2019 who were employed in pharmacy or in a pharmacy-related field were in the medication provider who also provides patient care segment. In 2009/2014/2019, these pharmacists devoted an average of 65%/60%/63% of their time to medication providing and 19%/22%/16% to patient care services, as defined in this study. Table 2 shows that, in 2009, 48% percent of this segment were female, only 17% had a PharmD degree, and only 4% had residency training. In 2014, 59% were female, 48% had a PharmD degree, and 5% had residency training. By 2019, 62% were female, 59% had a PharmD degree, and 6% had residency training. In 2009, 67% of this segment of pharmacists worked in community pharmacy practice settings, 25% in hospital settings, and 7% in other pharmacy settings. In 2019, 64% worked in community pharmacy settings, 21% worked in hospital settings, and 13% worked in other pharmacy settings. For 2019, three questions were added to the survey and showed that this segment of pharmacists worked an average of 1.5 hours per week from home or remotely, worked at an average of 1.8 locations for their primary employment, and interacted with an average of 16.9 patients per day as a pharmacy care provider (second highest among the five segments).

4.3. Other Activity Pharmacists

In 2009, 16% of pharmacists who were employed in pharmacy or in a pharmacy-related field were in the other activity pharmacists segment. In 2014, the proportion was 18%, and, in 2019, the proportion was 14%. In 2009/2014/2019, these pharmacists devoted an average of 5%/6%/3% of their time to medication providing and 3%/5%/4% to patient care services, as defined in this study. Most of their time was devoted to other activities, such as business/organization management, research, education, and other health-system improvement activities. Table 2 shows that, in 2009, 40% were female, 42% had a PharmD degree, and 19% had residency training. In 2014, 54% were female, 58% had a PharmD degree, and 27% had residency training. By 2019, 60% were female, 60% had a PharmD degree, and 26% had residency training. This segment contributed the most hours worked per week of any segment in 2009, 2014, and 2019. In 2009, 45% of this segment of pharmacists worked in 'other, setting not licensed as a pharmacy', and 30% worked in a hospital setting. This remained consistent through 2019, with 50% of this segment of pharmacists working in 'other, setting not licensed as a pharmacy', and 27% working in a hospital setting. For 2019, this segment of pharmacists worked an average of 11.9 hours per week from home or remotely (highest among the five segments), worked at an average of 2.2 locations for their primary employment, and interacted with an average of 5.5 patients per day as a pharmacy care provider (lowest among the five segments).

4.4. Patient Care Providers Who also Provide Medication

This segment (12% of pharmacists in 2009, 13% of pharmacists in 2014, and 15% of pharmacists in 2019 who were employed in pharmacy or in a pharmacy-related field) devoted an average of 33%/29%/30% of their time to medication providing and 43%/49%/43% in 2009, 2014, and 2019, respectively, to patient care services, as defined in this study. Table 2 shows that they were the youngest of the five segments, on average, in both 2009 and 2014, and second youngest in 2019. In 2009, 64% were female, 40% had a PharmD degree, and 25% had residency training. In 2014, 66% were female, 59% had a PharmD degree, and 30% had residency training. In 2019, 65% were female, 75% had a PharmD degree, and 28% had residency training. In 2009, the hours worked per week by this segment were below the overall average. In 2014 and 2019, the hours worked per week were above the overall average. In 2009, 54% of this segment of pharmacists worked in hospital settings, 23% worked in community pharmacy practice settings, and 16% worked in 'other, licensed pharmacy settings'. In 2014, 70% worked in hospital settings, 13% in community settings, and 14% in 'other, licensed pharmacy settings'. In 2019, 57% worked in hospital settings, 15% in community settings, and 20% in 'other, licensed pharmacy settings'. For 2019, this segment of pharmacists worked an average of 2.7 hours per week from home or remotely, worked at an average of 1.6 locations for their primary employment, and interacted with an average of 10.4 patients per day as a pharmacy care provider.

4.5. Patient Care Providers

In 2009, 6% of pharmacists who were employed in pharmacy or in a pharmacy-related field were in the patient care provider segment. In 2014, the proportion was 7%, and, in 2019, it grew to 12%. In 2009/2014/2019, these pharmacists devoted an average of 5%/5%/5% of their time to medication providing and 82%/84%/81% to patient care services, as defined in this study. Table 2 shows that they were the second youngest of the five segments, on average, in both 2009 and 2014 and the youngest segment in 2019. In 2009, 59% were female, 53% had a PharmD degree, and 26% had residency training. In 2014, 68% were female, 61% had a PharmD degree, and 34% had residency training. In 2019, 74% were female, 81% had a PharmD degree, and 40% had residency training. In 2009, 64% worked in hospital pharmacy practice settings, 27% worked in 'other, pharmacy settings', and 8% worked in 'other, setting non-pharmacy'. In 2014, 49% worked in hospital settings, 36% worked in 'other, pharmacy settings', and 14% worked in 'other, setting non-pharmacy'. In 2019, 47% worked in hospital settings, 34% worked in 'other, pharmacy settings', and 17% worked in 'other, setting non-pharmacy'. For 2019, this segment of pharmacists worked an average of 6.0 hours per week from home or remotely (second highest among the five segments), worked at an average of 1.8 locations for their primary employment, and interacted with an average of 10.9 patients per day as a pharmacy care provider.

4.6. Year of Licensure Cohorts

Table 3 summarizes comparisons for U.S. pharmacists by year of licensure cohorts and provides insight regarding future pharmacy profession capacity as cohorts of pharmacists exit the workforce and newly trained pharmacists join the workforce. For example, Table 3 shows that pharmacists who were licensed before 1980 were typically male, not likely to hold a PharmD degree, and not likely to had residency training. This cohort comprised only 8% of the 2019 survey respondents (393 out of 4686). In comparison, pharmacists who were licensed from 2005 onward were much more likely to be female, over 95% held a PharmD degree, and over 20% had residency training in addition to a PharmD. In 2019, this cohort accounted for 49% of the pharmacist respondents (2300 out of 4686). Pharmacists who were licensed between 1980 and 2004 accounted for the remaining 43% of respondents and showed the transition from BSPharm to PharmD training during this time period.

Table 3. Comparison of U.S. Pharmacist Year of Licensure Cohorts in 2009, 2014, and 2019.

Year of Licensure Cohort (Year of First Licensure)	Female Gender	Age (years)	Hold PharmD Degree	Residency Training	Have Both PharmD and Residency	% (Medication Provider)	% (Medication Provider who also Provides Patient Care)	% (Other Activity Pharmacist)	% (Patient Care Provider who also Provides Medication)	% (Patient Care Provider)
2009 Survey Data										
2005 to 2006 (n = 23)	70%	30.9	96%	30%	30%	52%	4%	9%	13%	22%
2000 to 2004 (n = 101)	66%	33.7	75%	22%	21%	33%	23%	18%	20%	7%
1995 to 1999 (n = 136)	67%	38.2	46%	13%	13%	31%	27%	18%	19%	5%
1990 to 1994 (n = 142)	66%	42.0	30%	14%	14%	44%	23%	12%	11%	10%
1985 to 1989 (n = 141)	58%	47.0	17%	6%	6%	38%	26%	17%	15%	4%
1980 to 1984 (n =164)	50%	51.2	20%	7%	6%	35%	29%	21%	9%	6%
1975 to 1979 (n = 188)	39%	55.6	12%	6%	3%	47%	23%	16%	9%	5%
1970 to 1974 (n = 133)	22%	60.7	7%	3%	0%	39%	30%	17%	8%	6%
1965 to 1969 (n = 74)	10%	65.4	5%	7%	3%	47%	24%	18%	10%	1%
1960 to 1964 (n = 41)	10%	70.0	8%	3%	3%	71%	20%	7%	2%	0%
Before 1960 (n = 33)	6%	77.1	9%	0%	0%	73%	21%	6%	0%	0%
OVERALL (N = 1176)	47%	51.6	26%	9%	8%	41%	25%	16%	12%	6%
2014 Survey Data										
2010 to 2013 (n = 111)	63%	30.5	96%	28%	28%	37%	23%	8%	21%	11%
2005 to 2009 (n = 174)	71%	33.9	95%	22%	22%	35%	24%	15%	17%	9%
2000 to 2004 (n = 153)	71%	38.3	85%	27%	26%	34%	24%	17%	16%	9%
1995 to 1999 (n = 137)	72%	42.7	52%	16%	14%	39%	23%	21%	12%	5%
1990 to 1994 (n = 157)	66%	47.5	31%	13%	11%	41%	19%	20%	15%	5%
1985 to 1989 (n = 147)	61%	52.1	28%	8%	6%	40%	21%	22%	11%	7%
1980 to 1984 (n = 165)	51%	55.9	18%	8%	4%	38%	23%	19%	12%	9%
1975 to 1979 (n = 162)	36%	60.9	18%	10%	2%	48%	19%	20%	9%	6%
1970 to 1974 (n = 73)	21%	65.3	18%	5%	2%	41%	22%	19%	8%	10%
1965 to 1969 (n = 39)	18%	69.7	9%	16%	3%	49%	18%	21%	10%	3%

Table 3. Cont.

Year of Licensure Cohort (Year of First Licensure)	Female Gender	Age (years)	Hold PharmD Degree	Residency Training	Have Both PharmD and Residency	% (Medication Provider)	% (Medication Provider who also Provides Patient Care)	% (Other Activity Pharmacist)	% (Patient Care Provider who also Provides Medication)	% (Patient Care Provider)
1960 to 1964 (n = 15)	13%	74.5	0%	0%	0%	80%	13%	7%	0%	0%
Before 1960 (n = 5)	20%	78.0	0%	0%	0%	40%	0%	40%	0%	20%
OVERALL (N = 1338)	60%	48.1	50%	15%	13%	40%	22%	18%	13%	7%
2019 Survey Data										
2015 to 2019 (n = 842)	68%	30.4	97%	22%	22%	34%	28%	6%	17%	16%
2010 to 2014 (n = 1054)	69%	33.6	98%	22%	22%	32%	25%	11%	18%	14%
2005 to 2009 (n = 404)	75%	39.0	95%	23%	23%	31%	21%	16%	17%	16%
2000 to 2004 (n = 296)	73%	43.4	80%	11%	11%	33%	25%	17%	13%	12%
1995 to 1999 (n = 397)	74%	48.6	43%	9%	9%	39%	26%	12%	14%	9%
1990 to 1994 (n = 515)	70%	52.1	28%	8%	6%	35%	24%	19%	12%	10%
1985 to 1989 (n = 413)	62%	56.2	22%	7%	5%	34%	26%	20%	10%	10%
1980 to 1984 (n = 372)	55%	60.5	15%	10%	5%	35%	24%	19%	12%	10%
1975 to 1979 (n = 245)	37%	65.0	18%	5%	4%	40%	19%	25%	8%	8%
1970 to 1974 (n = 102)	28%	69.9	18%	10%	5%	38%	24%	20%	11%	9%
1965 to 1969 (n = 27)	7%	75.1	11%	4%	0%	37%	22%	19%	11%	11%
1960 to 1964 (n = 13)	31%	76.5	8%	0%	0%	62%	23%	8%	8%	0%
Before 1960 (n = 6)	0%	88.8	17%	17%	17%	17%	17%	17%	17%	33%
OVERALL (N = 4686)	65%	44.4	64%	15%	14%	34%	25%	14%	15%	12%

2009 Survey: N does not total 1200 due to missing data; 2014 Survey: N does not total 1382 due to missing data; 2019 Survey: N does not total 4766 due to missing data.

5. Discussion

The 2019 findings showed that 34% of U.S. pharmacists devoted their time primarily to medication providing (compared to 40% in 2009 and 2014), 52% contributed a significant portion of their time to patient care service provision (compared to 40% in 2009 and 2014), and the remaining 14% contributed most of their time to other health-system improvement activities. This is the first time in the modern pharmacy era that over half of all pharmacists (52%) spend considerable amounts of time in patient care service provision that is separate from patient care that accompanies medication providing. In addition, the segment of pharmacists who devote almost all of their time to patient care services, separate from medication providing, had doubled from 6% of pharmacists in 2009 to 12% of pharmacists in 2019. It should be noted that the data collection method for 2019 used an electronic survey, which was different than a mailed questionnaire approach that was used for 2009 and 2014. However, non-response bias was checked for each of the three survey years, and respondents were found to be representative of the overall pharmacist population of interest in terms of geographic distribution, gender, age, and year of the first licensure. Our confidence in the representativeness of each sample for each of the years was high, but this variation in the method should be considered when interpreting the findings.

These shifts have significant implications for the work system and process designs that will be needed for new ways of delivering products, managing inventory, and reimbursing for the product cost. At the same time, new ways for recruiting and connecting patients with practitioners, achieving patient outcomes, organizing space for patients to receive services, and being reimbursed for value-based outcomes are needed. We suggested that these significant changes in work systems and processes of care are now the most significant influences on the types of work activities performed by pharmacists and the time they devote to these activities [2]. Distinguishing characteristics of the segments suggested that recent growth in the pharmacist workforce has been in the patient care services, with more being provided through remote means in organizations that are not licensed as pharmacies (see Table 2). This not only has implications for the work system and process designs but also for updates that are needed for scope-of-practice regulations.

One of our goals was to interpret the findings within the context of the future scope of practice changes that could affect roles filled by pharmacists and pharmacy workforce support personnel. Whereas transitions in clinical training (PharmD, Residency) had contributed to increased capacity for pharmacist contributions to the U.S. Health Care System [1,2,5], the 2019 data showed that transitions in work systems and processes of care (including updates for regulation and roles for pharmacy support personnel) are likely necessary for increasing pharmacist contributions to the U.S. Health Care System in the next decade. As mentioned in the introduction of this paper, pharmacies are being organized by their capacity to operate as healthcare access points that provide patient care and public health services. Comprehensive integrated care models are being created through horizontal integration with clinics, medical centers, community centers, and even places of employment [8–12]. Vertical integration between insurance companies, wholesalers, manufacturers, integrated delivery networks, pharmacy benefit management companies, and health care centers are being formed to coordinate services, improve access, leverage data, and bear financial risk for health outcomes of patient populations [9,14–17]. As these transitions take place, new ideas for (1) tech-check-tech processes [34–36], (2) patient-tailored packaging and delivery [37], and (3) application of new technologies [37] are being applied.

As pharmacist work activities continue to evolve in the future, it is likely that pharmacy support personnel work activities will be impacted as well. A systematic review of pharmacy technician participation in support of medication therapy management service provision [42] has shown that they are most commonly provided assistance with medication reconciliation (70%), documentation (41%), and medication therapy review (30%). Actions least likely to be described include personal medication record development (5%), physical assessment (5%), follow-up (2%), and medication action plan development (0%). Another study [43] has shown that pharmacy technicians in the United States are regularly involved in calling prescribers for clarifications of orders, collecting information from patients, documenting pharmacy care in patient records, and calling patients regarding refills. Other tasks that are not regularly performed but for which technicians report that they are very willing to provide include preparing vaccinations for administration, taking orders from physicians over the phone, transferring a prescription to another pharmacy, and conducting medication reconciliation after a patient is discharged from a hospital [43]. That study has identified four work system and process changes that would help facilitate technicians embrace emerging tasks. They are related to adequate staffing, having time to complete additional tasks, classifying technicians based on specialized skills, and helping cope with stress in the work environment [43]. We highlighted these findings to make the suggestion that, as pharmacist work activities change, pharmacy support personnel work activities will change as well. Koehler and Brown reported that pharmacy technicians and other pharmacy support workforce cadres differ globally in terms of supervision, requirements, education systems, and regulations [44]. Similarly, a pharmacy technician stakeholder consensus conference in the United States [45] has shown variation among technicians in the United States and called for more uniform standards for pharmacy support personnel in terms of legal definition/licensing/regulation, education, entry-level competencies, certification, and advanced practice roles.

As such changes are made within the pharmacy profession, it must be noted that the U.S. Health Care System is filled with perverse incentives, financial pressures, documentation burdens, the pressure to meet production metrics, and a constant specter of litigation that are creating intensely competing drivers that are emotionally and morally exhausting for pharmacists and pharmacy support personnel as they try to deliver the care that their patients need [46,47]. Thus, there is also a need for a focus on training and system change related to work conditions for personnel, patient safety, payment models, organizational designs, wellbeing, and communications within the overall systems of health care. This will take collective action.

6. Limitations

The results and our interpretation of them should be tempered with the limitations of the study. Slightly different methods were used to obtain the data in each of the three data collection years. These differences might account for some of the findings of the current analyses. The results were based on respondents' self-reports, raising questions regarding the extent to which respondents gave socially desirable responses. Non-response bias was another limitation. It is possible that responders were more interested in the topic we studied or had stronger opinions about the questions we asked than those who chose not to respond. For our analysis, usable data from respondents working in a pharmacy or a pharmacy-related field were used. While our findings were representative of pharmacists working in a pharmacy or a pharmacy-related field, it should be noted that our analysis did not include licensed pharmacists who were outside of these domains (retired, unemployed, or working outside of a pharmacy-related field). Finally, patient care services might vary widely among responders in terms of specific activities and various roles served. This variable should be viewed as a broadly defined one when interpreting the findings.

7. Conclusions

The 2019 findings showed that 34% of U.S. pharmacists devoted their time primarily to medication providing (compared to 40% in 2009 and 2014), 52% contributed a significant portion of their time to patient care service provision (compared to 40% in 2009 and 2014), and the remaining 14% contributed most of their time to other health-system improvement activities. Distinguishing characteristics of the segments suggested that recent growth in the pharmacist workforce has been in the patient care services, with more being provided through remote means in organizations that are not licensed as pharmacies. The findings have implications for pharmacist training, continuing education, labor monitoring, regulations, work systems, and process designs. These changes will create new roles and tasks for pharmacy organizations and personnel that will be needed to support emerging patient care services provided by pharmacists.

Author Contributions: Conceptualization was completed by all co-authors; methodology, W.D., M.W.; software, W.D., M.W., J.S.; validation, all co-authors.; formal analysis, J.S.; investigation, J.S.; resources, W.D., M.W.; data curation, W.D., M.W.; writing—original draft preparation, J.S.; writing—review and editing was completed by all co-authors.; project administration, W.D., M.W.; funding acquisition, W.D., M.W. All authors have read and agreed to the published version of the manuscript.

Funding: This research was funded by a grant from the Pharmacy Workforce Center, Alexandria, VA and by the University of Iowa, College of Pharmacy, Iowa City, IA.

Acknowledgments: We appreciate the contributions to survey development, data collection, and data management by Scott Egerton, University of Iowa. An earlier version of this manuscript was accepted for presentation at the 2020 American Pharmacists Association Annual Conference.

Conflicts of Interest: The authors declare no conflict of interest. The funders had no role in the design of the study; in the collection, analyses, or interpretation of data; in the writing of the manuscript, or in the decision to publish the results.

References

1. Schommer, J.C.; Planas, L.; Johnson, K.A.; Doucette, W.R.; Gaither, C.A.; Kreling, D.H.; Mott, D.A. Pharmacist Contributions to the U.S. Health Care System. *Innov. Pharm.* **2010**, *1*, 16. [CrossRef]
2. Schommer, J.C.; Gaither, C.A.; Doucette, W.R.; Kreling, D.H.; Mott, D.A. Pharmacist Contributions to the U.S. Health Care System Reported in the 2009 and 2014 National Pharmacist Workforce Surveys. *Innov. Pharm.* **2015**, *6*, 14. [CrossRef]
3. 2017–2018 Profile of Pharmacy Students—AACP, American Association of Colleges of Pharmacy. Available online: www.aacp.org (accessed on 10 October 2019).
4. Maine, L.L. It Really Isn't That Simple. *Am. J. Pharm. Educ.* **2019**, *83*, 7593.
5. Lebovitz, L.; Eddington, N.D. Trends in the Pharmacist Workforce and Pharmacy Education. *Am. J. Pharm. Educ.* **2019**, *83*, 7051. [PubMed]
6. Baines, D.; Bates, I.; Bader, L.; Hale, C.; Schneider, P. Conceptualising production, productivity and technology in pharmacy practice: A novel framework for policy, education and research. *Hum. Resour. Health* **2018**, *16*, 51. [CrossRef] [PubMed]
7. Frogner, B.K.; Fraher, E.P.; Spetz, J.; Pittman, P.; Moore, J.; Beck, A.J.; Buerhaus, P.I. Modernizing Scope-of-Practice Regulations—Time to Prioritize Patients. *N. Engl. J. Med.* **2020**, *382*, 591–593. [CrossRef]
8. Olson, A.W.; Schommer, J.C.; Hadsall, R.S. A 15 Year Ecological Comparison for the Market Dynamics of Minnesota Community Pharmacies from 2002 to 2017. *Pharmacy* **2018**, *6*, 50. [CrossRef]
9. Schommer, J.C.; Olson, A.W.; Isetts, B.J. Transforming community-based pharmacy practice through financially sustainable centers for health and personal care. *J. Am. Pharm. Assoc.* **2019**, *59*, 306–309. [CrossRef] [PubMed]
10. Schommer, J.C.; Doucette, W.R.; Johnson, K.A.; Planas, L. Positioning and integrating medication therapy management. *J. Am. Pharm. Assoc.* **2012**, *52*, 12–24. [CrossRef] [PubMed]
11. Schommer, J.C.; Doucette, W.R.; Planas, L. Establishing pathways for access to pharmacist-provided patient care. *J. Am. Pharm. Assoc.* **2015**, *55*, 664–668. [CrossRef] [PubMed]
12. Knapp, K.K.; Olson, A.W.; Schommer, J.C.; Gaither, C.A.; Mott, D.A.; Doucette, W.R. Retail Clinics Co-Located with Pharmacies: A Delphi Study of Pharmacist Impacts and Recommendations for Optimization. *J. Am. Pharm. Assoc.* **2019**. [CrossRef]
13. Pedersen, C.A.; Schneider, P.J.; Ganio, M.C.; Scheckelhoff, D.J. ASHP National Survey of Pharmacy Practice in Hospital Settings: Monitoring and Patient Education—2018. *Am. J. Health Syst. Pharm.* **2019**, *76*, 1038–1058. [CrossRef]
14. Healthcare Financial Management Association. *Acquisition and Affiliation Strategies*; Healthcare Financial Management Association: Westchester, IL, USA, 2014; Available online: https://www.hfma.org/DownloadAsset.aspx?id=23451 (accessed on 4 September 2018).
15. Greaney, T.L.; Richman, B.D. *Consolidation in Provider and Insurer Markets: Enforcement Issues and Priorities*; American Antitrust Institute: Washington, DC, USA, 2018; Available online: https://www.antitrustinstitute.org/sites/default/files/AAI_Healthcare%20WP%20Part%20I_6.12.18.pdf (accessed on 4 September 2018).
16. Greaney, T.L.; Richman, B.D. *Promoting Competition in Healthcare Enforcement and Policy: Framing an Active Competition Agenda*; American Antitrust Institute: Washington, DC, USA, 2018; Available online: https:

//www.antitrustinstitute.org/sites/default/files/AAI_Healthcare%20WP%20Part%20II_6.18.18.pdf (accessed on 4 September 2018).
17. Madara, J.L. *The Acquisition of Aetna, Inc. by CVS Health Corporation*; Position Paper; American Medical Association: Chicago, IL, USA, 2018; Available online: https://searchlf.ama-assn.org/undefined/documentDownload?uri=%2Funstructured%2Fbinary%2Fletter%2FLETTERS%2F2018-8-7-Letter-to-Delrahim-CVS-Aetna-Merger.pdf (accessed on 4 September 2018).
18. Urick, B.Y.; Meggs, E.V. Towards a Greater Professional Standing: Evolution of Pharmacy Practice and Education, 1920–2020. *Pharmacy* **2019**, *7*, 98. [CrossRef]
19. Ascione, F. Preparing Pharmacists for Collaborative/Integrated Health Settings. *Pharmacy* **2019**, *7*, 47. [CrossRef]
20. Goode, J.-V.K.R.; Owen, J.A.; Page, A.; Gatewood, S. Community-Based Pharmacy Practice Innovation and the Role of the Community-Based Pharmacist Practitioner in the United States. *Pharmacy* **2019**, *7*, 106. [CrossRef]
21. Doucette, W.R. Innovative Collaboration between a Medical Clinic and a Community Pharmacy: A Case Report. *Pharmacy* **2019**, *7*, 62. [CrossRef]
22. Knapp, K.; Yoshizuka, K.; Sasaki-Hill, D.; Caygill-Walsh, R. Co-located Retail Clinics and Pharmacies: An Opportunity to Provide More Primary Care. *Pharmacy* **2019**, *7*, 74. [CrossRef]
23. Neves, C.D.M.; Nascimento, M.M.G.D.; Silva, D.; Álvares, M.; Ramalho-De-Oliveira, D. Clinical Results of Comprehensive Medication Management Services in Primary Care in Belo Horizonte. *Pharmacy* **2019**, *7*, 58.
24. Twigg, G.; David, T.; Taylor, J. An Improved Comprehensive Medication Review Process to Assess Healthcare Outcomes in a Rural Independent Community Pharmacy. *Pharmacy* **2019**, *7*, 66. [CrossRef]
25. Took, R.L.; Liu, Y.; Kuehl, P.G. A Study to Identify Medication-Related Problems and Associated Cost Avoidance by Community Pharmacists during a Comprehensive Medication Review in Patients One Week Post Hospitalization. *Pharmacy* **2019**, *7*, 51. [CrossRef]
26. Schullo-Feulner, A.; Krohn, L.; Knutson, A. Reducing Medication Therapy Problems in the Transition from Hospital to Home: A Pre- & Post-Discharge Pharmacist Collaboration. *Pharmacy* **2019**, *7*, 86.
27. Liu, Y.; Guthrie, K.D.; May, J.R.; DiDonato, K.L. Community Pharmacist-Provided Wellness and Monitoring Services in an Employee Wellness Program: A Four-Year Summary. *Pharmacy* **2019**, *7*, 80. [CrossRef] [PubMed]
28. Abraham, O.; Morris, A. Opportunities for Outpatient Pharmacy Services for Patients with Cystic Fibrosis: Perceptions of Healthcare Team Members. *Pharmacy* **2019**, *7*, 34. [CrossRef] [PubMed]
29. Safitrih, L.; Perwitasari, D.A.; Ndoen, N.; Lestari, K. Health Workers' Perceptions and Expectations of the Role of the Pharmacist in Emergency Units: A Qualitative Study in Kupang, Indonesia. *Pharmacy* **2019**, *7*, 31. [CrossRef]
30. Maes, K.A.; Ruppanner, J.A.; Imfeld-Isenegger, T.L.; Hersberger, K.E.; Lampert, M.L.; Boeni, F. Dispensing of Prescribed Medicines in Swiss Community Pharmacies-Observed Counselling Activities. *Pharmacy* **2018**, *7*, 1. [CrossRef]
31. Kaae, S.; Nørgaard, L.S.; Sporrong, S.K.; Almarsdottir, A.B.; Kofoed, M.; Daysh, R.F.; Jowkar, N. Patients', Pharmacy Staff Members', and Pharmacy Researchers' Perceptions of Central Elements in Prescription Encounters at the Pharmacy Counter. *Pharmacy* **2019**, *7*, 84. [CrossRef]
32. Schindel, T.J.; Breault, R.R.; Hughes, C.A. "It Made a Difference to Me": A Comparative Case Study of Community Pharmacists' Care Planning Services in Primary Health Care. *Pharmacy* **2019**, *7*, 90. [CrossRef]
33. Redmond, S.; Paterson, N.; Shoemaker, S.J.; Ramalho-De-Oliveira, D. Development, Testing and Results of a Patient Medication Experience Documentation Tool for Use in Comprehensive Medication Management Services. *Pharmacy* **2019**, *7*, 71. [CrossRef]
34. Frost, T.P.; Adams, A.J. Pharmacist and Technician Perceptions of Tech-Check-Tech in Community Pharmacy Practice Settings. *J. Pharm. Pract.* **2017**, *31*, 190–194. [CrossRef]
35. Miller, R.F.; Cesarz, J.; Rough, S. Evaluation of community pharmacy tech-check-tech as a strategy for practice advancement. *J. Am. Pharm. Assoc.* **2018**, *58*, 652–658. [CrossRef]
36. Andreski, M.; Myers, M.; Gainer, K.; Pudlo, A. The Iowa new practice model: Advancing technician roles to increase pharmacists' time to provide patient care services. *J. Am. Pharm. Assoc.* **2018**, *58*, 268–274.e1. [CrossRef] [PubMed]

37. Loria, K. A Look Ahead: What to Expect from the Pharmacy Landscape in 2020. Drug Topics. 2020. Available online: https://www.drugtopics.com/latest/look-ahead-what-expect-pharmacy-landscape-2020 (accessed on 29 January 2020).
38. Doucette, W.R.; Matthew, J.W.; Vibhuti Arya, B.K.; Bakken, C.A.; Gaither, D.H.; Kreling, D.A.; Schommer, J.C. *2019 National Pharmacist Workforce Survey*; Pharmacy Workforce Center: Washington, DC, USA, 2019; Available online: https://www.aacp.org/article/national-pharmacist-workforce-studies (accessed on 10 January 2020).
39. Schommer, C.J.; Doucette, W.R.; Gaither, C.A.; Kreling, D.H.; Mott, D.A. *Final Report of the 2009 National Pharmacist Workforce Survey*; Pharmacy Manpower Project, Inc.: Alexandria, VA, USA, 2009; Available online: https://www.aacp.org/article/2009-national-pharmacist-workforce-study (accessed on 2 November 2009).
40. Gaither, A.C.; Schommer, J.C.; Doucette, W.R.; Kreling, D.H.; Mott, D.A. *2014 National Pharmacist Workforce Survey*; Pharmacy Workforce Center: Washington, DC, USA, 2014; Available online: https://www.aacp.org/article/2014-national-pharmacist-workforce-study (accessed on 31 January 2015).
41. Yim, O.; Ramdeen, K.T. Hierarchical Cluster Analysis: Comparison of Three Linkage Measures and Application to Psychological Data. *Quant. Methods Psychol.* **2015**, *11*, 8–21. [CrossRef]
42. Gernant, S.A.; Nguyen, M.-O.; Siddiqui, S.; Schneller, M. Use of pharmacy technicians in elements of medication therapy management delivery: A systematic review. *Res. Soc. Adm. Pharm.* **2017**, *14*, 883–890. [CrossRef] [PubMed]
43. Doucette, W.R.; Schommer, J.C. Pharmacy Technicians' Willingness to Perform Emerging Tasks in Community Practice. *Pharmacy* **2018**, *6*, 113. [CrossRef]
44. Koehler, T.; Brown, A. A global picture of pharmacy technician and other pharmacy support workforce cadres. *Res. Soc. Adm. Pharm.* **2017**, *13*, 271–279. [CrossRef]
45. Zellmer, W.A.; McAllister, E.B.; Silvester, J.A.; Vlasses, P.H. Toward uniform standards for pharmacy technicians: Summary of the 2017 Pharmacy Technician Stakeholder Consensus Conference. *Am. J. Health Pharm.* **2017**, *74*, 1321–1332. [CrossRef]
46. Schommer, J.C.; Gaither, C.; Goode, J.-V.K.R.; Owen, J.A.; Scime, G.M.; Skelton, J.B.; Cernasev, A.; Hillman, L. Pharmacist and student pharmacist views of professional and personal well-being and resilience. *J. Am. Pharm. Assoc.* **2019**, *60*, 47–56. [CrossRef]
47. Desselle, S.P.; Holmes, E.R. Results of the 2015 National Certified Pharmacy Technician Workforce Survey. *Am. J. Health Pharm.* **2017**, *74*, 981–991. [CrossRef]

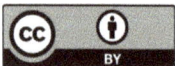

© 2020 by the authors. Licensee MDPI, Basel, Switzerland. This article is an open access article distributed under the terms and conditions of the Creative Commons Attribution (CC BY) license (http://creativecommons.org/licenses/by/4.0/).

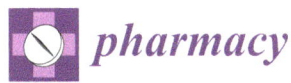

Communication

Perceived Benefit of Immunization-Trained Technicians in the Pharmacy Workflow

Taylor G. Bertsch * and Kimberly C. McKeirnan

Department of Pharmacotherapy, College of Pharmacy and Pharmaceutical Sciences, Washington State University, Spokane, WA 99202, USA
* Correspondence: tbertsch@wsu.edu

Received: 7 March 2020; Accepted: 13 April 2020; Published: 21 April 2020

Abstract: Clinical community pharmacists have continually restructured their workflow to serve the community by optimizing patient care outcomes. Defining the perceived benefits of having an immunizing pharmacy technician in the workflow can help to redefine the way community pharmacists operate during patient immunization. The purpose of this study is to share the opinions of supervising pharmacists that have an immunizing technician within their workflow model and highlight their contributions. Pharmacists involved in this novel workflow model were interviewed two times, once in 2017 and then in 2020, to gauge opinions over time. Findings in the results of this study included such themes as: (1) Pharmacists' perceived improvement in workflow flexibility; (2) The choice of the correct technician to immunize within the pharmacy; (3) Pharmacists' perceived improved workflow time prioritization; (4) Limited available training as a barrier to implementation; and (5) The initial apprehension and later acceptance of pharmacists with respect to the innovation. As technician immunization administration spreads beyond early adopter states, further research into the impact on pharmacy workflow is needed.

Keywords: immunizing pharmacy technicians (IPT); community-pharmacy immunizations; assessment of workflow in community pharmacy

1. Introduction

The Department of Health and Human Services supports the expansion of the role of the pharmacist, enhancing patient autonomy and providing competition within the current healthcare model [1]. Advancements in the role of the pharmacist in community-based practice to meet the needs of patients within the area they serve have been largely successful [2]. The impact of pharmacy-based immunization services has resulted in millions of additional immunizations being given annually [3,4]. Given the increased need to provide continued vaccination efforts in the United States [5,6] and promote community-pharmacist role advancement, a transition of current workflow responsibilities could be considered in order to support this change.

When pharmacists move from traditional dispensing roles to increasingly clinical roles, the need for pharmacy technicians to take on advanced roles increases. According to Koehler and Brown, pharmacy technician roles have historically evolved when the role of the pharmacist has changed, creating gaps and a need for technicians to perform new tasks [7]. Literature supports advancing the role of pharmacy technicians to improve patient outcomes within the pharmacy, particularly when training is available and there is a clear and tangible benefit to the technician [8].

In recent years, pharmacy technicians have taken on several new roles, including accepting verbal prescriptions, performing prescription transfers, and checking prescriptions. Results show these new technician roles have had a positive impact on pharmacy workflow. Fleagle and colleagues piloted a tech-check-tech program in a community pharmacy setting and found technicians were at least as accurate as pharmacists in checking prescriptions, with the potential to save pharmacists approximately 23 working days per year by performing this task [9]. A qualitative study by Hohmeier and colleagues showed that high-performing pharmacy sites had pharmacy technicians engaged in both nonclinical and clinical support activities [10]. Clinical activities at high-performing pharmacies included responsibilities such as scheduling patient appointments with pharmacists, preparing patient charts for the pharmacists prior to appointments, and documenting patient communication [10].

A recent role for pharmacy technicians in the United States includes the administration of immunizations. Technician immunization advancement has gained momentum and support since it began in Idaho in 2017. Three states legally allow pharmacy technicians to administer immunizations [11–13]. Eid and colleagues assessed the regulatory nature of pharmacy technician vaccine administration with a nine-question survey sent to 51 state boards of pharmacy [14]. Findings demonstrated that, in addition to the three states where technicians were already allowed to immunize, nine other states did not expressly prohibit this advanced technician role [14].

Doucette and Schommer recently assessed pharmacy technician willingness to undertake new advanced roles and identified variables that could improve this willingness [15]. Administering immunizations was found to be one of the tasks technicians were least willing take on, but education and support from the pharmacy team were found to be variables that were most associated with improving willingness to perform these tasks [15]. The American Pharmacist's Association recently began offering an immunization training program specifically for pharmacy technicians [16]. McKeirnan and colleagues conducted a pilot study, training a small number of pharmacy technicians to administer immunizations, and found that immunizing technicians were competent, willing, and successful at this new role [17]. Time will tell how increased opportunity for technician education on this topic impacts technicians' willingness to administer immunizations.

One aspect of utilizing pharmacy technicians to administer immunizations that has not been explored is the impact on pharmacy workflow. Bertsch and colleagues showed that pharmacists who supervise immunizing technicians are supportive of this role, would encourage more technicians to become immunization-trained, and believe having immunizing technicians has increased the number of immunizations given at the pharmacy [18]. However, more information about how immunizing technicians are utilized in workflow may encourage the expansion of this new advanced role. This in mind, the objective of this work is to gather more information and provide additional insight on the topic of immunization and pharmacy workflow. Specifically, understanding how immunizing technicians are utilized in workflow, how often technicians are administering immunizations, and determining existing barriers to utilizing technicians in immunization workflow are the goals of this research.

2. Materials and Methods

This research was designed as a two-phase qualitative descriptive study utilizing key informant interviews. The first phase was conducted in 2017 [18]. Pharmacists within one pharmacy chain were contacted to participate in a key informant interview. These pharmacists supervised the first group of immunizing technicians in the United States trained during the pharmacy technician immunization training pilot project conducted by McKeirnan and colleagues in 2016. A description of the 2016 training pilot project can be found elsewhere [17]. The pharmacists from this chain were chosen as participants because they had more experience supervising immunizing technicians than any other pharmacists in the United States at the time of the first phase due to their technicians' participation in this pilot project.

2.1. Study Phase One

During phase one, pharmacists from the Albertsons corporation were contacted if at least one pharmacy technician employed at their pharmacy was included in the 2016 training pilot project. Pharmacy technicians were trained in December of 2016; key informant interviews were conducted six months later (May 2017). Researchers aimed to understand the perspective of these supervising pharmacists when incorporating trained immunizing technicians into their pharmacy. Two sets of interview questions were developed during this project. One was related to pharmacists' perceptions of the implementation ("perceptions questions"), and the second was created to inquire further into the impact on pharmacy workflow ("workflow questions"). Rogers' Diffusions of Innovations theoretical framework was utilized to help researchers disseminate this novel information to others wishing to adopt this practice. The perception questions were coded to the Five Stages of the Adoption Process and the workflow questions were coded to Rogers' 5 Factors [19]. Rogers' 5 Factors are intrinsic characteristics of innovation that influence the decision regarding whether to adopt a new idea or innovation [19].

The perception questions were created to specifically target supervising pharmacists' initial trust and utilization of immunizing technicians, perceptions about the training program, and recommendations to other pharmacists who are considering having immunization-trained technicians [18]. The workflow questions focused on embedding immunizing technicians into pharmacy workflow. These workflow questions best paired with the theoretical framework of Rogers' 5 Factors in the Diffusion of Innovation [19]. In this theoretical framework, Rogers defines five characteristics of innovation that influence the adoption or rejection of an innovation by an individual. Rogers describes these characteristics as interrelated but conceptually distinct. These five characteristics include:

1. Relative Advantage: the degree to which the new option is improved (or not) over a previous version or standard.
2. Compatibility: the degree to which the new option fits in with existing values and needs and can be assimilated into the potential adopter's life.
3. Complexity or Simplicity: the degree to which an innovation is perceived as difficult or simple to understand and implement.
4. Trialability: the degree to which an innovation may be trialed and customized during the implementation process.
5. Observability: the degree to which the results are visible to adopters or others.

These characteristics were utilized to develop five of the seven survey questions, as displayed in Table 1.

Table 1. Key informant interview questions.

Key Informant Interview Questions	Rogers' 5 Factors Characteristic
(1) How long have you been working as a pharmacist?	Demographics
(2) How many immunizing technicians do you currently have at your pharmacy?	Complexity or Simplicity
(3) How has the addition of immunizing technicians impacted pharmacy workflow?	Trialability
(4) What did you find was the best way to utilize your pharmacy technician(s) when administering immunizations?	Compatibility
(5) Describe all barriers or challenges that you felt you had to overcome in introducing technicians in the immunization workflow.	Complexity or Simplicity
(6) Would you recommend having immunizing technicians to other pharmacists? Why or why not?	Relative Advantage (or lack thereof)
(7) What percentage of the time does your technician(s) administer the immunizations? *	Observability
(8) Do you have any additional feedback that was not addressed by this questionnaire?	General

* Question used from 2017 [18] and 2020 only.

The key informant interview question script was developed by the primary investigator (TB), a licensed pharmacist who had experience providing the WSU Pharmacy Technician Immunization Training program but was not involved in training any of the technicians who were supervised by the participating pharmacists. The interview questions were peer-reviewed by colleagues. Key informant interviews were offered to supervising pharmacists at all 20 Albertsons pharmacies in Idaho State that had at least one pharmacy technician who attended the initial 2016 immunization training program. Initially, each pharmacy was emailed a copy of both sets of study interview questions by the district clinical coordinator. The intent of emailing the questions ahead of the phone interviews was to provide opportunity for the participants to give the questions thoughtful consideration and to minimize disruption of workflow.

The primary investigator (TB) called each pharmacy during normal business hours and both sets of interview questions were asked. If the participant was not available or did not have time to answer all of the questions, the researcher offered to call back at a more convenient time. Pharmacists who were willing and available to participate were informed that participation was voluntary and that the decision whether or not to participate would not be shared with pharmacy management. Pharmacists were also told the conversation would be audio-recorded but individual participant names and locations would be removed prior to analysis and the dissemination of results. These study methods were found to be exempt from the need for review by the Washington State University Institutional Review Board (WSU IRB, #16030).

After all of the interviews were completed, the audio files were transcribed using an online transcription service (https://www.rev.com/) and redacted of information that could identify the participant or specific store. The transcriptions were reviewed, and each set of questions was coded separately using qualitative coding methods. Qualitative coding procedures, as described by Miles et al., were performed by two researchers [20]. First-level coding, the systematic labeling of items or concepts that appeared repeatedly in the text, was completed by hand independently. The researchers then met to discuss and cluster the codes into higher-level categories, performing second-level coding to create themes. Disagreements were resolved through discussion. Results from the perception questions demonstrated that saturation had been reached on this topic and a manuscript was published [18]. After reviewing the results from the workflow questions, researchers decided that saturation had not been reached on this topic. In order to achieve a more in depth understanding of the integration of immunizing pharmacy technicians into workflow further research would need to be conducted.

2.2. Study Phase Two

Phase two was conducted in January and February of 2020. Initially, the intent was to contact all 19 pharmacies that had participated in phase one of the study. However, permission was only given to contact five pharmacies located in northern Idaho. The same key informant workflow interview questions as shown in Table 1 were utilized again with the addition of one question previously included in the perceptions question list: "What percentage of the time does your technician(s) administer the immunizations?" The researchers believed comparing previous results of this question would help future adopters discern how immunizing technician utilization had varied over time in the workflow.

Key informant interviews were held by the same researcher (TB) who conducted the initial interviews in 2017. Individual pharmacies were called during normal business hours with consideration given to which times of the day would likely be less busy. Willing participants were informed this was a follow-up study for pharmacists who supervised immunizing pharmacy technicians. Following the same methods as phase one, all interviews were audio-recorded and transcribed, and identifying information was redacted. First-level and second-level coding were performed using the same methods described during phase one. After coding was complete, 2017 interview findings were compared with 2020 findings and mapped to corresponding domains in Rogers' 5 Factors of the Diffusion of Innovation [19]. An integral component associated with Rogers' theory of innovation is time; innovations need to be tested over time in order to determine value [19]. The second set of interviews were conducted three years later with the same set of pharmacies, minus those who were unable to participate. Researchers determined that a saturation point in thematic findings had been met, as the outcomes were similar enough between the two sets of interviews. The 2020 responses repeated the majority of comments recorded previously in 2017. The research yielded no new data after this specific lapse in time.

3. Results

During phase one in 2017, 19 pharmacists, each from a separate individual pharmacy within the same chain, agreed to participate in the key informant interviews. One pharmacist declined to participate during the interview. During phase two in 2020, five of the original pharmacies that were contacted had a pharmacist who was willing to participate, and all five pharmacies still employed pharmacy technicians who administered immunizations. Participant demographics from 2017 [18] and 2020 are included in Tables 2 and 3.

Table 2. Demographics for 2017 [18] and 2020.

Pharmacist ID and Store Number	Gender	Would Recommend Technician Immunization Training	Percentage of Time the Technician Administers Immunizations vs. the Pharmacist
\multicolumn{4}{c}{2017 Demographics [18]}			
1	M	Y	70%
2	F	Y	50%
3	F	Y	85%
4	F	Y	75%
5	F	Y	80%
6	M	N	100%
7	M	Y	75%
8	F	Y	60%
9	M	Y	100%
10	F	Y	80%
11	M	Y	100%
12	M	Y	10%
13	F	Y	80%
14	F	Y	50%
15	M	Y	95%
16	M	Y	70%
17	F	Y	50%
18	F	Y	100%
19	M	Y	100%
			Est Average: 74%
\multicolumn{4}{c}{2020 Demographics}			
Pharmacist ID and Store #	Gender	Would Recommend Technician Immunization Training	Percentage of Time the Technician Administers Immunizations vs. the Pharmacist
1	F	Y	50%
2	M	Y	80%
3	M	Y	100%
4	F	Y	70%
5	F	Y	35%
			Est. Average: 67%

Table 3. Key informant interview demographics continued.

Pharmacist ID and Store Number	2020 Demographics	
	How long have you been working as a pharmacist?	Current Immunizing Technicians
1	16 years	0 *
2	N/A	2
3	16 years	1
4	N/A	1
5	2 years	1

* No active immunizing technician for one month.

Qualitative analysis led to the following themes mapped back to each of Rogers' 5 Factors, which are intrinsic components associated with the adoption of an innovation. Specifics on Rogers' 5 Factors, relative advantage, compatibility, complexity or simplicity, trialability, and observability are described within the Methods section.

3.1. Factor 1: Relative Advantage

The relative advantage domain had one theme: improved flexibility towards creating a continuous workflow associated with immunizations administered within the pharmacy. This was reported by pharmacists in 2017 and confirmed by similar responses from 2020.

Theme 1. *Pharmacists believe having immunizing technicians improved the pharmacy workflow flexibility involved with immunizations.*

- "For us specifically, the way that our system's designed it's been great during busy times. We'll send the technician in to do the immunizations so that we can continue to keep the workflow moving in the pharmacy. In that respect it's been really positive, and just having the extra person in the store that can give [immunizations]. It's going to be great during flu season." (2017 Pharmacist 1)
- "The pharmacist doesn't feel too overburdened, especially during flu season and they feel like they can defer some of those responsibilities to somebody else." (2017 Pharmacist 2)
- "It's kind of amazing because if you are stuck counseling or verifying something or on the phone due to an issue, [the immunizing technicians] are able to help with the immunization aspect of it." (2020 Pharmacist 5)
- "It helps free me up. As long as I'm trusting [my technician] to do the shot because I feel like I'm getting pulled in a million directions, it just helps and is paying off." (2020 Pharmacist 1)

3.2. Factor 2: Compatibility

Compatibility is described as the assimilation of an innovation into a particular model. In this model the pharmacy technicians' compatibility with the newly provided service was highlighted by their supervising pharmacists.

Theme 2. *Pharmacists believe in choosing a confident and friendly technician to provide immunizations.*

- "I think technicians who are very people-friendly will do better doing this, technicians who can go back and talk to the patient and put them at ease. It helps to have them be the person who starts them at the window and actually gives the shot, too. I think that having that person through the process helps." (2017 Pharmacist 3)
- "I have a technician who is confident in herself ... you've got different personalities, and she's definitely one of the appropriate personality types for that." (2017 Pharmacist 4)
- "I would only do it if a technician is a go-getter and wants to do it. I would never put a technician on the spot if they weren't comfortable with it. I would never want them to have to feel that they were being pushed into doing it because they were a technician." (2020 Pharmacist 4)

- "I think a lot of it's the technician's personality. I try and pick technicians who are really comfortable with it, and if they'll own it, those are the ones who are going to be most successful at it. That's what I would say to look for, when you choose technicians to do it look for ones that that's going to fit their personality type." (2020 Pharmacist 3)

3.3. Factor 3: Complexity or Simplicity

The complexity or simplicity of introducing a newly immunization-trained pharmacy technician into the workflow should be considered by stakeholders. The level of effort required to train and observe does not immediately improve workflow. However, after comfort is established by the supervising pharmacist the level of complexity for each immunization is reduced.

Theme 3. *Supervising pharmacists believe the innovation of having a technician capable of immunizing within the workflow helps to better prioritize their time.*

- "Having to stop workflow to go and give a whole family of five people flu shots tends to be difficult. Once [my technicians] were able to [immunize], it saves a lot of time. It makes it so that workflow doesn't have to stop if I'm the only pharmacist here. I can say we need an injection and we keep on rolling. (2017 Pharmacist 5)
- "Having that extra hand if we need it is very helpful, so we don't get overrun. Because I don't know about you, but in my flu shot season, we're doing upwards of 40 a day." (2020 Pharmacist 5)
- "Especially during flu season, there are times where we have multiple people getting immunizations. And so during those times, both myself and the technician will be giving shots, at the same time." (2020 Pharmacist 2)
- "I'm the pinch point, and again, I mean it just depends what's going on, and a lot of times, if I'm busy verifying or doing something, I'll just ask the technician, 'would you please give this person their immunization?' " (2020 Pharmacist 1)

3.4. Factor 4: Trialability

Trialability helps stakeholders to determine how easily an innovation can be adopted. By testing for this factor, adopters can anticipate certain pitfalls to avoid. After implementation and trial, the barriers of the new innovation should be considered to determine whether stakeholders should adopt the new practice. Ultimately, one recurrent theme was highlighted by the key informant interviews.

Theme 4. *Pharmacists wanted more immunization-trained pharmacy technicians in their pharmacies.*

- "I mean that was the biggest roadblock is that we had individuals that we wanted to get certified, but the program just wasn't available to be able to get them to do that." (2020 Pharmacist 2)
- "Yeah. I think everybody's going to eventually see the benefit in it. We've got a second technician going through the training course next week. We'll have two technician immunizers in our pharmacy here soon. It's pretty easy to see the benefits of it though when you look at the workflow." (2017 Pharmacist 2)
- "[The biggest challenge is] the ease of getting the training." (2020 Pharmacist 5)

3.5. Factor 5: Observability

Transparency and the observability of the opinions of supervising pharmacists or early adopters provide an effective way to create either positive or negative communication channels to drive decisions. Pharmacists communicated that having an immunization-trained pharmacy technician as part of the workflow was positive.

Theme 5. *Pharmacists as observers were initially hesitant, then accepting of the added member to the immunization team.*

- "So I only have one full time that is eligible that went through the training so pretty much any vaccination that came up, I pretty much put a tech to go vaccinate. So I would still have to check the prescription and go over the paperwork first but ... We would go, prepare all the gloves and everything and get all the side work done, and then go administer the vaccination." (2017 Pharmacist 7)
- "Take advantage of it. I mean, I'm sure that some of them might feel hesitant allowing the tech to be able to do that, because we've all [thought], 'Oh, no, it's the pharmacist's job'. But you have to jump onboard and trust your teammates." (2020 Pharmacist 5)

4. Discussion

Rogers' 5 Factors should help community pharmacy stakeholders determine the rate at which this innovation should be adopted [19]. Reflecting on the results and themes produced in terms of relative advantage, compatibility, complexity, or simplicity, trialability, and observability is necessary to make an informed decision. In summation, the perception of the supervising pharmacists was that having an immunizing technician improved workflow and allowed for improved time prioritization. However, some concerns were highlighted: The choice of the appropriate technician to receive the training was considered important, and the current low offer of immunization training was perceived to be a barrier towards implementation. In addition, initial hesitation and temporarily increased workload were expressed as challenges by supervising pharmacists who introduced an immunizing technician into the workflow.

Pharmacy technicians have a palpable impact on community pharmacy workflow, and advanced technician roles have been shown to positively affect technician job satisfaction [8]. In addition, patient care aspects in pharmacy technician roles contribute to increased self-actualization [21]. Providing pharmacy technicians with perceivably meaningful activities, such as involving them in patient care, can benefit their work performance [22]. Fostering innovations that can produce new workplace environments such as this can improve the traditional community pharmacy paradigm.

There were limitations to this research. During phase 1, interview questions were emailed to staff pharmacists prior to the interviews with the goal of providing opportunity for thoughtful consideration of the questions and minimizing disruption to workflow. While these goals may have been achieved, providing the questions ahead of time may have created bias since the participants had the opportunity to provide responses that were formulated rather than giving the reactionary responses expected during interviews where the participant cannot prepare ahead of time.

Although researchers were not able to contact and interview all 20 pharmacies in phase 2, researchers believed saturation was reached after conducting the 2020 interviews because the 2020 responses repeated the majority of the comments recorded in 2017, and because all five of the 2020 interviews yielded similar results. One pharmacy in 2020 had no current immunizing pharmacy technician, which was a recent change that had occurred less than one month prior to the interview (Table 3). As pharmacy technician immunization administration becomes more widespread, conducting similar research on pharmacy workflow with a larger and more diverse key informant group could lead to different results.

This project was conducted in one state and within one pharmacy chain. Information about individual pharmacy prescription volumes, number of patients, and number of employees was not available to the research team, but could provide valuable insight into how immunizing technicians are utilized in workflow in stores with varying degrees of staff support and time available to engage with each patient. This pharmacy chain was a very early adopter of this new advanced technician role and chain leadership was very supportive. Results of similar work in a chain where pharmacists or pharmacy leadership are less supportive of immunizing technicians would likely lead to different results. Results may also differ with pharmacists that are not comfortable with immunizing patients. All the pharmacists interviewed in this study already administered immunizations before immunizing technicians were added into the workflow. Additionally, because of the way the research was conducted, the pharmacists interviewed in 2017 were not necessarily the same pharmacists who were interviewed in 2020. Conducting a similar project longitudinally with the same subset of pharmacists may provide a more detailed picture of the impact on workflow.

There is still much research to be done on this topic. Although pharmacists' perceive an increase in the number of immunizations administered [18] when immunizing technicians are integrated into pharmacy workflow, actual immunization data comparing stores with immunizing technicians to similar stores without immunizing technicians would strengthen these results. Similarly, pharmacists perceive that workflow is improved and pharmacist time is saved by utilizing technicians to administer immunizations, but conducting a study similar to that of Fleagle and colleagues in 2019 where workflow hours were analyzed would lead to definitive results about the amount of time saved for pharmacists. Additionally, the training available for pharmacy technicians to learn to administer immunizations is being expanded from a small program at Washington State University [23] to a program offered on a national level through the American Pharmacists Association [16]. Since one of the challenges identified by the study pharmacists was lack of availability of the training program because they had willing technicians who were not able to attend to date, the implications of broader access to the program have not yet been realized. This training expansion will lead to a multitude of additional research opportunities as technicians in more geographic regions of the country with varying needs for additional immunizers begin undertaking this role.

5. Conclusions

Rogers' 5 Factors from the Diffusion of Innovation provide insight into ideal characteristics for encouraging adoption of an innovation. Immunizing is a relatively new role for pharmacy technicians, and consideration of factors that can encourage and ease implementation into pharmacy workflow can aid in future application. The findings of this study included themes such as: (1) Pharmacists' perceived improvement in workflow flexibility; (2) The choice of the correct technician to immunize within the pharmacy; (3) Pharmacists' perceived improved workflow time prioritization; (4) Limited available training as a barrier to implementation; and (5) The initial apprehension and later acceptance of pharmacists with respect to the innovation. Pharmacists are able to focus on the task at hand rather than facing interruptions and delays in checking prescriptions caused by providing walk-in immunizations. The biggest barrier identified by the participant pharmacists was the challenge of getting more technicians trained. Technicians were interested in immunizing and pharmacists supported them in becoming immunizers, but the training was not being offered in their area as frequently as they would prefer. As technician immunization administration spreads beyond early adopter states, further research into the impact on pharmacy workflow is needed.

Author Contributions: T.G.B. and K.C.M. contribute equally. All authors have read and agreed to the published version of the manuscript.

Funding: This research received no external funding.

Acknowledgments: The Albertsons (Sav-on) Pharmacy team®.

Conflicts of Interest: The authors declare no conflict of interest.

References

1. US Department of Health and Human Services Reforming America's Healthcare System through Choice and Competition. Available online: https://www.hhs.gov/sites/default/files/Reforming-Americas-Healthcare-System-Through-Choice-and-Competition.pdf (accessed on 23 February 2020).
2. Good, J.V.; Owens, J.; Page, A.; Gatewood, S. Community-Based Pharmacy Practice Innovation and the Role of the Community-Based Pharmacist Practitioner in the United States. *Pharmacy* **2019**, *7*, 106. [CrossRef] [PubMed]
3. Patel, A.; Breck, A.; Law, M. The Impact of Pharmacy-Based Immunization Services on the Likelihood of Immunization in the USA. *J. Am. Pharm. Assoc.* **2018**, *58*, 505–514. [CrossRef] [PubMed]
4. McConeghy, K.W.; Wing, C. A national examination of pharmacy-based immunization statues and their association with influenza vaccinations and preventative health. *Vaccine* **2016**, *34*, 3463–3468. [CrossRef] [PubMed]

5. Ventola, C.L. Immunization in the United States: Recommendations, Barriers, and Measures to Improve Compliance: Part 1: Childhood Vaccinations. *Pharm. Ther.* **2016**, *41*, 426–436.
6. Kao, C.M.; Schneyer, R.J.; Bocchini, J.A. Child and adolescent immunizations: Selected review of recent U.S. recommendations and literature. *Curr. Opin. Pediatr.* **2014**, *26*, 383–395. [CrossRef] [PubMed]
7. Koehler, T.; Brown, A. Documenting the evolution of the relationship between the pharmacy support workforce and pharmacists to support patient care. *RSAP* **2017**, *13*, 280–285. [CrossRef]
8. Mattingly, A.N.; Mattingly, T.J., II. Advancing the role of the pharmacy technician: A systematic review. *J. Am. Pharm. Assoc.* **2018**, *58*, 94–108. [CrossRef]
9. Fleagle Miller, R.; Cesarz, J.; Rough, S. Evaluation of community pharmacy tech-check-tech as a strategy for practice advancement. *JAPhA* **2018**, *58*, 652–658. [CrossRef] [PubMed]
10. Hohmeier, K.C.; McDonough, S.; Rein, L.J.; Brookhart, A.L.; Gibson, M.L.; Powers, M.F. Exploring the expanded role of the pharmacy technician in medication therapy management service implementation in the community pharmacy. *JAPhA* **2019**, *59*, 187–194. [CrossRef] [PubMed]
11. Idaho State Board of Pharmacy Pharmacy Code & Administrative Rules. Available online: https://bop.idaho.gov/pharmacy-code-administrative-rules/ (accessed on 24 February 2020).
12. Pharmacists, Pharmacies, and Manufacturers, Wholesalers, and Distributors (216-RICR-40-15-1). Available online: https://rules.sos.ri.gov/regulations/part/216-40-15-1 (accessed on 24 February 2020).
13. State of Utah Department of Commerce Vaccine Administration Protocol. Available online: https://dopl.utah.gov/pharm/vaccine_administration_protocol.pdf (accessed on 24 February 2020).
14. Eid, D.; Osborne, J.; Borowicz, B. Moving the Needle: A 50-State and District of Columbia Landscape Review of Laws Regarding Pharmacy Technician Vaccine Administration. *J. Pharm.* **2019**, *7*, 168. [CrossRef]
15. Doucette, W.R.; Schommer, J.C. Pharmacy Technicians' Willingness to Perform Emerging Tasks in Community Practice. *Pharmacy* **2018**, *6*, 113. [CrossRef]
16. Pharamcy-based Immunization Administration by Pharmacy Technicians. Available online: https://www.pharmacist.com/pharmacy-based-immunization-administration-pharmacy-technicians-1 (accessed on 6 March 2020).
17. McKeirnan, K.; Frazier, K.; Nguyen, M.; MacLean, L. Training Pharmacy Technicians to Administer Immunizations. *J. Am. Pharm. Assoc.* **2018**, *58*, 174–178. [CrossRef]
18. Bertsch, T.G.; McKeirnan, K.C.; Frazier, K.R.; VanVoorhis, L.; Shin, S.; Le, K. Supervising Pharmacists' Opinions About Pharmacy Technicians as Immunizers. *J. Am. Pharm. Assoc.* **2019**, *59*, 527–532. [CrossRef] [PubMed]
19. Rogers, E. *Diffusion of Innovations*, 5th ed.; Free Press: New York, NY, USA, 2003.
20. Miles, M.; Huberman, A.M.; Saldaña, J. *Qualitative Data Analysis: A Methods Sourcebook*, 3rd ed.; Sage: Thousand Oaks, CA, USA, 2014.
21. Desselle, S.P. An in-depth examination into pharmacy technician worklife through an organizational behavior framework. *RSAP* **2016**, *12*, 722–732. [CrossRef] [PubMed]
22. Peiró, J.M.; Kozusznik, M.W.; Soriano, A. From Happiness Orientations to Work Performance: The Mediating Role of Hedonic and Eudaimonic Experiences. *Int. J. Environ. Res. Public Health* **2019**, *16*, 5002. [CrossRef]
23. Pharmacy Technician Immunization Training. Washington State University. Available online: https://pharmacy.wsu.edu/pharmacy-technician-immunization-training/ (accessed on 24 March 2020).

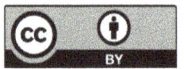

© 2020 by the authors. Licensee MDPI, Basel, Switzerland. This article is an open access article distributed under the terms and conditions of the Creative Commons Attribution (CC BY) license (http://creativecommons.org/licenses/by/4.0/).

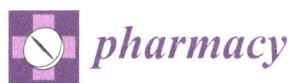

Article

T.E.A.M.S.Work: Leveraging Technicians to Enhance ABM Med Sync in Community Pharmacies

Tamera D. Hughes, Lana M. Minshew, Stacey Cutrell and Stefanie P. Ferreri *

UNC Eshelman School of Pharmacy, University of North Carolina, Chapel Hill, NC 27599, USA; tamera_hughes@unc.edu (T.D.H); minshew@live.unc.edu (L.M.M.); scutrell@live.unc.edu (S.C.)
* Correspondence: stefanie_ferreri@unc.edu

Received: 6 March 2020; Accepted: 24 March 2020; Published: 27 March 2020

Abstract: The expansion of pharmacy technicians' roles in community pharmacies allows pharmacists the opportunity to focus on providing clinical services to patients. This study explores the tasks pharmacy technicians' perform to support Med Sync programs in community pharmacies. Pharmacy staff members at North Carolina pharmacies with more than fifty percent of their prescription volume being dispensed as part of a Med Sync program were recruited to participate in semi-structured interviews. Inductive coding and summary analysis were used to analyze the interview data. Study participants described pharmacy technicians' roles in identifying patients for marketing and enrollment, reviewing patients' medications list, choosing alignment dates based on patient preference, contacting patients in preparation for dispensing and, lastly, engaging in pickup or delivery of medications. This study highlights technicians' vital role in completing tasks that support Med Sync programs in community pharmacies.

Keywords: medication synchronization; community pharmacy; pharmacy technicians; pharmacy workforce

1. Introduction

In response to value-based payment structures, community pharmacies recognize the expansion of pharmacy technicians' roles for achieving optimal patient care [1]. Both medication dispensing support and clinical service support have been adopted by pharmacy technicians [2]. Technicians' roles have expanded to include taking and transferring prescriptions and "tech-check-tech" duties with no statistically significant differences detected in the accuracy or error-detection rates between pharmacists and technicians [3]. Advanced roles, such as, immunization administration have also emerged in some states to include technicians, further encouraging the advancement of their roles [1]. The evolution of technician roles better positions pharmacy technicians to support and free up pharmacists to focus on providing patient care services [4].

Medication nonadherence is estimated to account for nearly $300 billion of the annual healthcare cost in the United States [5]. In an effort to improve adherence and reduce unnecessary spending, medication synchronization (Med Sync) programs have been adopted by community pharmacies [6]. Studies show medication adherence improves when patients are enrolled in a Med Sync program; however, considerable variability in the implementation of this service exists between community pharmacies [7–11]. Med Sync, as described by the American Pharmacists' Association (APhA) in their white paper, is designed to improve consumers' adherence to medications and build efficiencies in pharmacy operations. The white paper establishes how community pharmacies can integrate the Appointment Based Model (ABM) Med Sync into pharmacy workflow and business models [12]. The 10 steps outlined in the white paper were summarized in a systematic review of the Med Sync process conducted by Patti and colleagues [12,13]. The systematic review revealed 5 core components:

(1) pharmacy staff identifying and enrolling patients, (2) pharmacy staff reviewing and assessing medication, (3) pharmacy staff working with patients to synchronize medication refills, (4) pharmacy staff contacting patients or designated care providers to identify medications for fill, and (5) patients meeting with pharmacy staff for pick up or delivery of medication [13]. The white paper and the systematic review demonstrate key roles that must take place to perform Med Sync services, yet neither document mentions which pharmacy staff members should perform these services.

Across the country, community pharmacies have implemented Med Sync to promote medication adherence and improve patient outcomes. The National Community Pharmacists Association (NCPA) *Digest* reports 79% of independent pharmacies currently offer Med Sync to combat nonadherence [14]. Researchers identified several pharmacies in North Carolina who dispense more than fifty percent of their prescriptions as part of a Med Sync program. To explore how these community pharmacies operate Med Sync, a qualitative study was undertaken with the aim to reveal strategies that incorporate technicians' roles into Med Sync. Determination of these roles and responsibilities will provide insight into specific pharmacy operations employing technicians for successfully operating a Med Sync program.

2. Materials and Methods

The research team consisted of two pharmacists, one pharmacy student, and a qualitative research methodologist. The study reported here is a part of a larger multi-phase project examining adoption of Med Sync programs in community pharmacies. For the purposes of the study reported here, the data that focuses on the role of pharmacy technicians is highlighted. This observational study utilized a semi-structured interview guide with the initial goal of identifying the barriers and facilitators to adoption and explored community pharmacies practical solutions to ensure successful adoption of Med Sync services. Purposeful sampling was used to identify North Carolina community pharmacies with greater than 50% of their prescriptions in a Med Sync program and the leads of the Med Sync program were invited to participate in an interview. Interviews were conducted by three members of the research team via Zoom Client for Meetings [computer program] Version 4.6.7. (Zoom Video Communications Inc., San Jose, CA, USA). The semi-structured interview guide focused on all aspects of adoption of Med Sync. Each interview lasted approximately 60 min and were transcribed verbatim.

The analysis of interview data used an inductive approach to coding, and codes were derived from the data in order to reflect participants' perspective [15,16]. As a group, the team read and discussed participant responses and through these discussions created codes and corresponding definitions. Memos were written during and after each coding session to capture the analytic process and any themes or patterns that were emerging in the data [15,16]. Preliminary analysis revealed heavy involvement of non-pharmacist staff, leading the research team to further investigate the roles and tasks of technicians in Med Sync. After initial coding, cluster analysis was used to focus on the data that emphasized the roles of and tasks completed by technicians [15,16]. This process involved creating a summary matrix of the data and reviewing the data iteratively to identify key ideas expressed by participants regarding the role and tasks of technicians in the Med Sync program. At least two members of the research team analyzed the qualitative data at a given time and agreed on the application of codes and the identified themes. A third researcher, a pharmacist, verified all themes. This study (IRB# 19-1832) was determined to be exempt by the university's IRB.

3. Results

Twelve community pharmacies met the inclusion criteria of having greater than 50% of their prescriptions in a Med Sync program and were invited to participate in the study. Seven pharmacies responded and agreed to be interviewed, Table 1 displays their demographic characteristics. The recruitment email requested to interview an individual who was the primary leader of the Med Sync program at the pharmacy. Six pharmacists and one pharmacy technician were interviewed.

Table 1. Participating Community Pharmacy Characteristics.

Characteristics	Exemplar 1	Exemplar 2	Exemplar 3	Exemplar 4	Exemplar 5	Exemplar 6	Exemplar 7
Geographic Region	Rural	Urban	Urban	Rural	Rural	Urban	Urban
Average Prescription volume per week	1750	900	650	4500	750	2000	250
Years of Reported MedSync Services	4–5	7	3	3-5	5	4	2

Analysis of the seven community pharmacies revealed technicians' support of Med Sync through various roles and tasks. Participants described technicians' roles in identifying patients for marketing and enrollment, reviewing patients' medications list to establish a plan for synchronization, choosing alignment dates based on patient preference, contacting patients in preparation for dispensing, and lastly, engaging in pickup or delivery of medications.

Program leaders from each store described varying levels of technician involvement in all aspects of the Med Sync Program. Each pharmacy recounted technician responsibilities in at least three of the tasks mentioned above. One pharmacy acknowledged technician involvement in all Med Sync tasks, and another pharmacy had a technician involved in four. All pharmacies detailed involvement in both documentation of patient information as part of the Med Sync process and preparation and packaging of prescriptions. Two pharmacies discussed technician involvement in addressing additional interventions, such as, delivery. Six of the seven pharmacies described technician assistance with patient enrollment.

Tasks mentioned in the marketing and enrollment of Med Sync patients included identifying nonadherent patients via performance information management systems and communicating with new and frequent patients during face to face and telephonic encounters. For instance, one participant shared they have technicians *"run a report of everybody who is less than 80% adherent"* as a way to target patients for enrollment in Med Sync. Patient assessments and medication review tasks included technicians identifying low, medium, and high-risk patients for medication nonadherence based on medication burden and prior incidence with adherence. One participant, a pharmacist, when asked to "Walk me through how you synchronize your prescriptions once they are enrolled", responded, *"That's probably a better question for the techs."* In addition, technicians also documented patient information, such as, counting refills and patient's "at home stock". For example, one participant stated that technicians *"tally up how many pills of each medication we need to give to the [patient] . . . and short fill whatever needs to be short filled to get [the patient] lined up."* Technicians interacted with patients to set synchronization dates that accommodated finances, transportation and other patient limiting preferences. One participant noted their technicians set sync dates based upon patient preference, *"we leave it up to the individual [patient] . . . they tell us when [they] want it, what day or what week and we kind of go from there."* During the preparation of the medications for dispensing, technicians conducted routine patient interviews and packaging of prescriptions using multi-dose packaging systems. Lastly, technicians were either present for pickup or addressed additional services, such as, delivery when necessary.

Additional corresponding participant quotes capturing technician roles, responsibilities, and tasks are matched with the identified 5 major themes in Table 2.

Table 2. Quotes Discussing Technician Activities in Medication Synchronization.

Activity—Major Themes	Participant Quote
Market and Enroll Creation of a structured system to target and enroll patients who are most likely to benefit from a medication synchronization program.	"And so, our analytics technician, she would go in and run a report of everybody who is less than 80% adherence." (Exemplar 1) "Technicians market the program" (Exemplar 4) "I mean, it's more of just like a technician says, hey, listen, this person isn't on a Med Sync that they'd be a prime candidate." (Exemplar 6) "If they're on monthly medications . . . . the maintenance medications that they need to be on all the time . . . . we [the technicians identify] for our sync program." (Exemplar 7)
Medication review and patient assessment Assessment and review of patients' medication prior to synchronization.	"The technician who's working sync that day, they'll take those forms and then you know tally up you know how many pills of each med we need to give to the customer." (Exemplar 1) "So, our categories are green, yellow, red, and those are what our technicians [review] . . . . And so sometimes it is like a pharmacist or technician referral . . . we kind of watch them a little closer make sure they're getting what they need." (Exemplar 6) "I'm [technician] the main one that does the initial contact and then the initial drop of the prescriptions . . . If there's any issues, we let them know." (Exemplar 7)
Align refills Selection of a synchronization date	"You'll get a phone call from one of our technicians who call you to set everything up [set date] and go from there." (Exemplar 1) "Then we'll [the technicians] set their sync date based off the last time that they got that bulk medication . . . we try to like let the patient know that we're going to short [fill]. That way we can get it lined up so they can get all their medications at the same time each month." (Exemplar 7)
Preparations for medication pick-up and delivery Initiating contact with patient prior to preparation of prescriptions for pick-up. This communication is essential to ensure that the appropriate medications are refilled and to guide topics for discussion at the appointment. Preparation of the medications for the patient.	"When it [queue] actually pops up in the queue, that's when the technician will go through and they fill all those medications." (Exemplar 1) "So, whenever the technicians call for the monthly Med Sync call when they talk to the patient and they kind of get a feel that, you know, the patient does not know what's going on, or they're being picky of their medication, they [the technician] tend to triage the call to the pharmacist." (Exemplar 2) "And so, there's four workstations, three for technicians and one for pharmacists that are all kind of simultaneously being used to both make synchronization calls as well as fill prescriptions." (Exemplar 3) "The technicians are supposed to process a certain amount of baskets each day to keep us up ahead of the Med Sync pick up date." (Exemplar 6) "Mostly I'm [the technician] the main one that does the initial contact and then the initial drop of the prescriptions. So, we attempt to reach out to the patient, let them know that we're working on their medications for the week." (Exemplar 7)
Pick up or delivery of medication and other services Receipt of medication in person or via delivery. Additional services/interventions may be addressed.	"We've had technicians that would offer to deliver their medications too." (Exemplar 2) "By the point the prescriptions are all filled and ready to go out to the patient. We'll [technicians] reach out to them again to set up pickup date or delivery date." (Exemplar 7)

4. Discussion

In this study, pharmacy technicians were identified as having varying assignments in Med Sync programs in community pharmacies who had 50% or more prescriptions in the program. Our results demonstrate that technicians can support Med Sync programs by marketing and enrolling patients, reviewing patient prescriptions, selecting medication synchronization dates, and assisting in the delivery or pick up of medications. These results help to close the gap on the conversation as to whether Med Sync services fall on pharmacists and initiate the capturing of non-pharmacist staff participation in the Med Sync process [13]. This study demonstrates that technicians can be engaged in all tasks of the Med Sync process.

The APhA white paper establishes the steps to improve consumers' adherence to medication and the systematic review conducted by Patti and colleagues summarizes the white paper to help standardize Med Sync within community pharmacies. [13,16]. The white paper and the systematic review demonstrate key roles that must take place to perform Med Sync services, yet neither document mentions which pharmacy staff members should perform these services. The five activities that technicians participated in that emerged from our data are reflective of the Patti and colleagues 5 core components. Participant responses alluded to technicians' practicality in performing most, if not all tasks. This suggests that technicians are and can be integral components for effective Med Sync implementation.

According to the results, technicians have constant engagement with patients and are in a great position for involvement in all steps of a Med Sync program from initiation to pick up and/or delivery. In fact, one of the pharmacies mentioned technician involvement in all 5 core components of the

Med Sync process, and the technician was the primary lead on the service. This demonstrates that technicians are capable of participating in all steps of the Med Sync process, and technicians are also in a great position to take the lead of the service. Recent studies have shown having a dedicated Med Sync technician assists in supporting clinicians [17,18]. In the current study, one participant, a pharmacist, deferred their question regarding patient synchronization and enrollment responding, *"That's probably a better question for the techs."* This suggests the pharmacist trusted the technician to be the leader of the Med Sync program.

Not only are technicians in a great position to lead the program, they are also able to assume increased responsibility. Two recent workforce surveys suggest technician responsiveness and eagerness in assuming increased responsibility [1,19]. When the lone pharmacy technician was asked how they became involved in the program they responded, *"I have an eye for organization, and I just started taking it over, little by little."* This represents the increased responsibility the technician was willing to take on to lead the program. In addition, to leading the Med Sync program, the technician also attended a national meeting to learn more about the service. This further solidified the technician's commitment as a leader and their continued involvement in Med Sync.

In other observations of pharmacies struggling to implement new services, underutilization of pharmacy technicians is a common theme. Given the challenging practice environment that community pharmacists are faced with, efficiently involving all staff members in Med Sync operation is key. Participant responses were consistent in leveraging the technician workforce in support of Med Sync success. Though this study focused on the role of technicians, future research needs to investigate the roles of additional non-pharmacist staff. Clerks and cashiers were mentioned in multiple steps in the Med Sync process. One participant acknowledged the importance of the cashiers in their Med Sync enrollment process stating *"cashiers… would get a lot more [enroll more patients] because they were talking face to face with people"*.

Finally, this study expands the literature regarding advancing the roles for pharmacy technicians in community pharmacies. By allowing technicians to have more advanced technical roles, it provides community pharmacist opportunities to become more involved in direct patient care. This transition allows pharmacists to participate in activities that use their expertise in medication optimization services and improves medication outcomes. Inevitably, advancing pharmacy practice depends on elevating the roles and responsibilities of pharmacy technicians.

Study Limitations

The current study focused solely on community pharmacies in North Carolina that had 50% or more of their prescriptions enrolled in a Med Sync program. More knowledge could be gained by broadening the participant sample to include community pharmacies in other states. Despite the small sample, the current study does include both urban and rural community pharmacies and a range of prescription volume per week indicating technicians can support Med Sync utilization in a variety of contexts. Furthermore, expanding this research to determine how technicians' roles affect patients' outcomes may be beneficial and is warranted.

5. Conclusions

Effective leveraging of pharmacy technician roles is important to the success of Med Sync programs. This study highlights technicians' ability to support Med Sync programs in community pharmacies. The roles of pharmacy technicians and other workforce personnel must continually expand in an attempt to meet the needs of an ever-changing healthcare landscape. Continuous advancements in the responsibilities of pharmacy technicians will undoubtedly advance community pharmacy practice.

Author Contributions: Conceptualization, T.D.H., L.M.M., S.C., and S.P.F.; methodology, T.D.H., L.M.M., and S.C.; formal analysis, T.D.H., L.M.M., S.C., and S.P.F.; investigation, T.D.H., L.M.M., S.C., and S.P.F.; data curation, T.D.H. and S.C.; writing—original draft preparation, T.D.H., L.M.M., and S.C.; writing—review and editing, T.D.H., L.M.M., S.C., and S.P.F.; supervision, T.D.H. and S.P.F.; project administration, T.D.H. All authors have read and agreed to the published version of the manuscript.

Funding: This research received no external funding.

Acknowledgments: The authors thank Patrick Brown for his insight and critical review as a member check. The authors thank Mutual Drug Company pharmacies for their commitment to providing enhanced patient services.

Conflicts of Interest: The authors declare no conflict of interest.

References

1. Boughen, M.; Sutton, J.; Fenn, T.; Wright, D. Defining the Role of the Pharmacy Technician and Identifying Their Future Role in Medicines Optimisation. *Pharmacy* **2017**, *5*, 40. [CrossRef] [PubMed]
2. Adams, A.J.; Desselle, S.P.; McKeirnan, K.C. Pharmacy Technician-Administered Vaccines: On Perceptions and Practice Reality. *Pharm. Basel Switz.* **2018**, *6*, 124. [CrossRef] [PubMed]
3. Sasser, J. The First Pharmacy Technicians to Give Immunizations: How Idaho Did It. Available online: https://info.nhanow.com/learning-leading-blog/the-first-pharmacy-technicians-to-give-immunizations-how-idaho-did-it (accessed on 29 February 2020).
4. McKeirnan, K.C.; McDonough, R.P. Transforming pharmacy practice: Advancing the role of technicians. *Pharm. Today* **2018**, *24*, 54–61. [CrossRef]
5. Bosworth, H.B.; Granger, B.B.; Mendys, P.; Brindis, R.; Burkholder, R.; Czajkowski, S.M.; Kimmel, S.E. Medication adherence: A call for action. *Am. Heart J.* **2011**, *162*, 412–424. [CrossRef] [PubMed]
6. Bonner, L. Med Sync Catching on Across Nation. Available online: https://www.pharmacist.com/article/med-sync-catching-across-nation (accessed on 29 February 2020).
7. Patterson, J.A.; Holdford, D.A.; Saxena, K. Cost-benefit of appointment-based medication synchronization in community pharmacies. *Am. J. Manag. Care* **2016**, *22*, 587–593. [PubMed]
8. Barnes, B.; Hincapie, A.L.; Luder, H.; Kirby, J.; Frede, S.; Heaton, P.C. Appointment-based models: A comparison of three model designs in a large chain community pharmacy setting. *J. Am. Pharm. Assoc.* **2018**, *58*, 156–162.e1. [CrossRef] [PubMed]
9. Clifton, C.L.; Branham, A.R.; Hayes, H.H.; Moose, J.S.; Rhodes, L.A.; Marciniak, M.W. Financial impact of patients enrolled in a medication adherence program at an independent community pharmacy. *J. Am. Pharm. Assoc. JAPhA* **2018**, *58*, S109–S113. [CrossRef] [PubMed]
10. Holdford, D.A.; Inocencio, T.J. Adherence and persistence associated with an appointment-based medication synchronization program. *J. Am. Pharm. Assoc. JAPhA* **2013**, *53*, 576–583. [CrossRef] [PubMed]
11. Doshi, J.A.; Lim, R.; Li, P.; Young, P.P.; Lawnicki, V.F.; State, J.J.; Troxel, A.B.; Volpp, K.G. A Synchronized Prescription Refill Program Improved Medication Adherence. *Health Aff. Proj. Hope* **2016**, *35*, 1504–1512. [CrossRef] [PubMed]
12. APhA Foundation. *White Paper on Pharmacy's Appointment Based Model: A Prescription Synchronization Program that Improves Adherence*; APhA Foundation: Washington, DC, USA, 2013.
13. Patti, M.; Renfro, C.P.; Posey, R.; Wu, G.; Turner, K.; Ferreri, S.P. Systematic review of medication synchronization in community pharmacy practice. *Res. Soc. Adm. Pharm.* **2019**, *15*, 1281–1288. [CrossRef] [PubMed]
14. NCPA. NCPA Releases 2019 Digest. Available online: https://www.ncpanet.org/newsroom/news-releases/2019/10/29/ncpa-releases-2019-digest (accessed on 4 March 2020).
15. Bhattacharya, K. *Fundamentals of Qualitative Research*, 1st ed.; Routledge: New York, NY, USA, 2017.
16. Miles, M.B.; Huberman, A.M. *Qualitative Data Analysis: An Expanded Sourcebook*; SAGE: Thousand Oaks, CA, USA, 1994.
17. Hinson, J.L.; Garofoli, G.K.; Elswick, B.M. The impact of medication synchronization on quality care criteria in an independent community pharmacy. *J. Am. Pharm. Assoc. JAPhA* **2017**, *57*, 236–240. [CrossRef] [PubMed]

18. Kadia, N.K.; Schroeder, M.N. Community Pharmacy–Based Adherence Programs and the Role of Pharmacy Technicians. *J. Pharm. Technol. JPT Off. Publ. Assoc. Pharm. Tech.* **2015**, *31*, 51–57. [CrossRef]
19. Borchert, J.S.; Phillips, J.; Thompson Bastin, M.L.; Livingood, A.; Andersen, R.; Brasher, C.; Lee, J.C. Best practices: Incorporating pharmacy technicians and other support personnel into the clinical pharmacist's process of care. *JACCP J. Am. Coll. Clin. Pharm.* **2019**, *2*, 74–81. [CrossRef]

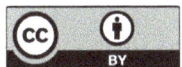

© 2020 by the authors. Licensee MDPI, Basel, Switzerland. This article is an open access article distributed under the terms and conditions of the Creative Commons Attribution (CC BY) license (http://creativecommons.org/licenses/by/4.0/).

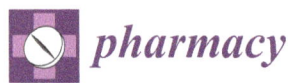

Article

Exploring Pharmacy Technician Roles in the Implementation of an Appointment-Based Medication Synchronization Program

Chelsea Renfro [1], Davis Coulter [1], Lan Ly [1], Cindy Fisher [2], Lindsay Cardosi [3], Mike Wasson [2] and Kenneth C. Hohmeier [4],*

[1] Department of Clinical Pharmacy and Translational Science, University of Tennessee Health Science Center College of Pharmacy, Memphis, TN 38163, USA; crenfro@uthsc.edu (C.R.); dcoulter@uthsc.edu (D.C.); lly2@uthsc.edu (L.L.)
[2] Kroger Pharmacy, Memphis, TN 38103, USA; cindy.fisher@kroger.com (C.F.); mike.wasson@kroger.com (M.W.)
[3] Methodist South Bedside Delivery Program, Memphis, TN 38116, USA; linbblan@uthsc.edu
[4] Department of Clinical Pharmacy and Translational Science, University of Tennessee Health Science Center College of Pharmacy, Nashville, TN 37211, USA
* Correspondence: khohmeie@uthsc.edu

Received: 1 November 2019; Accepted: 25 February 2020; Published: 3 March 2020

Abstract: The objective of this study was to qualitatively explore the role of pharmacy technicians in the implementation of an appointment-based model (ABM) medication synchronization program. The purposeful sampling of technicians working within six different locations of a supermarket chain pharmacy in Mississippi and Tennessee was carried out, and the technicians were interviewed between January and April 2018. A semi-structured interview guide was developed based on the Consolidated Framework for Implementation Research (CFIR). Questions gathered information around pharmacy technician demographics and CFIR domains (process, inner setting, outer setting and intervention characteristics). Interviews were audiotaped and transcribed. Two members of the research team performed thematic content analysis. Six full-time, certified pharmacy technicians with 8.3 ± 2.7 years of experience were interviewed. Findings suggest that including hands-on experience with program software is needed during training to successfully implement ABM. A barrier to implementation was the time needed to complete ABM tasks as compared to other tasks. Although some barriers exist regarding implementation, technicians believe that overall, this program has positive benefits for patients. Results from this study signify that ABM implementation can be challenging. Better ABM portal integration with the pharmacy patient profile and appropriate workforce budgeting are key to continued success.

Keywords: medication synchronization; service implementation; community pharmacy; pharmacy technicians

1. Introduction

According to the Centers for Disease Control and Prevention (CDC), one in four adults suffer from at least two or more chronic diseases such as diabetes, dyslipidemia, and hypertension [1]. The World Health Organization (WHO) found that only 50% of patients, on average, in developed countries with chronic diseases are adherent to their medications [2]. Medication nonadherence in patients with chronic conditions escalates direct health care costs nearly $100–$300 billion dollars each year [3]. Medication synchronization is a program proven to increase adherence, reduce emergency department visits and reduce hospitalizations for these patients [4,5]. Community pharmacies have incorporated medication synchronization into their workflow to improve quality of care and medication adherence.

Medication synchronization is the alignment of a patient's medication refills to a single date each month. Other features can be added in conjunction, such as comprehensive medication reviews (CMRs) and delivery [6,7].

The Appointment Based Model (ABM), one type of medication synchronization, is a patient care model where patients have one or two appointed days per month to pick up all medications [7]. The pharmacist performs additional patient care services, such as a comprehensive medication review (CMR), on that day to evaluate therapy and answer any questions or concerns from the patient [8]. Approximately 20,000 community pharmacies have implemented this service in the United States, and it is predicted to expand [9]. The medication synchronization component of ABM may be implemented by personnel at the patient's pharmacy, or via a call center that identifies appropriate patients to enroll and places medication orders into pharmacy workflow. These programs allow pharmacies to clarify medication regimens, for stakeholders to enable optimization of medications while improving predictability of workflow and workload [6–9].

Successful process implementation requires buy-in from all members of the healthcare team [10]. Given the demands on pharmacist time, new service implementation in community pharmacy is frequently met with barriers [11–13]. While pharmacists deliver the clinical components of ABM, pharmacy technicians have a vital role in the implementation process for this service. The exploration of the pharmacy technician perspectives is crucial to understand how to overcome the hurdles facing ABM and medication adherence. There is limited research on roles, responsibilities, and challenges faced by pharmacy technicians in ABM implementation. The objective of this study was to qualitatively explore the role of pharmacy technicians in the implementation of an appointment-based medication synchronization program.

2. Materials and Methods

2.1. Recruitment and Participants

Pharmacy technicians working one regional division of a large community pharmacy chain in either Mississippi or Tennessee were recruited. A purposeful sampling approach was used to recruit participants, whereby key informants were selected based on their exposure to ABM implementation, rather than selected randomly. The researchers were provided with a list of pharmacies from which subjects could be contacted, and researchers subsequently contacted and consented participants via telephone. Participants were stratified based on their pharmacy's type of ABM used (in-store technician call model or an off-site call center model) and ABM performance (as defined by internal pharmacy measures of ABM implementation) within the supermarket chain pharmacy's division. Participants had no prior experience with ABM prior to the study. This study was approved by the Institutional Review Board at the researchers' university. All subjects gave their informed consent for inclusion before they participated in the study. The study was conducted in accordance with the Declaration of Helsinki, and the protocol was approved by the Ethics Committee of the University of Tennessee Health Science Center (18-05758-XM).

2.2. Data Collection

One member of the research team, with training in qualitative research, conducted 6 in-depth, semi-structured interviews from January to April 2018. Interviews lasted approximately 60 minutes and were conducted either via telephone or in person at the workplace. To best understand individual technician perspectives about ABM implementation, semi-structured interviews were chosen as compared to other methods, such as focus groups, which have the potential to obtain a consensus. [14].

A semi-structured interview guide was developed (Table 1) based on the Consolidated Framework for Implementation Research (CFIR) [10]. The interview guide was pilot tested with technicians at the same supermarket chain in a different division. CFIR consists of 37 constructs developed to synthesize a unified typology of implementation and dissemination theories and frameworks. The interview guide included questions categorized within four CFIR domains: (1) process (i.e., champion, engaging, innovation participants; (2) inner setting (i.e., relative priority, readiness for implementation, access to knowledge and information; (3) outer setting (i.e., needs and resources of those served by the organization); and (4) intervention characteristics (i.e., adaptability). A verbal consent statement was gathered prior to conducting the interview. The interviews were audiotaped and transcribed in their original format. Field notes were made during the interviews and added to the transcripts.

Table 1. Interview guide.

Section 1: Participant Demographics
1. Are you a certified technician?
2. How long have you been working as a technician?
• [PROBE] How long have you been working at this store?   • [PROBE] How long have you been working for Kroger?
3. On average, how many hours do you work per week?
4. Describe your roles and responsibilities in executing the medication synchronization program at your store.
Section 2: Adaptability
5. What changes, if any, would you like to make to the program?
Section 3: Patient Needs and Resources
6. What is your perception of patient satisfaction with the medication synchronization program?
7. What are the benefits, if any, of medication synchronization to the pharmacy?
Section 4: Access to Knowledge and Information
8. Explain the training, if any, that you received to carry out the roles and responsibilities you described above.   • [PROBE] Do you feel the training prepared you to carry out the roles and responsibilities expected of you?   • [PROBE] Why or why not?
Section 5: Relative Priority
9. Walk me through your process for adding medication synchronization into your workflow.   • [PROBE] Do you feel that you have adequate time to implement this program?
10. What are some of the barriers, if any, your pharmacy has faced when implementing medication synchronization?   • [PROBE] How has your pharmacy worked to overcome these barriers?
Section 6: Champion
11. Does your store have a designated champion for the medication synchronization program?
Section 7: Intervention Participants
12. Tell me an example of how you are informing patients about this program?   • [PROBE] What promotional materials, if any, do you use to communicate the availability of this program?   • [PROBE] How do you select which patients to promote this program to?

2.3. Data Analysis

Using the CFIR codebook, two members of the research team (CR and DC) analyzed thematic content [10]. The initial session consisted of both researchers identifying preliminary codes and subthemes and resolving differences through active discussion. Afterwards, the researchers independently translated the remaining transcripts and met for a second session to identify any further emerging codes or subthemes that surfaced. Transcripts were analyzed using NVivo12 (QSR International Pty Ltd., 2018). Consistent themes observed were mapped to the constructs of the CFIR. The Consolidated Criteria for Reporting Qualitative Studies checklist was used to guide the reporting of qualitative methods and findings [15].

3. Results

A total of six participants were interviewed. Recruitment was stopped after six technicians since theme saturation (i.e., occurrence of similar themes with no new information collected) was reached [16]. Participants were full-time, certified pharmacy technicians with 8.3 ± 2.7 years of experience. Participants worked an average of 39.5 ± 1.1 hours per week. All participants interviewed had been employed at the supermarket chain studied for their entire career.

3.1. Inner Setting of ABM Implementation

Questions exploring the Access to Knowledge and Information construct found that while training effectively described the utility of the program, technicians were not always familiarized with the ABM support software adequately (Table 2). One participant expressed that the overall training was "useless" due to the lack of specific ABM user interface training. Technicians preferred the hands-on instruction. Technician training consisted of a presentation by a pharmacist or shadowing a pharmacist during the enrollment process for one training session. Repeat sessions were available if needed.

Table 2. Interview constructs, definitions, and illustrative quotations.

Construct	Definition	Illustrative Quotation
Access to Knowledge and Information	Ease of access to digestible information and knowledge about the innovation and how to incorporate it into work tasks.	"Yeah, I mean we went, but that's no good until you're in Med Sync, it doesn't explain it in any way. It's useless."
Relative Priority	Individuals' shared perception of the importance of the implementation within the organization.	"With the recent cuts and hours, no we don't. Because the 30 minute enrollment visits take away the pharmacists and we used to have two pharmacists at all times, but now some days we only have one. To take the pharmacist out of the work flow is very detrimental to the actual work flow." "...they have us with so many things...I am trying to get the MedSync people 90 days at the same time, make one phone call and do all my phone calls. I don't know if that's right or wrong."
Patient Needs and Resources	The extent to which the needs of those served by the organization (e.g., patients), as well as barriers and facilitators to meet those needs, are accurately known and prioritized by the organization.	"I think more middle aged and younger people are satisfied with the program, but the elderly seem to get very confused, and don't understand."
Adaptability	The degree to which an innovation can be adapted, tailored, refined, or reinvented to meet local needs.	"I make sure I get a list of the medications they do want to be included on Med Sync and try not to mark the ones that they don't want because that saves a lot of time, and money, and headache for the patients when they come in." "Since our patients are older here, their medicines change all the time. They get here and they pick up medicines and it's not what they want. Then they wanna bring it back but our policy is you can't bring it back, therefore they get a little mad at us."

Table 2. *Cont.*

Construct	Definition	Illustrative Quotation
Champions	"Individuals who dedicate themselves to supporting, marketing, and 'driving through' an [implementation]", overcoming indifference or resistance that the innovation may provoke in an organization.	"I kind of pay attention to patients who are voices their concerns on making multiple trips, and also patients who have five or more medications that are falling on different dates. I go back and look at their profile and then I'll say, "Oh, hey, we've got this new program called Med Sync where we can synchronize your prescription. That way, you'll make one trip, get all your prescriptions right then," and most of the time we can get 90-day supplies, which really saves a lot of time, and in some cases, it saves a lot of money."
Innovation Participants	Individuals served by the organization that participate in the innovation, e.g., patients in a prevention program in a hospital.	"We tell people, we have some little flyers that we pass out, and we have people, anybody that seems to benefit from it, that if they normally have a caregiver that picks up for them and they don't get out, so it's not as convenient for them to make five trips a month ... So we're just talking to the patients, and I have called several people that are on the recommended list and some people were not very receptive to that. She told me I was trying to get all of her money, so we did not, we deleted her. We have had a list of insurances that will pay and work with this, and so we've pulled patients from that, patients we know could benefit from the service."

Relative Priority of the program was a barrier because participants often felt they did not have enough time allocated to complete this task. Other time-consuming duties and initiatives in the pharmacy technicians stressed the already limited workforce hours allocated. This program was of secondary importance to the core operations of the pharmacy due to time constraints.

3.2. Outer Setting of the ABM Implementation Environment

The Patient Needs and Resources construct exploration in the technician interviews found that technicians perceived that patients benefit from the simplification of their medication regimens and the convenience of having to pick up once per month or once per quarter. Notably, adherent patients on a stable regimen were said to benefit the most from the program. The convenience of ABM was reported to allow patients to make fewer trips to the pharmacy. Technicians reported that some elderly patients had an aversion to change and a desired to remain on their current schedule of medication orders. Technicians perceived patient concerns about the increased single, monthly cost per pharmacy visit, as the cost of their monthly medication regimen would no longer be spread out over the entire month.

3.3. Intervention Characteristics Enabling ABM Success

The inability to adapt the ABM program to local needs was described as a barrier by technicians. The lack of integration of the ABM platform with the pharmacy dispensing software system caused prescriptions to "fall off" or old prescriptions to be filled. There was no dynamic update to accurately reflect the patient profile in the ABM portal, so technicians reported frustration managing medications manually (calculate the days' supply on hand and fill the corresponding, appropriate quantity) to fit the ABM profile. The lack of ABM integration to the patient profile was identified as a critical issue with the program by pharmacy team members, that led to disrupted workflow and unneeded fills. The listing of every medication a patient has had on the ABM profile was described as a "busy" distraction that was a source of confusion when technicians are attempting to enroll patients with multiple medications.

3.4. Process ABM Follows for Success

For the construct of champion, having a technician responsible for leading ABMS implementation and working with the team to achieve ABM goals was perceived to yield successful goal achievement and increased pharmacy staff buy-in. Roles reported included; taking the initiative to engage patients on the ABM enrollment list and managing the existing patient fills. These champions would actively listen to patients and suggest ABM to those individuals who expressed that travel to the pharmacy or complexity of regimen was a concern for them. Teams with a champion reported an increase in successful enrollments.

Enrollment of Innovation Participants happened one of three ways: a patient would ask to have medications synchronized for convenience's sake, a technician would identify the need based upon a past relationship with a patient, or the ABM program or sync center would (central location with telephonically available pharmacy technicians trained in medication synchronization) generate a list of patients to enroll. Here was an identified need for better communication from the sync center to the pharmacy, so that the correct patients could be identified. The ABM program is structured to automatically generate appropriate patients, but technicians reported making judgement calls on eligible patients who would likely benefit the most. The automatically generated call list, that was described as helpful by technicians, also caused unnecessary calls to unwilling patients. Promotional materials, such as flyers, were not always reported to be in use, but were always reported to be helpful by technicians when they did have them. The most frequent goal for enrollment of new patients within the program was stated to be two patients per week. Two pharmacies had no goal for patient enrollments and one pharmacy had a goal of 5–10 enrollments/week.

4. Discussion

This qualitative study explored pharmacy technician perspectives of their role in ABM and found that they felt the program increases adherence and convenience for patients, but there were hurdles to effective implementation remaining. Establishing the role of the technician in ABMS services is critical as pharmacist-extender involvement in clinical service delivery is associated with a service implementation success, for frequent and diverse clinical service offerings, and improved quality of work life for both pharmacists and pharmacy technicians [17–24]. However, integration of technicians into advanced or clinical support roles can prove challenging [21,24–26]. Understanding their unique perspectives on these new roles can be instrumental in designing training programs and assisting pharmacy leadership in the selection of technicians for these advanced roles [27].

Some important takeaways were uncovered in this exploratory study related to technician work life. The semi-structured interviews found that technicians felt their help to patients was appreciated. This team member buy-in of the ABM process is key for pharmacists to leverage the workflow efficiencies generated to enable clinical interventions such as CMR [17]. Downstream, this may have important implications for technicians' perceived quality of work life (QOWL), which has previously reported to be low among pharmacy technicians practicing in a community pharmacy [25,28,29]. Moreover, such advanced roles may decrease technician turnover and further improve QOWL, as lack of career advancement is a known QOWL issue among pharmacy technicians [28].

Evaluation of the content within the Adaptability and Relative Priority constructs found that siloed prescriptions in the ABM portal could be a source of time-consuming erroneous fills. Housing the platform used for ABM within the pharmacy management system or enabling dynamic profile updating is necessary. The ABM interface must reflect the most current version of the patient profile to ensure that erroneous fills do not occur. This is a patient care concern that reduces pharmacy team support. Also, the report that too little time was budgeted to implement the program and complete other duties that must take priority worsened technician perceptions of the program. To prevent this, it is critical that new projects are integrated into existing workflows appropriately through accurate modeling of the workforce hours required.

The Champion construct emerged during the interviews as a successful aspect of implementation. Pharmacy technicians who recognized the importance of the program and took initiative to implement it were associated with success. By tailoring each ABM encounter to the specific needs of the patient, these champions generated more process buy-in from patients and team members. This generated synergy and reduced unnecessary prescription fills. Interviews found the champions were well-informed about the intervention process and felt comfortable integrating it into workflow. Our study indicates that empowering technicians on the local level to take initiative when patients are struggling with a high volume of prescriptions and poor adherence is an effective approach to circumventing the inefficiencies around the automated enrollment processes.

The variability in training reported by technicians is another barrier to implementation identified. Some team members felt that although they had a great explanation of ABM conceptually, they had little exposure to the actual interface. Training specific to the ABM user interface is needed to ensure the success of the program. Hands-on training will reduce the likelihood of erroneous fills and wasted time in the enrollment process.

Significant improvements to the ABM program may be made to better patient care and increase efficiency in the business operations of pharmacies that implement it. Effective implementation of medication synchronization core components within ABM is key to ensure that this program is effective. These components include the identification and enrollment of patients, inclusion of a medication review and patient assessment, the alignment of refills, a formal process for preparation of medications, and the delivery of medications and other services [7,30]. There is support in the literature for implementing a vaccination assessment program with ABM also. The CMR component of ABM has been proven to detect medication errors and successfully promote vaccination for patients [31]. The patients who benefit most are older adult patients with multiple medications, or have a chronic condition such as diabetes, COPD, or asthma [32]. The medical complications associated with medication nonadherence are worsening. Without proper management, nonadherence will continue to increase hospitalizations and raise costs in the health care system. This study contributes important data on pharmacy technicians, an understudied stakeholder whose perspectives are key to effectively implement patient care initiatives in a community pharmacy [7,30].

Study Limitations

Analysis of the relative success of each program was limited due to the lack of enrollment statistics for each pharmacy and direct indicators of patient opinion. This study was limited to supermarket chain pharmacies and may not have generalizability to all other pharmacies in the community setting. A small number of interviews occurred due to saturation of themes which may limit external validity of the study, as technicians were from only one grocery store chain representing a small geographical area. These qualitative results may also have limited generalizability to other countries, due to ABM not being implemented in the community pharmacy setting. However, the study's findings provide a helpful understanding of affective factors that are important to consider in the pre-implementation phase for any service implemented in the community pharmacy setting. Expanding this research to personnel in multiple settings may be beneficial and is warranted to discover new themes. The information technology (IT) issues specific to this supermarket chain may limit generalizability to some extent. However, most chain pharmacies contract with third party vendors to automate the enrollment process, so IT issues may persist.

5. Conclusions

Results from this study signify that ABM implementation can be challenging. Better ABM portal integration with the pharmacy patient profile, the promotion of champions, and appropriate workforce budgeting are key to the continued success for the program.

Author Contributions: Conceptualization, L.L., C.F., M.W., L.C., and K.C.H.; methodology, K.C.H. and L.L.; formal analysis, C.R. and D.C.; investigation, L.L., C.F., M.W., L.C., and K.C.H.; data curation, L.L.; writing—original draft preparation, C.R. and D.C.; writing—review and editing, C.R. and K.C.H.; supervision, K.C.H., C.F., and M.W.; project administration, L.L. and K.C.H. All authors have read and agreed to the published version of the manuscript.

Funding: This research received no external funding.

Acknowledgments: In this section you can acknowledge any support given which is not covered by the author contribution or funding sections. This may include administrative and technical support, or donations in kind (e.g., materials used for experiments).

Conflicts of Interest: The authors declare no conflict of interest.

References

1. Chronic Disease Overview. CDC.gov. Available online: https://www.cdc.gov/chronicdisease/index.htm (accessed on 8 August 2017).
2. Chapter II: The magnitude of the problem of poor adherence. In: World Health Organization. 2003. Available online: http://www.who.int/chp/knowledge/publications/adherence_full_report.pdf. (accessed on 20 July 2018).
3. Neiman, A.B.; Ruppar, T.; Ho, M.; Garber, L.; Weidle, P.J.; Hong, Y.; George, M.G.; Thorpe, P.G. CDC Grand Rounds: Improving Medication Adherence for Chronic Disease Management—Innovations and Opportunities. *MMWR. Morb. Mortal. Wkly. Rep.* **2017**, *66*, 1248–1251. [CrossRef] [PubMed]
4. Krumme, A.A.; Glynn, R.J.; Schneeweiss, S.; Gagne, J.J.; Dougherty, J.S.; Brill, G.; Choudhry, N.K. Medication Synchronization Programs Improve Adherence To Cardiovascular Medications And Health Care Use. *Heal. Aff.* **2018**, *37*, 125–133. [CrossRef] [PubMed]
5. Bernard, K.; Cowles, B.; McCall, K.; Henningsen, R.M.; O'Toole, M.; Tu, C. Impact of medication synchronization programs on proportion of days covered (PDC) scores and Medicare Part D medication-related adherence metrics. *J. Am. Pharm. Assoc.* **2019**, *59*, 343–348. [CrossRef] [PubMed]
6. Chater, R.W. Improving Quality Care: The Appointment-Based Model. Available online: https://www.pharmacytimes.com/publications/directions-in-pharmacy/2015/march2015/improving-quality-care-the-appointment-based-model (accessed on 7 August 2019).
7. Patti, M.; Renfro, C.; Posey, R.; Wu, G.; Turner, K.; Ferreri, S.P. Systematic review of medication synchronization in community pharmacy practice. *Res. Soc. Adm. Pharm.* **2019**, *15*, 1281–1288. [CrossRef] [PubMed]
8. Watson, L.L.; Bluml, B.M. Pharmacy's Appointment Based Model Implementation Guide for Pharmacy Practice Distributed in partnership with APhA and NASPA. American Pharmacists Association Foundation Website. 2013. Available online: www.aphafoundation.org (accessed on 8 August 2019).
9. Bonner, L. Med Sync Catching on across Nation. American Pharmacists Association Website. 2015. Available online: https://www.pharmacist.com/article/med-sync-catching-across-nation?is_sso_called=1 (accessed on 8 August 2019).
10. Consolidated Framework for Implementation Research (CFIR): Codebook Template. Available online: https://cfirguide.org/constructs/ (accessed on 20 July 2018).
11. Lewis, S.B.; Price, H.K.; Stafford, R.A. The Effect of Appointment-Based Medication Synchronization on Clinical Services in a Community Pharmacy. *Pharmacy* **2008**, *6*, 44.
12. Holdford, D. Simplify My Meds®Appointment-based Medication Synchronization Pilot Study Report: Prepared for National Community Pharmacists Association. Available online: http://www.ncpa.co/pdf/ncpa-ABM-report.pdf (accessed on 15 July 2018).
13. Patterson, J.A.; Holdford, D.A.; Saxena, K. Cost-benefit of appointment-based medication synchronization in community pharmacies. *Am. J. Manag. care* **2016**, *22*.
14. Ulin, P.R.; Robinson, E.T.; Tolley, E.E. Qualitative Methods in Public Health: A Field Guide for Applied Research. *Med. Sci. Sports Exerc.* **2005**, *37*, 1249. [CrossRef]
15. Tong, A.; Sainsbury, P.; Craig, J. Consolidated criteria for reporting qualitative research (COREQ): A 32-item checklist for interviews and focus groups. *Int. J. Qual. Heal. Care* **2007**, *19*, 349–357. [CrossRef]
16. Guest, G.; Bunce, A.; Johnson, L. How Many Interviews Are Enough? *Field Methods* **2006**, *18*, 59–82. [CrossRef]
17. Gernant, S.A.; Nguyen, M.-O.; Siddiqui, S.; Schneller, M. Use of pharmacy technicians in elements of medication therapy management delivery: A systematic review. *Res. Soc. Adm. Pharm.* **2017**, *14*, 883–890. [CrossRef]

18. Mattingly, A.; Mattingly, T.J. Advancing the role of the pharmacy technician: A systematic review. *J. Am. Pharm. Assoc.* **2018**, *58*, 94–108. [CrossRef] [PubMed]
19. Hohmeier, K.C.; Garst, A.; Adkins, L.; Yu, X.; Desselle, S.P.; Cost, M. The Optimizing Care Model: A novel community pharmacy approach to enhance patient care delivery by leveraging the technician workforce through technician product verification. *J. Am. Pharm. Assoc.* **2019**, *59*, 880–885. [CrossRef] [PubMed]
20. Hohmeier, K.C.; McDonough, S.L.; Rein, L.J.; Brookhart, A.L.; Gibson, M.L.; Powers, M.F. Exploring the expanded role of the pharmacy technician in medication therapy management service implementation in the community pharmacy. *J. Am. Pharm. Assoc.* **2019**, *59*, 187–194. [CrossRef] [PubMed]
21. Hohmeier, K.C.; Desselle, S.P. Exploring the implementation of a novel optimizing care model in the community pharmacy setting. *J. Am. Pharm. Assoc.* **2019**, *59*, 310–318. [CrossRef]
22. Lengel, M.; Kuhn, C.H.; Worley, M.; Wehr, A.M.; McAuley, J.W. Pharmacy technician involvement in community pharmacy medication therapy management. *J. Am. Pharm. Assoc.* **2018**, *58*, 179–185.e2. [CrossRef]
23. Bright, D.; Klepser, M.E.; Murry, L.; Klepser, D.G. Pharmacist-Provided Pharmacogenetic Point-of-Care Testing Consultation Service: A Time and Motion Study. *J. Pharm. Technol.* **2018**, *34*, 139–143. [CrossRef]
24. Justis, L.; Crain, J.; Marchetti, M.L.; Hohmeier, K.C. The Effect of Community Pharmacy Technicians on Industry Standard Adherence Performance Measures After Cognitive Pharmaceutical Services Training. *J. Pharm. Technol.* **2016**, *32*, 230–233. [CrossRef]
25. Desselle, S.P. Job Turnover Intentions Among Certified Pharmacy Technicians. *J. Am. Pharm. Assoc.* **2005**, *45*, 676–683. [CrossRef]
26. Desselle, S.P.; Holmes, E.R. Structural model of certified pharmacy technicians' job satisfaction. *J. Am. Pharm. Assoc.* **2007**, *47*, 58–72. [CrossRef] [PubMed]
27. Moya, A.; Unni, E.; Montuoro, J.; Desselle, S.P. Engaging pharmacy technicians for advanced clinical support tasks in community pharmacies: A cluster analysis. *J. Am. Pharm. Assoc.* **2019**, *59*, S32–S38.e1. [CrossRef]
28. Desselle, S.P. Survey of certified pharmacy technicians in the United States: a quality-of-worklife study. *J. Am. Pharm. Assoc.* **2005**, *45*, 458–465. [CrossRef] [PubMed]
29. Desselle, S.P.; Holmes, E.R. Results of the 2015 National Certified Pharmacy Technician Workforce Survey. *Am. J. Heal. Pharm.* **2017**, *74*, 981–991. [CrossRef] [PubMed]
30. Renfro, C.; Patti, M.; Ballou, J.; Ferreri, S.P. Development of a medication synchronization common language for community pharmacies. *J. Am. Pharm. Assoc.* **2018**, *58*, 515–521. [CrossRef] [PubMed]
31. Ariyo, O.; Kinney, O.; Brookhart, A.; Nadpara, P.; Goode, J.-V. "Kelly" R. Medication therapy problems and vaccine needs identified during initial appointment-based medication synchronization visits. *J. Am. Pharm. Assoc.* **2019**, *59*, S67–S71. [CrossRef]
32. Luder, H.; Kunze, N.; Heaton, P.C.; Frede, S.M. An appointment-based model to systematically assess and administer vaccinations. *J. Am. Pharm. Assoc.* **2018**, *58*, 290–295. [CrossRef]

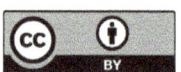

© 2020 by the authors. Licensee MDPI, Basel, Switzerland. This article is an open access article distributed under the terms and conditions of the Creative Commons Attribution (CC BY) license (http://creativecommons.org/licenses/by/4.0/).

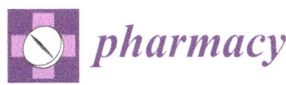

Article

Moving the Needle: A 50-State and District of Columbia Landscape Review of Laws Regarding Pharmacy Technician Vaccine Administration

Deeb Eid *, Joseph Osborne and Brian Borowicz

Department of Pharmacy Practice, Ferris State University, Grand Rapids, MI 49503, USA; osborj14@ferris.edu (J.O.); borowib@ferris.edu (B.B.)
* Correspondence: deebeid@ferris.edu

Received: 25 November 2019; Accepted: 5 December 2019; Published: 10 December 2019

Abstract: Pharmacy technicians are essential for inner workings of pharmacy teams and their depth of involvement in roles continues to evolve. An innovative role for pharmacy technicians, administration of vaccines, has emerged. With Idaho, Rhode Island, and Utah recently implementing changes that allow pharmacy technicians to safely perform this role, the need arose for a detailed examination of the law climate in all 50 states and the District of Columbia. A nine-question survey was sent out to all 51 state boards of pharmacy inquiring to legislative and regulatory environment of pharmacy technician vaccine administration. Additionally, a protocol driven, peer-reviewed process of state-specific regulations and statutes revealed categorized trends pertaining to this topic. Each state was classified per protocol into four different categories. The categorization resulted in identification of nine states in which pharmacy technician administered vaccination may be considered "Not Expressly Prohibited". A majority of states were categorized as prohibited (either directly or indirectly). Board of pharmacy respondents (43%) reported varying viewpoints on technician administered vaccines. While three states (Idaho, Rhode Island, Utah) have already made changes to allow for pharmacy technician administered vaccinations, opportunities exist for other states to consider changes to statutes or rules.

Keywords: pharmacy technician; vaccination; delegation; regulations; statutes; board of pharmacy; practice of pharmacy

---

1. Introduction

Vaccines remain one of the most cost-effective preventative health measures available and have been estimated to reduce direct financial burden on healthcare by $9.9 billion [1]. Additionally, pharmacies represent the second most common location for an adult to receive an influenza vaccination [2]. With an estimated 42,000 adult and 300 child deaths per year on average attributable to influenza alone, opportunity exists to improve access to this crucial preventative health intervention through expansion of patient access to vaccinations [1]. The World Health Organization (WHO) estimated that vaccinations prevent between two and three million deaths each year [3]. Kamal et al. identified various factors that may contribute to low rates of vaccination such as apathy, misconceptions, cost, distance to clinics, wait times, and inconvenient hours [4]. When it comes to barriers to receiving immunizations, less talked about or mentioned are the statutes and regulations surrounding them or who may be authorized to provide them. Given that pharmacies are one of the most accessible health destinations for the general public, they have served as a gateway to increase vaccination rates and improve access to care. According to data reported by the American Pharmacist Association (APhA) and National Alliance of State Pharmacy Associations (NASPA), pharmacists are authorized legally to administer vaccines in all 50 states and D.C. [5]. Pending a couple of states that have worked on recent law changes (New

Jersey, New York), student pharmacists (interns) will soon be able to administer vaccines in all states as well [5–7].

As pharmacist roles continue to evolve over time, so will those of pharmacy technicians. Pharmacists' professional delegation has become a key shift towards ensuring workload allocations and safe practices can remain intact. Working together with pharmacists and student pharmacists, pharmacy technicians play a critical role in impacting public health. Technicians represent a key opportunity to add a team member to help attribute to the public health initiative of increasing access to vaccinations. More recently, a technical but seemingly innovative role for pharmacy technicians, administration of vaccines, has emerged. With recent outbreaks of vaccine preventable diseases, and patient safety at the forefront of missions of boards of pharmacy, the public may benefit from adding another pharmacy team member to help increase access to vaccinations.

In 2016–17, Idaho actively underwent a rule rewrite which included adding language that directly permitted pharmacy technicians to administer immunizations [8]. With this, they became the first state within the U.S. to do so and also became the first state to actively involve pharmacy technicians in a training program and administration at local pharmacies. More recently in 2018, Idaho broadened language to allow for delegation utilizing professional judgement and therefore laws became "silent" on the topic. Seeing that statutes and regulations are silent, this could be interpreted as technically not an illegal task to delegate and perform, or in legal terminology; permissive. This also raises an interesting concept of silence within law and how state agencies or others may interpret these findings. Rhode Island became the second in late 2018 to promulgate rules and Utah made changes to their statewide vaccine protocol shortly after [9,10].

To date, three states have made changes within scope of practice to include pharmacy technician administration of vaccinations, including Idaho, Rhode Island, and Utah with others pending [8–11]. What may not be as apparent are the statutes and regulations surrounding allowance, prohibition, or silence in all 50 states and D.C. The purpose of this survey was to review and compile data surrounding the statutes and regulations pertaining to pharmacy technician administration of immunizations. With the data analyzed, the goal of the project was to provide a national overview of state specific language, citations, and examples of law variations. This report may serve as an informative reference for discussion or changes that could be made to either statutes or regulations per respective states.

2. Materials and Methods

Data collection consisted of a two-pronged approach in which a state-specific board of pharmacy survey and a peer-reviewed classification process were conducted. This project was found to be exempt from Institution Review Board (IRB) approval by the Ferris State University IRB (IRB-FY18-19-58).

In October 2018, a nine-question survey constructed in QuestionPro was emailed to 50 state boards of pharmacy, including the District of Columbia. Contact information for each board of pharmacy had been identified using a publicly available compiled contact list collected via the website www.stateside.com. Any failure to deliver notices or kickback messages required direct communication with that specific board for updated contact information. Instructions for completion of the survey along with consent were included in an introduction with a given time estimate of 5–15 minutes. Those contacted were informed that participation in the survey was voluntary, and that all responses, including non-response, would be recorded and published. No personal or demographic information was collected, and all respondents remained anonymous. Representatives were asked to indicate the state agency their response represented. See Table A1 in Appendix A, for a comprehensive list of survey questions.

The survey was disseminated 24th October 2018, with a two-week timeline of 6th November 2018. Reminders to complete the survey were sent 29th October 2018, one week before the deadline via email to the same contact address used initially. Data was assimilated from QuestionPro into a shared data collection program for evaluation. The classification process contained two-steps: 1) manual review of state-specific statutes and regulations, and, 2) group peer review of manual review results. The peer-review classification process began in November 2018 and concluded in May 2019.

While the manual survey categorization methods could be considered somewhat unique, a review of methodology from Tzanetakos et al. and Stewart et al. helped build the foundation [12,13]. The manual review of state-specific statute began with the division of 50 states (and the District of Columbia) alphabetically (Alabama through Missouri; Montana through Washington D.C.) into two sets consisting of 25 and 26 states. One author was then selected to review each of these divisions, with selection of author review of these groups arbitrarily chosen. The protocol in Figure 1 was used as a standardized approach to research, identify, and document state-specific results: State-specific statutes (Public Health Code, Revised Code, and "State Code") were reviewed through the use of the following key words: "Practice of pharmacy", "Pharmacy Technician", "Immunizations [or] Vaccines", "Delegate [or] Delegation", "Professional Judgement", and "Administration". If language was found in state-specific statute after the search using these keywords, it was documented into one of four categories discussed in the Results section (Section 3). If no language was found in state-specific statute, that same search protocol was directed at the matching state's Board of Health and Board of Medicine. At this step, regardless of if language had been identified or not, it would be categorized per protocol and documented into the shared data collection program into one of the following categories: Not Expressly Prohibited, Prohibited Directly, Prohibited Indirectly, and Permissive. This process was then repeated for that identical state's regulations (Board of Pharmacy Rules or Administration Code) with categorization and documentation occurring in an equal fashion. After both statutes and regulations had been documented for a state, this entire procedure was repeated until all states had been categorized. Upon completion of data collection, the author assigned to one set subsequently peer reviewed the opposite set via the same protocol, ensuring that every data point had received equal analysis. A color-coded system (red, yellow, green) was used to compare agreement in findings (complete disagreement, agreement with discourse, and complete agreement) to facilitate the group peer-review process.

The group peer-review process began shortly after the conclusion of the manual review. A final step of the peer review process involved having the primary investigator review all entries to confirm categorization or settle differences identified. All authors met and discussed results of data collection using citations documented in the shared data collection program. Discussion occurred until every data point had been finalized to facilitate bias mitigation and settle any discrepancies. This peer review methodology known as triangulation was adopted from Farmer et al. [14]. The primary investigator also reconciled survey data as another comparator. Final data categorization was then recorded.

Definitions of Permissive, Prohibited Directly, Prohibited Indirectly, and Not Expressly Prohibited are encapsulated in Table A2 in Appendix A.

3. Results

3.1. Board of Pharmacy Survey Results

Of the 50 states and the District of Columbia polled, 22 (43%) states successfully completed the survey. State boards of pharmacy who finished the survey included the following: Arizona, Hawaii, Idaho, Iowa, Kansas, Kentucky, Louisiana, Maryland, Massachusetts, Minnesota, Nevada, New Hampshire, North Carolina, North Dakota, Ohio, Oregon, Rhode Island, Texas, Vermont, Virginia, Washington and Washington D.C. One state submitted past the 6th November deadline (submitted 9th November). Of the states responding, 16 (72%) reported that there were statutes (state legistlation, public health code ... etc.) that prohibit pharmacists from delegating the task of vaccine administration to a properly trained pharmacy technician. For the similar question regarding regulation, 13 (59%) states reported prohibition via rule. Eight (36%) respondent states answered "yes" to if there had been any discussion from their board on this topic to date. Table A3 in Appendix A outlines a few selected free responses from the survey. For both question eight and question nine of the survey, six (27%) of the responding states gave an answer equivalent to "no comment". When asked about initial impressions in question eight, 17 (77%) free responses were recorded. In question nine, when asked about risks, 15 free responses were recorded (68%). All 22 states (100%) provided statute or regulation citation when required. Overall, there were also multiple free responses that respondents declined to answer or did not directly answer the question(s). For those purposes, Table A3 includes free responses that were thought provoking and/or provided insight based on the question asked.

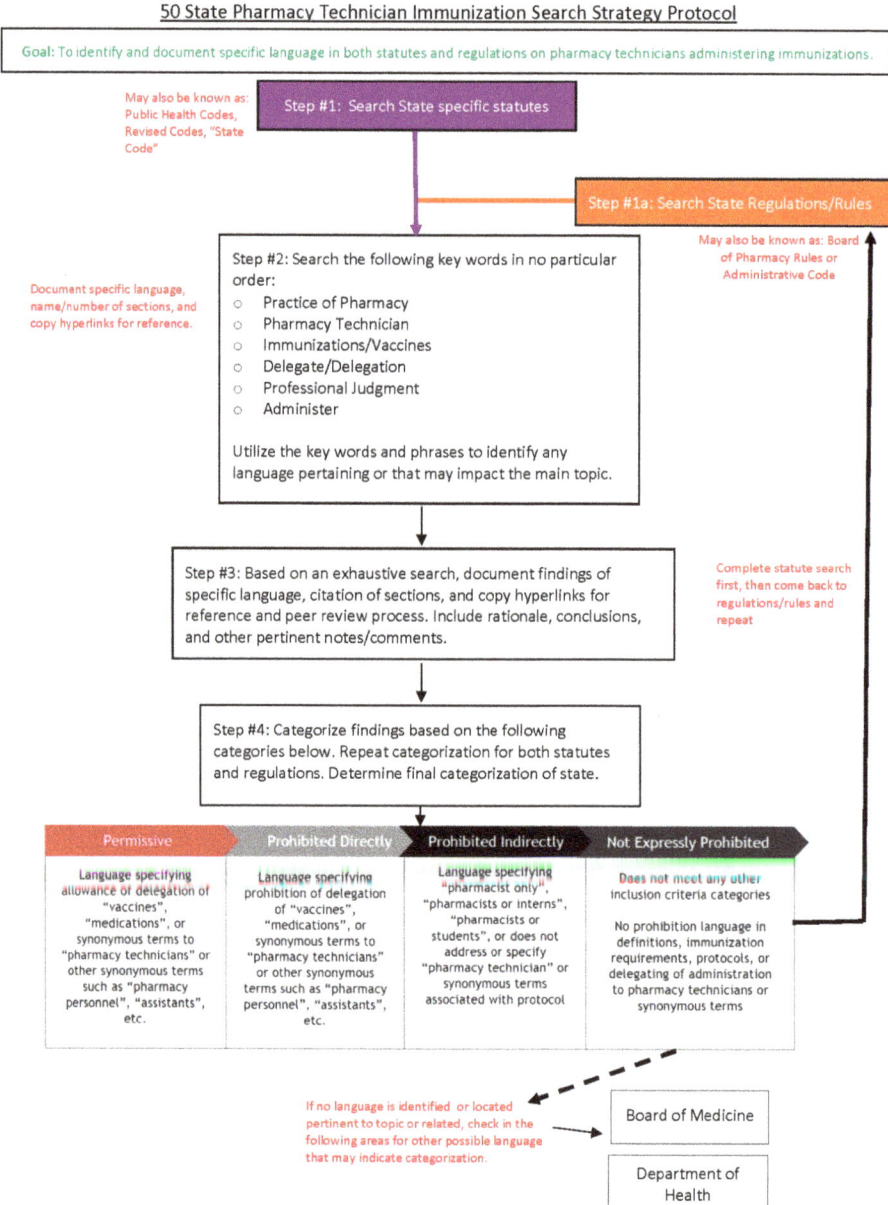

Figure 1. Manual Review Search Protocol.

3.2. Peer-Review Classification Results

The following data was collected per protocol from all 50 states and D.C.: overall, one (2%) state was found to be Permissive, 21 (41%) states were classified as Prohibited Directly, 20 (39%) states were classified as Prohibited Indirectly, and nine (17%) states were classified as Not Expressly Prohibited. The above classification considered both statute and regulation and the stricter of the two findings per state (including D.C.). Regarding statute only, zero (0%) states were found to be Permissive, 11 (21%) states were classified as Prohibited Directly, 15 (29%) were classified as Prohibited Indirectly, and 25 (49%) of states were classified as Not Expressly Prohibited. When regulations were examined, 1 (2%) state was classified as Permissive, 14 (27%) states were found to be Prohibited Directly, 23 (45%) states were classified as Prohibited Indirectly, and 13 (25%) were classified as Not Expressly Prohibited. See Figure 2 for a graphical representation of the data. To further provide examples of how the categorization occurred, selected examples that were most transparent are provided below.

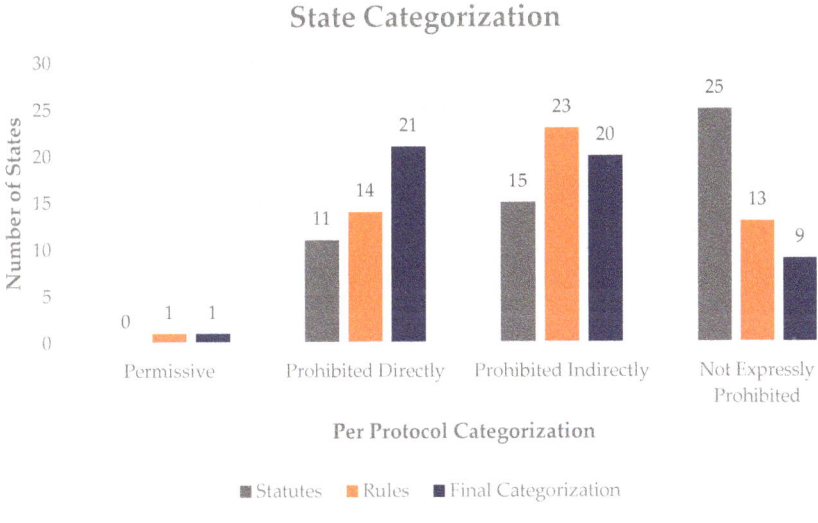

Figure 2. State Categorization (including D.C.).

Rhode Island, being the only state to expressly permit pharmacy technicians to administer immunizations within rules, is the example of a Permissive state. Statute contains no explicit prohibitions when examining the definitions of "pharmacist" or "pharmacy technician" and includes the following definition of "practice of pharmacy" found in RI Gen L 5-19.1-2(x): "Practice of pharmacy...includes...administration of adult immunizations in accordance with regulations and training requirements promulgated by the department of health" [15]. Considering regulation, administrative code 216-RICR-40-15-1.11 (8, b.) outlines "A technician II who has completed a recognized certificate training course on appropriate immunization administration technique and holds a current basic cardiopulmonary resuscitation (CPR) training certificate, shall be permitted to administer vaccinations under the direct supervision and with the authorization of an immunizing pharmacist ... " [16]. Rhode Island's responses to the survey also indicated answers of "no" to questions two and four. The above language is an example of Permissive categorization.

South Carolina provides example of a state in which pharmacy technicians are Prohibited Directly. Within statutes, Section 40-43-190 (B,3) clearly prohibits with the following language: "A pharmacist may not delegate the administration of vaccines to a pharmacy technician or certified pharmacy technician" [17]. Seeing that a majority of pertinent language relating to pharmacy technicians or vaccines are within statute, there were no prohibitions found within regulations, therefore deeming Not Expressly Prohibited. Interestingly, prohibition is further reinforced through the Pharmacy Policies and Procedures document within Approved Technician Duties Policy and Procedure #140 which states "The pharmacy technician is prohibited from performing the following functions:...administering immunizations" [18]. Although no clear indication, authors assumed Policy #140 is referring back to Section 40-43-190 (B,3), as the document often cited other specific statutes. South Carolina additionally prohibits technician immunization through language within statewide protocol: "A pharmacist may not delegate the administration of vaccines to a pharmacy technician ... " [19]. According to survey results, South Carolina started a response but failed to complete the survey, therefore there was no data to reconcile during the peer review process. As documented in South Carolina law, this state was categorized as Prohibited Directly.

North Carolina illustrates the Prohibited Indirectly category. NC Gen Stat § 90-85.3.i1 outlines that "'Immunizing pharmacist' means a licensed pharmacist who meets all of the following qualifications.[lists qualifications]" [20]. This statute does not implicitly disallow pharmacy technicians, yet it does specifically list a pharmacist. Regulations in North Carolina also provided Prohibited Indirectly language as seen in 21 NCAC 46.2507: Administration of Vaccines by Pharmacists with "A) an Immunizing Pharmacist or a Pharmacy Intern who is under the direct, in-person supervision of an Immunizing Pharmacist;" [21]. It is worth noting that while pharmacy technicians may be technically prohibited via exclusion, a regulatory artifact exists that permits "(B) the patient at the direction of either an Immunizing Pharmacist or a health care provider" to administer their own immunization [21]. This indicates that a pharmacist or other healthcare professional may teach a layperson to administer their own vaccine, yet a trained pharmacy technician may not qualify. Because of the lack of specific prohibition of pharmacy technician immunization administration combined with the explicit listing of those who can administer, North Carolina was classified as Prohibited Indirectly.

Idaho was found to be an example of Not Expressly Prohibited categorization, being that pharmacy technician immunization was not defined within their statute or regulation per the protocol defined. In both statutes ID Code 54-1704 and regulations IDAPA Rule 27.01.01.100 no mention was made to pharmacy technicians being able, or unable, to provide immunization administration [22–24]. Rather within 27.01.01.100, it states "To evaluate whether a specific act is within the scope of pharmacy practice in or into Idaho, or whether an act can be delegated to other individuals under their supervision, a licensee or registrant of the Board must independently determine whether: ... " and then lists a few lines of guidance. According to survey results, Idaho also answered questions two and four with "no", indicating similarities with peer review findings.

Only one state was found to be categorized as Permissive (Rhode Island), which both the survey and peer-reviewed classification agreed upon. A total of 41 states (80%) were classified as Prohibited Directly or Prohibited Indirectly through statute or regulation. This finding was not surprising considering the minority of states (three) in which pharmacy technicians currently can administer immunizations [0–11]. The remaining two states (Idaho, Utah) which currently have pharmacy technician administration of immunizations are classified as Not Expressly Prohibited. This peer-review classification was in agreement with the results from the Idaho Board of Pharmacy survey. Utah board survey data was unavailable.

3.3. Comparison of Survey to Peer-Review

When comparing survey respondent states to their collected peer-review data, the authors were in agreement with the state board of pharmacy 16 out of 22 times (73%) regarding statutes. When comparing data for regulation, the authors were in agreement with survey respondents 16 out of 22 times (73%). Of the disagreements, the authors disagreed with the categorization of both statute and regulation with four states of the 22 states who completed the survey. Four state board survey findings (Kentucky, Louisiana, Minnesota, and Washington) were misaligned with the results from the peer-reviewed classification. Of note, three of these states (Kentucky, Minnesota, and Washington) reported board survey information that was more conservative (i.e., the authors found their state to be Not Expressly Prohibited rather than Prohibited Indirectly) than the peer-review classification, while Louisiana reported a more liberal interpretation (i.e., the authors found their state to be Prohibited Indirectly rather than Not Expressly Prohibited) than the peer-review classification. An encompassing state-specific compilation of both survey results and peer-reviewed classifications complete with rationale is available in Table A4 in Appendix A.

4. Discussion

The vision for the project was to be eventually used as a tool for all interested parties. Stakeholders may consider findings, elicit discussion, and spread awareness across the nation in the future. State agencies or other stakeholders may enter discussions on the topic and want to better understand the landscape of laws from a national overview. This project does not serve as legal interpretation or was not meant to be misinformed or misconstrued as so.

As mentioned prior, three states, Idaho, Rhode Island, and Utah have expanded practice by making regulatory or protocol changes. From the federal level, the Commissioned Corps of the U.S. Public Health Service announced that credentialed pharmacists have the chance to provide federal pharmacy technicians an opportunity to obtain training to administer vaccines [24]. In Whiteriver, Arizona within the Indian Hospital, pharmacy technicians have administered vaccines to patients of all ages (including children) with oversight from a federal pharmacist [25]. With change on the horizon and precedent set, investigation and categorization of laws in other states were identified as gap areas within published literature.

The topic itself does not lend to an array of literature examples or studies to draw from, therefore this presents as a novel area to provide insight. A comparator study would be the 2015 study by Stewart and colleagues which examined the state laws and standing orders for immunization services. Within this study, authors did not examine pharmacy technicians specifically, but looked more broadly at non-physician health professionals. Interestingly, it was found that medical assistants (comparable to pharmacy technicians in training, education, and roles) had delegated authority to administer vaccines in fourteen (14) states, own authority in one (1) state and laws were silent within thirty-six (36) states and D.C. [13]. State laws also varied, but a general trend noted was that physicians are able to delegate the task of vaccine administration to medical assistants in many states. The study by Stewart and colleagues had conceptual similarities but did not endure a triangulation peer review methodology. Of note, training and education requirements of medical assistants and pharmacy technicians also vary from state to state, which can make it challenging to argue that education requirements are mandatory for one to succeed outside of a training program designed specifically for the task.

When considering the topic of pharmacy technician administered vaccines within law, there arose a few theme areas investigators identified for state agencies and others to consider after completion of data analysis and discussing results. One area includes the training requirements and availability of a training program. McKeirnan et al. and Washington State University (WSU) developed a training program that is specific for pharmacy technicians [26]. The program was designed to be less time intensive or in-depth (2-hour self-study, 4 hour live) compared to the pharmacist/student program (~20 hours) with a clear separation of the technical versus clinical aspects of vaccine administration [27]. There have also been speculations as to if the WSU program has been recently acquired by a national association and may soon be featured as a nationally recognized program.

The second theme to consider includes the platform by which changes would need to occur. Would the state require rule promulgation or amendments, a statute change, or both? Are amendments to statewide protocols or collaborative practice agreements needed? Maybe a state currently has no true prohibitions and it may be up to employers to kickstart the practice model? While there were (9) states identified in the categorization of Not Expressly Prohibited, readily available opportunities may exist to begin implementation of technician vaccine administration within these states. It serves important for stakeholders to work closely with state agencies, boards, and others on moving initiatives forward. If rules or statutes need to be amended or changed, states could also consider utilizing a pharmacist delegatory model. This model would allow for pharmacists to use professional judgement to delegate technical tasks such as immunization administration to support personnel. Similar to physician, optometry, or dentistry models, it may enable pharmacists to practice and manage their practices at a level that may be conducive to the public and patient safety. This model also supports the recent NABP Task Force developed to investigate moving pharmacy to a "Standard of Care" model [28]. To continue to evolve, the profession of pharmacy must evolve as a team and utilize teamwork to provide patient care that is safe and effective.

A third and final theme to consider involves fears and emotions that arise when considering any type of changes. Atkinson et al. describes in depth the typical fears and emotions brought up whenever having discussions on the topic as deliberated in initial discussions in Idaho [29]. Many points of concern highlighted within Atkinson et al. are theories based on precautionary principle, and lack evidence to support rationale. To properly evaluate the topic, it is crucial to consider what concerns are present, but to not let theories supersede and prohibit positive public health initiatives backed by evidence. Within the survey, when asked about safety concerns or risks, comments trended towards being majorly positive on the topic. Boards mentioned key phrases such as "with the same training", "if properly trained" or "just as untrained lay persons have", indicating a sense that proper training is key. A minority of respondents mentioned phrases such as "clinical education", "clinical judgement", or "the medical community may not be accepting". Therein lies the differentiation of clinical versus technical knowledge and roles. McKeirnan et al. demonstrated safety data which showcased 953 immunizations delivered by technicians with zero adverse events [26]. Three other studies, Burgess et al., Zahn et al., and Coleman et al. all demonstrated that even laypersons exhibited positive safety data when taught to administer their own vaccines [30–32]. Bertsch et al. surveyed pharmacists who supervise immunizing technicians and showed that opinions revealed positive morale of teams and can help to increase the number of vaccinations given by the pharmacy [33]. Not only has this practice shown safe data, but also has demonstrated another route to increasing public access to vaccines, a highly impactful public health initiative. Similar fears or emotions often arise when other expanded roles of pharmacy technicians are discussed. Within other well studied roles such as Technician Product Verification (Tech-Check-Tech), Verbals, Transfers, Clarifications, or, Point of Care Testing, evidence suggests similar affirmations around positive safety data and historical success in various jurisdictions for over 40 years for some roles [34–39].

Findings from the manual scanning of all states may have been subject to investigator expectations. Naturally, a majority of states were expected to include language that directly or indirectly may prohibit pharmacy technicians from administering immunizations. The survey responses helped to provide investigators with a comparator for the manual survey. Seeing that all states did not participate in the survey, this is an obvious limitation. Another limitation was the search protocol may not have encompassed all possible language included in regulations or statutes. While the protocol was designed to include as many relevant keywords or areas as possible, there was a chance that areas may have been missed. Free responses provide a snapshot of thoughts, discussions, and considerations by various boards across the country. Overall, respondents seemed to showcase the notion that the topic has been of interest or brought up, therefore validating that law changes or continued discussions may come in the near future.

5. Conclusions

Overall, a majority of states (41) were found to include language that prohibits administration of immunizations by pharmacy technicians. Nine (9) states were found to be Not Expressly Prohibited by the peer-review triangulation process. Two (2) (Idaho, Utah) of these nine (9) states currently allow pharmacy technician immunization administration with others undergoing discussion. This is of paramount importance when considering the seven remaining Not Expressly Prohibited states: Kentucky, Michigan, Minnesota, Nebraska, New Mexico, Tennessee, and Washington. Proponents of pharmacy technician administration of immunizations may consider these key states to explore implementation with opportunities for expansion of practice. Given the legal judgement needed to navigate the proximity of Prohibited Indirectly and Not Expressly Prohibited, stakeholders of pharmacy technician administered immunizations may wish to closely examine the wording in both statute and regulation in these states. Boards of Pharmacy have mixed responses when asked about the topic and discussions seem to be growing in prevalence throughout the country.

Author Contributions: Conceptualization D.E.; methodology, D.E.; software, D.E.; validation, D.E., J.O., B.B.; formal analysis, D.E., J.O., B.B.; investigation, J.O., B.B.; resources, D.E.; data curation, D.E., J.O., B.B.; writing—original draft preparation, D.E., J.O., writing—review and editing, D.E., B.B.; visualization, D.E.; supervision, D.E.; project administration, D.E.

Funding: This research received no external funding.

Acknowledgments: Michael E. Klepser, PharmD, FCCP, FIDP: for administrative support and guidance. Stephanie Zagordo, PharmD: for support with protocol development. Andrew Saul, PharmD: for administrative support.

Conflicts of Interest: The authors declare no conflict of interest.

Appendix A

Table A1. State-Specific Board of Pharmacy Survey Questions.

Question	Response Field
1. What State Board of Pharmacy do you represent?	Free Response
2. In your state, are there statutes (state legislation, public health code ... etc.) that prohibit pharmacists from delegating the technical task of vaccine administration to a properly trained pharmacy technician?	Yes (if answered logic guided to #3) No (skip to #4)
3. Please provide citation to the specific statute(s) (state legislation, public health code ... etc.) that prohibit pharmacists from delegating the technical task of vaccine administration to a properly trained pharmacy technician.	Free Response
4. In your state, are there regulations (rules, BOP rules ... etc.) that prohibit pharmacists from delegating the technical task of vaccine administration to a properly trained pharmacy technician?	Yes (if answered logic guided to #5) No (skip to #6)
5. Please provide citation to the specific regulation(s) (rules, BOP rules ... etc.) that prohibit pharmacists from delegating the technical task of vaccine administration to a properly trained pharmacy technician.	Free Response
6. Have there been any discussions from your board on this topic to date?	Yes (if answered, logic guided to #7) No (skip to #8)
7. Please briefly describe discussions that have occurred from your board on this topic.	Free Response
8. What initial impressions do you have about pharmacy technicians administering vaccinations?	Free Response
9. Do you believe there are any risks that can occur from a pharmacy technician administering a vaccine relative to a student pharmacist? Please explain:	Free Response

Table A2. Categorization Guidance Protocol.

Permissive	Prohibited Directly	Prohibited Indirectly	Not Expressly Prohibited
Language specifying allowance of delegation of "vaccines", "medications", or synonymous terms to "pharmacy technicians" or other synonymous terms such as "pharmacy personnel", "assistants", etc.	Language specifying prohibition of delegation of "vaccines", "medications", or synonymous terms to "pharmacy technicians" or other synonymous terms such as "pharmacy personnel", "assistants", etc.	Language specifying "pharmacist only", "pharmacists or interns", "pharmacists or students", or does not address or specify "pharmacy technician" or synonymous terms associated with protocol	Does not meet any other inclusion criteria categories. No prohibition language in definitions, immunization requirements, protocols, or delegating of administration to pharmacy technicians or synonymous terms

Table A3. Thought Provoking Open Responses to Survey Questions.

Survey Question	Survey Response(s)	Valid Responses
Please briefly describe discussions that have occurred from your board on this topic.	A: The concept is interesting but we are trying to gauge the public health impact of such a move. (would it increase immunization rates) Although we have no issue with allowing properly trained technicians to give immunizations/injections, we need to have better participation from pharmacies on providing immunization services as well as other extended services that the Board has championed (CLIA waived tests, collaborative agreement, tech check tech, etc.) A: This has been discussed recently and the Board voted to pursue legislation that would permit a pharmacist with the ability to delegate the administration of a vaccine to properly trained pharmacy staff. While no law currently exists that specifically prohibits the delegation of the administration, all laws pertaining to vaccine administration are specific to pharmacists.	8/22 (36%)
What initial impressions do you have about pharmacy technicians administering vaccinations?	A: The administration of an immunization is a technical task that has been successfully performed by lay persons. There is no reason to deny patients access to this. A: We follow the law. A: Surprise/shock. Followed by a dose of reality: Physicians, NPs, and PA-Cs don't typically perform the administrations of vaccines. That's typically done by a CNA or a CMA. A: There is a lack of standardized training of all pharmacy technicians. Many have never completed a pharmacy technician training program, and were 'grandfathered' in after the training requirement went into effect. If allowed by the Board, there would need to be standardized training and validation or certification, with ongoing continuing education for those technicians. A: Staff have had discussion on whether this might be allowed as a non-discretionary function of a specialized function under the current statutory and regulatory framework.	17/22 (77%) **
Do you believe there are any risks that can occur from a pharmacy technician administering a vaccine relative to a student pharmacist? Please explain:	A: We have never heard anyone say they think it would be unsafe for technicians to administer a vaccine; we have, however, heard various boards raise concerns about what it would do to pharmacist employment and how it could upset the medical profession. Neither of those reasons are appropriate decision points for boards of pharmacy to consider. Safety and safety alone, should be the consideration, and studies have been published demonstrating trained technicians can safely and appropriately take on this task, just as untrained lay persons have. A: With the same training, no I do not see any additional inherent risks merely because they are a technician. A: No follow the law. A: I believe that a properly trained technician can perform the technical administration of a vaccine just as safely as any other properly trained individual. Possible risk within the pharmacy environment are potential missed opportunities for the pharmacist to dialogue with their patients during the administration process. A: No. Anyone is capable of giving a bad shot whether it is a pharmacist, student or technician. A: The risks would be the same for both technicians and students.	15/22 (68%) **

** Responses were omitted if answers to the question were not given or "N/A", "no comment", were provided.

Table A4. Comprehensive Peer Review Results.

State	Statutes	Regulations	Conclusion	Documented Regulations or Statutes	Survey Results
Alabama	NEP	PRI	PRI	1) ALB Code Title 34-23-130 Pharmacy Technicians 2) 680-X-2-.14 (1),(2) (a,b)-The Role Of Technicians In Pharmacies In Alabama.	N/A
Alaska	PRI	NEP	PRI	1) Title 8 Ch 80 Article 2. Sec 08.80.168 2) Alaska Stat. § 08.80.168a	N/A
Arizona	PRI	PRI	PRI	1) AAC R-4-23-411 C1: non-delegation allowed 2) 32-1901-defines "administer" 3) 32-1974 defines immunization and states "pharmacist" multiple times	AZ –> Statute, cited 32-1974 as Prohibited, but missed definition of "Administer" which includes "by the practitioner's authorized agent". 4-23-411 cited in survey
Arkansas	PRD	PRI	PRD	1) A.C.A 17-92-101-16-xi-C-i 2) Regulation 3-Pharmacy Technicians: 03-00-0005 a,b	N/A
California	PRI	PRI	PRI	1) 4052.8. Initiation and Administration of Vaccines; Requirements 2) 1746.4 Pharmacists Initiating and Administering Vaccines.	N/A
Colorado	PRI	PRI	PRI	1) 12-42.5-102 (31)(b) 2) 12-42.5-102 (30) 3) 12-42.5-116 (5) 4) 3 CCR 719-1.19.01.10 5) 3 CCR 719-1.19.01.20	N/A
Connecticut	PRI	PRI	PRI	1) Chapter 400j. Sec. 20-633 2) 20-633-Administration of Vaccine By Pharmacist	N/A
Delaware	NEP	PRI	PRI	1) 24 Del.C. 2502 Definitions-(23)(h) 2) 24 Del.C. 2507 License required (b) 3) 14.0 DE Regs Administration of Injectable Medications, Biologicals and Adult Immunizations 4) 14.1 DE Regs, 14.2 DE Regs	N/A
Florida	PRI	PRI	PRI	1) Title XXXII, Chapter 465.014 Pharmacy technician 2) Title XXXII, Chapter 465.003 Definitions 3) Title XXXII, Chapter 465.189 Administration of vaccines and epinephrine auto injection 4) 64B16-27.420 Pharmacy Technician—Delegable and Non-Delegable Tasks.	N/A

Table A4. Cont.

State	Statutes	Regulations	Conclusion	Documented Regulations or Statutes	Survey Results
Georgia	NEP	PRD	PRD	1) OCGA Title 26-4-82: Duties requiring professional judgment; responsibilities of licensed pharmacist 2) Title 26-4-4: Definition of "practice of pharmacy" 3) Title 26-4-5 (1),(10),(32): Definitions 4) Rule 360-34-.01 Definitions 5) Rule 360-34-.02 Qualifications for Physician to enter a protocol 6) Rule 360-34-.03 Qualifications for a Pharmacist to enter a protocol 7) 360-34-.05 (6) Requirements of the Vaccine Protocol Agreement	N/A
Hawaii	PRI	PRI	PRI	1) §461-1 (2) (E. Administering) Definitions. 2) §16-95-86: Scope of practice of a pharmacy technician	§461-9 Pharmacist in charge; pharmacy personnel HAR §16-95-2: §16-95-86 Scope of practice of a pharmacy technician.
Idaho	NEP	NEP	NEP	1) Idaho Code Title 54-1704: Practice of Pharmacy 2) IDAPA Rule 27.01.01.100: Practice of Pharmacy: General Approach	Answered "No" to both Statute and Rule questions
Illinois	NEP	PRI	PRI	1) 225 ILCS 85/3 (4,b)-Definitions 2) 225 ILCS 85/9 (a)-Licensure as registered pharmacy technician. 3) Title 68-1330.50 (a)(b): Vaccinations/Immunizations (Qualifications, Protocols, Policies, and Procedures)	N/A
Indiana	PRI	PRD	PRD	1) IC 25-26-13-31.2: Administration of immunizations; emergency immunizations; immunization data 2) IC 25-26-13-31.5: Immunizations by pharmacist interns and pharmacist students; rules 3) IC 25-26-19-8: Prohibited activities of a licensed pharmacy technician 4) 856 IAC 4-1-1: Pharmacist Vaccinations Administered Via Protocol Authority 5) 856 IAC 4-1-3 Delegation of protocol authority	N/A

Table A4. Cont.

State	Statutes	Regulations	Conclusion	Documented Regulations or Statutes	Survey Results
Iowa	NEP	PRD	PRD	1) 155A.3 (1,12): Definitions 2) 155A.4 (c): Prohibition against unlicensed persons dispensing or distributing prescription drugs-exceptions. 3) 155A.44: Vaccine and immunization administration 4) 155A.46 (3-6): Statewide protocols 5) 155A.33: Delegation of technical functions 6) 657-39.10 (155A): Vaccine administration by pharmacists–physician-approved protocol 7) 657-39.11(155A): Vaccine administration by pharmacists—statewide protocol. Others to consider: 8) 657-3.22(155A) Technical functions. 9) 657-3.21(155A) Delegation of functions.	Answered "No" to both Statute and Rule questions Also provided comments on pursuing legislation
Kansas	PRD	NEP	PRD	1) 65-1635a (c). Administration of vaccine; education and reporting requirements; delegation of authority prohibited; "pharmacist" defined. 2) 68-2-20 Pharmacist function in filling a prescription.	Statutes –> KSA65-1635a Rules –> Answered "No"
Kentucky	NEP	NEP	NEP	1) 315.010 (21,22): Definitions for chapter. 2) 315.020 (4): Only pharmacists to supervise manufacturing of pharmaceuticals or practice pharmacy-Exceptions 3) 315.205: Notification of immunization to minor's primary care provider 4) 201 KAR 2:045. Technicians.	Answered KRS 315.010(22) for both
Louisiana	PRI	PRI	PRI	1) RS 37:1218: Administration of influenza immunization 2) RS 37:1218.1: Administration of immunizations and vaccines other than influenza immunizations 3) Title 46, Chapter 5: 521: Prescription Orders to Administer Medications 4) Title 46, Chapter 9: 907: Scope of Practice (Technicians)	Answered "No" to for both
Maine	PRD	PRI	PRD	1) Title 32, Chapter 117: 13834 Prohibited Acts 2) 13831: Authority 3) 02-392-4A: Administration of Drugs and Vaccines 4) 02-382-7: Licensure and Employment of Pharmacy Technicians	N/A

Table A4. Cont.

State	Statutes	Regulations	Conclusion	Documented Regulations or Statutes	Survey Results
Maryland	PRD	PRD	PRD	1) 12-6B-06: Authorized and prohibited acts 2) Code of Maryland Regulations: 10.34.34.03 (7): Delegated Pharmacy Acts 3) 10.34.32.03: Requirements to Administer Vaccinations	Referenced 10.34.32.03 (specific to immunization education, requirements for pharmacists) for both questions
Massachusetts	NEP	PRD	PRD	1) Section 24B1/2: Pharmacist collaborative practice agreements; collaborative drug therapy management 2) 247 CMR 8.00 (.04-4e): Pharmacy Interns and Technicians	247 CMR 8.04 referenced, nothing for Statute
Michigan	NEP	NEP	NEP	1) MCL 333.17739: Pharmacy technician functions; licensure 2) MCL 333.16215: Delegation of acts, tasks, or functions to licensed or unlicensed individual; supervision; rules; immunity; third party reimbursement or worker's compensation benefits. 3) R 338.3665 Performance of activities and functions; delegation. 4) R 338.486: "Medical institution" and "pharmacy services" defined; pharmacy services in medical institutions. 5) R 338.490 (5): Professional responsibility; "caregiver" defined.	N/A
Minnesota	NEP	NEP	NEP	1) 151.01 Subd.27 DEFINITIONS (Practice of pharmacy) 2) 151.102 Subd.1. Pharmacy Technician 3) 6800.3850 Subp.2 Pharmacy Technicians-Permissible Duties 4) Subp.4. Written Procedures 5) Subp.5. Supervision	Statute: Vaccine administration is defined in MN Statute 151.01, 27(5) as the practice of pharmacy, and practicing pharmacy without being licensed to do so is a violation of MN Statute 151.34 (13); see also MN Rule 6800.3850. Rule: Vaccine administration is considered the practice of pharmacy, and must be done by a licensed pharmacist per MN Statute 151.01, subds. 3, 15a., and 27(5); see also MN Rule 6800.3850.

Table A4. Cont.

State	Statutes	Regulations	Conclusion	Documented Regulations or Statutes	Survey Results
Mississippi	NEP	PRI	PRI	1) 73-21-73. Definitions 2) 73-21-83 Board to regulate practice of pharmacy; 3) 73-21-111. Personnel 4) Title 30, Part 3001: Pharmacy Practice Regulations, Definitions.1, 54, 59, 61 5) Title 30, Part 3001, Article XXIX, 8: Regulations Governing Institutional Pharmacy-Pharmacy Technicians 6) Article XL: Pharmacy Technicians (1) and (4) Board of Medicine: 7) Miss. Code Ann. §73-43-11 (1972, as amended). 8) Rule 9.2 Position.	N/A
Missouri	NEP	PRD	PRD	1) Title XXII Occupations and Professions: 338.010 Practice of pharmacy defined…etc. (1,7,12) 2) 20 CSR 2220-6.050 Administration of Vaccines Per Protocol	N/A
Montana	NEP	PRD	PRD	1) 37-7-105. Administration of immunizations 2) 24.174.503 (5) Administration of Vaccines by Pharmacists	N/A
Nebraska	NEP	NEP	NEP	1) NRS 38-2891, 38-2837, 38-2866.01 2) 28-013 Pharmaceutical Care Requirements, Title 175, Chapter 8: 8-002 Definitions	N/A
Nevada	NEP	PRD	PRD	1) NRS 639.0113, NRS 639.0124, NRS 639.1371 2) NAC 639.2971 Authorization; contents of and deviation from written protocol.	Yes –> NRS 639 No (Rules)
New Hampshire	PRI	PRD	PRD	1) 318:16-b Pharmacist Administration of Vaccines, 2) 318:16-d Pharmacist Administration of Additional Vaccines. 3) Part Ph 1303 Pharmacist Administration of Vaccines Qualifications and Application (c)	Yes –> 318:16-b Yes –> Refer to statute
New Jersey	PRI	PRI	PRI	1) 45:14-63 Administration of prescription medication directly to patient, immunization. 2) 13:39-11.13 pharmacy technicians, pharmacy interns, and pharmacy externs; required supervision 3) 13:39-4.21 procedures for physician ordered or government sponsored immunizations performed by pharmacists 4) 13:39-4.21a requirements for pharmacists to administer influenza vaccine to patients under 18 years of age	N/A

Table A4. Cont.

State	Statutes	Regulations	Conclusion	Documented Regulations or Statutes	Survey Results
New Mexico	NEP	NEP	NEP	1) 61-11-11.1. Pharmacy technician; qualifications; duties. (Repealed effective July 1, 2024.) 2) 16.19.22.11 improper activities of pharmacy technicians	N/A
New York	PRI	PRI	PRI	1) §6801. Definition of practice of pharmacy, 6803. Practice of pharmacy and use of title "pharmacist". 2) §63.9 Immunizations and emergency treatment of anaphylaxis pursuant to patient specific and non-patient specific orders and protocols.	N/A
North Carolina	PRI	PRI	PRI	1) § 90-85.3. Definitions (i1), 2) § 90-85.3A. Practice of pharmacy. (c) 3) § 90-85.15B. Immunizing pharmacists. 4) 21 NCAC 46.2507 administration of vaccines by pharmacists	Yes –> NCGS 90-85.15B only authorizes pharmacists to administer vaccines. There is no grant of authority for pharmacy technicians to do so. No (Rules)
North Dakota	PRD	PRI	PRD	1) 43-15-31.5. Injection of drugs - Rules, 43-15-01. Definitions (23, 24) 2) Chapter 61-04-11 Administration of medications and immunizations 3) 61-04-11-01. Definitions (1) 4) 61-04-11-02. 5) 61-02-07.1-06. Tasks pharmacy technicians may not perform 6) 61-02-07.1-05. Tasks pharmacy technicians may perform.	Yes –> NDCC 43-15-31.5 No (Rules)
Ohio	PRD	PRI	PRD	1) ORC 4729.41 Adult immunizations. (1, 2, 3 D,b) 2) 4729-5-38 Immunization and vaccine administration. 3) OAC 4729-5-38 Immunization and vaccine administration.	Yes –> Ohio Administrative Code 4729-5-38 Yes –> Same response for Rules
Oklahoma	NEP	PRI	PRI	1) §59-353.30. Use of agreements - Training requirements and administration of immunizations and therapeutic injections. 2) 535:10-9-13. Administer 3) 535:10-11 (1-6) Pharmacist Administration of Immunizations 4) 535:10-11-4. Immunization registration (a,d)	N/A

Table A4. *Cont.*

State	Statutes	Regulations	Conclusion	Documented Regulations or Statutes	Survey Results
Oregon	NEP	PRI	PRI	1) 689.005 Definitions. (1), (31) 2) 689.645 Vaccines, patient care services, drugs and devices; formulary; rules 3) 689.655 Power to administer drugs and devices; rules. 4) 855-019-0200: General Responsibilities of a Pharmacist 5) 855-019-0270: Qualifications 6) 855-025-0040 Certified Oregon Pharmacy Technician and Pharmacy Technician Tasks and Guidelines	Yes –> ORS 689.005 ORS 689.155 ORS 689.645 ORS 689.655 Yes –> OAR 855-019-0200 OAR 855-019-0270
Pennsylvania	PRD	PRD	PRD	1) Section 9.2. Authority to Administer Injectable (b) 2) 27.403. Conditions for administration. (b)	N/A
Rhode Island	NEP	PERM	PERM	1) § 5-19.1-31. Administration of influenza immunizations to individuals between the ages of nine (9) years and eighteen (18) years, inclusive. 2) § 5-19.1-2. Definitions. (w, x) 3) 216-RICR-40-15-1.11 Administration of Immunizations and Performance of Limited-Function Tests by Pharmacists	No No
South Carolina	PRD	NEP	PRD	1) 40-43-190 (B.3) Protocol for pharmacists to administer vaccines without order of practitioner; informed consent; records. 2) Board of Pharmacy Approved Technician Duties Policy and Procedure #140 Protocol for administration of vaccines by pharmacists (South Carolina Board of Medical Examiners)-language directly prohibits	N/A
South Dakota	NEP	PRD	PRD	1) 36-11-2.2. Practice of pharmacy defined. 2) 36-11-11. Promulgation of rules 3) 36-11-19.1. Authority of registered pharmacists 4) 20:51:28:01. Authority to administer influenza immunizations. 5) 20:51:29:20. Delegation and supervision of technical functions 6) 20:51:29:21. Technical functions 7) 20:51:29:22. Tasks a pharmacy technician may not perform	N/A

Table A4. Cont.

State	Statutes	Regulations	Conclusion	Documented Regulations or Statutes	Survey Results
Tennessee	NEP	NEP	NEP	1) 63-10-204. Definitions 2) 1140-02-.01 pharmacists and pharmacy interns 3) 1140-02-.02 pharmacy technicians	N/A
Texas	PRD	PRD	PRD	1) Title 3, Subtitle J. Sec. A554.004. Administration of medication 2) Rule 295.15 Administration of Immunizations or Vaccinations by a Pharmacist under Written Protocol of Physician	Yes –> Sec. 554.004. Administration of medication Yes –> 295.1 Administration of Immunizations or Vaccinations by a Pharmacist under Written Protocol of Physician
Utah	NEP	NEP	NEP	1) 58-17b-102. Definitions 2) R156-17b-621. Operating Standards-Pharmacist Administration-Training.	N/A
Vermont	NEP	PRI	PRI	1) § 2042b. Pharmacy technicians; nondiscretionary tasks; supervision 2) 10.35 Immunizations 3) 19.6 Coordinating Pharmacist Duties 4) 55.5 "Pharmacy Technician"	No Yes –> Administrative Rules of the Board of Pharmacy 10.35
Virginia	PRI	NEP	PRI	1) § 54.1-3320. Acts restricted to pharmacists 2) § 54.1-3321. Registration of pharmacy technicians 3) § 54.1-3300. Definitions 4) 54.1.3401 (Drug Control Act) 5) 18VAC90-21-50 (10) Requirements for Protocols for Administration of Adult Immunizations. 6) 18VAC110-20-111. Pharmacy technicians	Yes –> The Drug Control Act is seen as a permissive act and pharmacy technicians are not authorized to administer vaccines. No –> Rule
Washington	NEP	NEP	NEP	1) RCW 18.64.011 (28) 2) RCW 18.64A.010 3) RCW 18.64A.030 4) WAC 246-901-020 Pharmacy ancillary personnel utilization. 5) WAC 246-863-095 Pharmacist's professional responsibilities. 6) WAC 246-901-100 Board approval of pharmacies utilizing pharmacy ancillary personnel and specialized functions 7) WAC 246-901-035 Pharmacy technician specialized functions.	Yes –> RCW 18.64 and 18.64A. Yes –> WAC 266-901-020
West Virginia	PRD	PRI	PRD	1) 30-5-7. Rule-making authority 2) 15-12-3 Immunizations 3) 15-12-4 Qualifications	N/A

Table A4. Cont.

State	Statutes	Regulations	Conclusion	Documented Regulations or Statutes	Survey Results
Wisconsin	PRD	PRD	PRD	1) 450.035 (2m) Administration of drug products and devices; vaccines. 2) Phar 7.015 Pharmacy technicians.	N/A
Wyoming	NEP	PRI	PRI	1) § 33-24-157. Immunization administration. 2) WPA Rules Ch 16 Immunization Regulations, Sec 7 Qualifications	N/A
Washington DC	PRI	PRD	PRD	1) § 3-1201.02. Definitions of health occupations. 2) § 3-1202.08. Board of Pharmacy and Advisory Committee on Clinical Laboratory Practitioners. 3) Chapter 99: Pharmacy Technicians-9910.3-Scope of Practice. 4) Chapter 65: Pharmacists-6512-Administration of immunizations and vaccinations by pharmacists	Yes –> District of Columbia Municipal Regulations 9910.3 (g) Yes –> same as above

Note: Permissive = PER, Prohibited Directly = PRD, Prohibited Indirectly = PRI, Not Expressly Prohibited = NEP.

References

1. Office of Disease Prevention and Health Prevention. Immunizations and Infection Diseases. Available online: https://www.healthypeople.gov/2020/topics-objectives/topic/immunization-and-infectious-diseases (accessed on 30 October 2019).
2. Centers for Disease Control and Prevention. National Early-Season Flu Vaccination Coverage, United States. November 2016. Available online: https://www.cdc.gov/flu/fluvaxview/nifs-estimates-nov2016.htm (accessed on 30 October 2019).
3. World Health Organization. Health Topics: Immunizations. Available online: https://www.who.int/topics/immunization/en/ (accessed on 30 October 2019).
4. Kamal, K.M.; Madhavan, S.S.; Amonkar, M.M. Determinants of adult influenza and pneumonia immunization rates. *J. Am. Pharm. Assoc.* **2003**, *43*, 403–411. [CrossRef] [PubMed]
5. American Pharmacists Association/National Alliance of State Pharmacy Associations. Types of Vaccines Authorized to Administer. 2018. Available online: https://www.pharmacist.com/sites/default/files/files/IZ_Authority_012018.pdf (accessed on 28 September 2019).
6. New Jersey Senate Bill 724. Signed/Enacted 17 December 2018. Available online: https://www.billtrack50.com/BillDetail/919014 (accessed on 30 October 2019).
7. New York Senate Bill 1043. Signed/Enacted 17 December 2018. Available online: https://www.nysenate.gov/legislation/bills/2017/s1043/amendment/original (accessed on 30 October 2019).
8. Bright, D.; Adams, A.J. Pharmacy technician–administered vaccines in Idaho. *Am. J. Health Syst. Pharm.* **2017**, *74*, 2033–2034. [CrossRef] [PubMed]
9. Pharmacists, Pharmacies, and Manufacturers, Wholesalers, and Distributors (216-RICR-40-15-1) (1.11.1.B.8). 2018. Available online: https://rules.sos.ri.gov/regulations/part/216-40-15-1 (accessed on 28 September 2019).
10. State of Utah Department of Commerce: Vaccine Administration Protocol. Approved 26 March 2019. Available online: https://dopl.utah.gov/pharm/vaccine_administration_protocol.pdf (accessed on 15 September 2019).
11. Adams, A.; Desselle, S.; McKeirnan, K. Pharmacy technician-administered vaccines: On perceptions and practice reality. *Pharmacy* **2018**, *6*, 124. [CrossRef] [PubMed]
12. Tzanetakos, G.; Ullrich, F.; Mueller, K. Telepharmacy rules and statutes: A 50-state survey. *Am. J. Med. Res.* **2018**, *5*, 7–23. [CrossRef]
13. Stewart, A.M.; Lindley, M.C.; Cox, M.A. State law and standing orders for immunization services. *Am. J. Prev. Med.* **2016**, *50*, e133–e142. [CrossRef] [PubMed]
14. Farmer, T.; Robinson, K.; Elliott, S.J.; Eyles, J. Developing and implementing a triangulation protocol for qualitative health research. *Qual. Health Res.* **2006**, *16*, 377–394. [CrossRef] [PubMed]
15. Rhode Island General Laws 2019, RI Gen L 5-19.1-2(x). Available online: http://webserver.rilin.state.ri.us/Statutes/TITLE5/5-19.1/5-19.1-2.HTM (accessed on 1 November 2019).
16. Rhode Island Regulations: Pharmacists, Pharmacies, and Manufacturers, Wholesalers, and Distributors, 216-RICR-40-15-1.11(8b). Available online: https://rules.sos.ri.gov/regulations/part/216-40-15-1. (accessed on 1 November 2019).
17. South Carolina Code of Laws, SC Code § 40-43-190, B, 3. 2019. Available online: https://www.scstatehouse.gov/code/t40c043.php (accessed on 1 November 2019).
18. South Carolina Board of Pharmacy Policies & Procedures, Approved Technician Duties Policy and Procedure #140. Available online: https://llr.sc.gov/bop/PFORMS/BOP%20Policies%20Procedures.pdf (accessed on 1 November 2019).
19. South Carolina Board of Medical Examiners: Protocol for administration of vaccines by pharmacists. 2016. Available online: https://llr.sc.gov/bop/PFORMS/Joint_Pharmacist_Administered_Immunization_Protocol.pdf (accessed on 1 November 2019).
20. North Carolina General Statutes, NC Gen Stat § 90-85.3.i1. Available online: https://www.ncleg.net/EnactedLegislation/Statutes/PDF/ByArticle/Chapter_90/Article_4A.pdf (accessed on 1 November 2019).
21. North Carolina Administrative Code, 21 NCAC 46.2507. Available online: http://reports.oah.state.nc.us/ncac/title%2021%20-%20occupational%20licensing%20boards%20and%20commissions/chapter%2046%20-%20pharmacy/chapter%2046%20rules.pdf (accessed on 1 November 2019).

22. Idaho Code, ID Code 54-1704. Available online: https://legislature.idaho.gov/statutesrules/idstat/title54/t54ch17/sect54-1704/ (accessed on 1 November 2019).
23. Idaho Regulations, IDAPA Rule 27.01.01.100. Available online: https://adminrules.idaho.gov/rules/current/27/270101.pdf (accessed on 1 November 2019).
24. PEVA: Pharmacy Expanding Vaccine Access. Commissioned CORPS of the U.S. Public Health Service/Pharmacist Professional Advisory Committee Website. Available online: https://dcp.psc.gov/OSG/pharmacy/pevahomepage.aspx (accessed on 30 October 2019).
25. NIIW (National Infant Immunization Week) Champion Award Winners. CDC Website. Available online: https://www.cdc.gov/vaccines/events/niiw/champions/profiles-2018.html (accessed on 30 October 2019).
26. McKeirnan, K.C.; Frazier, K.R.; Nguyen, M.; MacLean, L.G. Training pharmacy technicians to administer immunizations. *J. Am. Pharm. Assoc.* **2018**, *58*, 174–178. [CrossRef] [PubMed]
27. Berger, K. Vaccines administered by certified pharmacy technicians in idaho. *Pharmacy Times*. 28 March 2018. Available online: https://www.pharmacytimes.com/contributor/karen-berger/2018/03/vaccines-administered-by-certified-pharmacy-technicians-in-idaho (accessed on 30 October 2019).
28. National Association of Boards of Pharmacy. Report of the Task Force to Develop Regulations Based on Standards of Care. 2018. Available online: https://nabp.pharmacy/wp-content/uploads/2018/12/Task-Force-to-Develop-Regulations-Based-on-Standards-of-Care-December-2018.pdf (accessed on 24 October 2019).
29. Atkinson, D.; Adams, A.; Bright, D. Should pharmacy technicians administer immunizations? *Innov. Pharm.* **2017**, *8*, 16. [CrossRef]
30. Burgess, T.H.; Murray, C.K.; Bavaro, M.F.; Landrum, M.L.; O'Bryan, T.A.; Rosas, J.G.; Cammarata, S.M.; Martin, N.J.; Ewing, D.; Raviprakash, K.; et al. Self-administration of intranasal influenza vaccine: Immunogenicity and volunteer acceptance. *Vaccine* **2015**, *33*, 3894–3899. [CrossRef] [PubMed]
31. Zahn, M.; Pursiful, P.; Carrico, R.; Woods, C.; Troutman, A. Self-immunization with live attenuated influenza vaccine in a mass vaccination clinic. *Disaster Med. Public Health Prep.* **2013**, *7*, 215–217. [CrossRef] [PubMed]
32. Coleman, B.L.; McGeer, A.J.; Halperin, S.A.; Langley, J.M.; Shamout, Y.; Taddio, A.; Shah, V.; McNeil, S.A. A randomized control trial comparing immunogenicity, safety, and preference for self-versus nurse-administered intradermal influenza vaccine. *Vaccine* **2012**, *30*, 6287–6293. [CrossRef] [PubMed]
33. Bertsch, T.G.; McKeirnan, K.C.; Frazier, K.; VanVoorhis, L.; Shin, S.; Le, K. Supervising pharmacists' opinions about pharmacy technicians as immunizers. *J. Am. Pharm. Assoc.* **2019**, *59*, 527–532. [CrossRef] [PubMed]
34. Frost, T.P.; Adams, A.J. Tech-check-tech in community pharmacy practice settings. *J. Pharm. Technol.* **2017**, *33*, 47–52. [CrossRef]
35. Frost, T.P.; Adams, A.J. Pharmacist and Technician Perceptions of Tech-Check-Tech in Community Pharmacy Practice Settings. *J. Pharm. Pract.* **2018**, *31*, 190–194. [CrossRef] [PubMed]
36. Adams, A.J.; Martin, S.J.; Stolpe, S.F. "Tech-check-tech": A review of the evidence on its safety and benefits. *Am. J. Health Syst. Pharm.* **2011**, *68*, 1824–1833. [CrossRef] [PubMed]
37. Frost, T.P.; Adams, A.J. Expanded Pharmacy Technician Roles: Accepting Verbal Prescriptions and Communicating Prescription Transfers. *Res. Soc. Adm. Pharm.* **2017**, *13*, 1191–1195. [CrossRef] [PubMed]
38. Klepser, D.; Dering-Anderson, A.; Morse, J.; Klepser, M.; Klepser, S.; Corn, C. Time and Motion Study of Influenza Diagnostic Testing in a Community Pharmacy. Time and motion study of influenza diagnostic testing in a community pharmacy. *Innov. Pharm.* **2014**, *5*. [CrossRef]
39. Bright, D.R.; Klepser, M.E.; Murry, L.; Klepser, D.G. Pharmacist-provided pharmacogenetic point-of-care testing consultation service: A time and motion study. *J. Pharm. Technol.* **2018**, *34*, 139–143. [CrossRef]

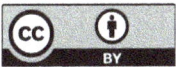 © 2019 by the authors. Licensee MDPI, Basel, Switzerland. This article is an open access article distributed under the terms and conditions of the Creative Commons Attribution (CC BY) license (http://creativecommons.org/licenses/by/4.0/).

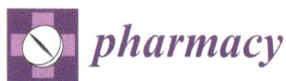

Article

The Value and Potential Integration of Pharmacy Technician National Certification into Processes That Help Assure a Competent Workforce

Shane P. Desselle [1,*], Kenneth C. Hohmeier [2] and Kimberly C. McKeirnan [3]

1. College of Pharmacy, Touro University California, Vallejo, CA 94592, USA
2. College of Pharmacy, University of Tennessee Health Sciences Center College of Pharmacy, Nashville, TN 37211, USA; khohmeie@uthsc.edu
3. College of Pharmacy, Washington State University, Pullman, WA 99202, USA; kimberly.mckeirnan@wsu.edu
* Correspondence: shane.desselle@tu.edu

Received: 20 September 2019; Accepted: 31 October 2019; Published: 5 November 2019

Abstract: The purposes of this study were: (1) to determine pharmacists' perceptions of the impact of certification on competence in specific job skills, its impact in combination with job experience, and its impact in combination with other types of vocational education/training; (2) to identify elements that could potentially enhance the value, or impact of national certification; and (3) to determine how pharmacists view certification in light of various personnel management and organizational behavior phenomena. A self-administered survey was constructed and delivered in spring of 2019 to a random sample of four U.S. states chosen for their geographic diversity and relatively high proportions of both certified and non-certified pharmacy technicians. Following multiple reminders, a response rate of 19.3% was obtained. The 326 responding pharmacists saw certification being less impactful alone than when combined with other types of education/training and previous job experiences. They saw the need for more skills-related and "soft skills" content on the certification examination and agreed that certification is a factor in hiring decisions and that it should be required for designation for advanced practice status. Taken together, respondents saw the need for pharmacy leaders to integrate certification with other aspects of preparation to make for a more competent and professional workforce support team.

Keywords: technician; pharmacy; certification; education; preparedness

1. Introduction

Pharmacy technicians and other workforce support personnel are recognized as essential in the evolution of pharmacy practice to a more patient-centric focus and public health orientation [1]. The previous few years are witness to considerable research into pharmacy technician roles, moving beyond descriptions of technician practice in one particular facility into broader examinations of roles that can be consistently delegated across organizations and even practice settings [2–5]. The growth in literature has helped spur recent systematic reviews of pharmacy technician practice. In one such review, Mattingly and Mattingly noted that approximately half of studies on pharmacy technician practice had been published in the previous decade and that on-the-job training was allowing them to assume more administratively based positions [6]. They found the benefits to technicians for these shifts in practice to be more indirect and/or intrinsic, thus associated with very little raises in pay. Another review centered more around uptake of specific roles associated with pharmacist provision of medication therapy management (MTM) services [7]. That review included 44 manuscripts describing pharmacy technician involvement with medication reconciliation (70% of papers reviewed), documentation (41%), medication therapy review (30%), medication record development (5%), physical assessment (5%), and patient follow-up (2%). The authors concluded that standardized training for pharmacy technicians that delineates administrative support from pharmacists' role of clinical decision making could help pharmacists achieve greater efficiency in MTM delivery.

These reports in the literature evince significant strides in technician practice but that which still stands much room for further growth and improvement. There have been a number of pleas for greater technician involvement in various roles such as telephonic prescription transfer [8], immunizations [9], and quality assurance [10]. However, technician work is already reported to be stressful [11] and for relatively little pay that does not improve with greater regulatory requirements for registration and/or licensure in the United States (U.S.) [12] Aside from assistance with medication reconciliation, much of the attention and growth of technician practice responsibilities have been under the auspices of re-engineering models such as "tech-check-tech" or "technician product verification" where technicians are delegated more tasks in the dispensing process and in some cases afforded a considerable amount of authority in supervising one another's work up to the point where the prepared medication order is provided to the patient [13]. Even while the presence of such "checking technicians" has been demonstrated to be safe, there is some reluctance in advancing technician roles much further [14].

At least a significant if not primary reason for this reluctance is the lack of standardization, even agreement, on the education, training, and professional development necessary for entry into practice and continued employment and advancement [15]. Leaders in pharmacy have long called for national (U.S.) standards for technician education, training, state licensure, as well as for properly defined "entry-level" versus "advanced" technicians [16,17]. The momentum for such clarity in standards has gained even more traction following a stakeholder consensus meeting of pharmacy leaders from various settings and from agencies with regulatory authority [18]. However, the current picture still sees wide variation in technician training and credentialing requirements from state to state. Entry-level practice requirements for technicians throughout the nation indicate that just over half of U.S. states require no education/training or certification of any type; five require certification, only; four require education/training only but not certification; seven require some sort of education/training and certification; another seven require either education/training or certification; and seven have no requirements for education, registration or licensure [19].

Given the lack regulatory authority by one national body, achieving further clarity on entry-level and advanced practice has remained elusive [20]. Moreover, various stakeholders, including some large employers might favor the status quo [21]. In addition to concern about rising labor costs in the face of tight profit margins, some employers might have preference for on-the-job training that fits their organization's specific requirements for the jobs they have designed.

Despite these factors, many stakeholders have embraced national certification as administered by either the Pharmacy Technician Certification Board (PTCB, administering the PTCE® examination) or through the National Healthcareer Association (NHA, administering the ExCPT examination). Several U.S. states now require certification for pharmacy technicians for registration and/or licensure. Other states are considering adopting the requirement for entry or for the designation of so-called "advanced" or similar such designations [22]. The state of Washington requires national certification in addition to experiential work in several, mandatory areas of knowledge [23]. Additionally, some employers have begun to mandate certification to coincide with in-house training, even requiring that PharmD students working as interns acquire certification, as well.

Both national certification procedures involve a self-study process culminating in an examination with components in the names and indications of common drugs, basic pharmacology, federal jurisprudence, dispensing processes, compounding, sterile intravenous admixture, medication safety/quality assurance, and issues surrounding controlled substances [24,25]. Impending changes examination suggest a more parsimonious set of domains, for example removal of sterile intravenous admixture from the PTCE [24].

The principle aims of certification have thusly been on imparting essential knowledge in carrying out the duties of a pharmacy technician. There is no experiential component or skills-based assessment.

However, evidence suggests that engagement in the certification process imbues a greater sense of professional identity and thus might spur greater professionalism and greater commitment to a pharmacy career [26].

While various stakeholders debate requirements for education and training of pharmacy stakeholders, it is important to discern the value of national certification. Previous studies on the value of certification were conducted approximately a decade ago [27,28]. These studies found modest contribution of certification toward various skills and attitudes. Much has changed since the publication of those studies, and that research was conducted in the absence of context, or consideration of other types of education and training. That is, those studies did not determine the extent to which certification might assist or be leveraged during other components or possible education training modalities, such as vocational education and on-the job training.

To that end, the overall aims of this study were to ascribe value to the certification process, and specifically: (1) to determine pharmacists' perceptions of the impact of certification on competence in specific job skills, its impact in combination with job experience, and its impact in combination with other types of vocational education/training; (2) to identify elements that could potentially enhance the value, or impact of national certification; and (3) to determine how pharmacists view certification in light of various personnel management and organizational behavior phenomena.

2. Materials and Methods

2.1. Survey Design

The study methods were deemed exempt from full evaluation and approved for conduct by the principal investigator's Institutional Review Board (IRB).

The study employed a cross-sectional design with use of a survey targeted to a sample of pharmacists from four U.S. states. The survey was comprised of several components. In the first component, pharmacist respondents were asked to identify the impact of certification, alone, on a technician's competence in performance of 21 different job functions and responsibilities in accordance with previous job analyses [29] but in this case job behaviors and roles that were not unique to a particular setting and that comported with components of professionalism and an organization behavior framework proposed by Roberts et al. [30] in pharmacy settings. This organizational behavior framework provides a useful perspective for recognizing the contributions of constituents within an organization, and in turn how their behaviors may affect each other and the organization as a whole. The items used for scaling, then, were items such as prescription/medication order entry, medication preparation, compounding, billing, supervision of other technicians, problem-solving, leadership, time management, basic pharmacology, math skills, and ability to adapt to organizational change. These items were evaluated on a five-point Likert-type scale ranging from 1 = Not all, to 5 = Very much. Participants then evaluated the impact of certification using the same scale and same items but this time in combination with experience on the job, and then also evaluated those same items using the same scale but for certification's impact in combination with other types training/education, such as vocational and on-the-job training.

The next component of the survey contained eight items representing possible actions taken to improve the utility or increase the value of certification. The items were scaled on importance on three points from "Not Important" to "Somewhat important" and "Very important". In this case, the investigators did not believe in the necessity of additional scale intervals and preferred to keep the scale simple and balanced between the intervals (hence, three points only). The items included various components such as more content in specific areas, more support from employers, more specialty certifications, better integration of the examination with vocational education, and more stringent criteria to be eligible to sit for the certification examination. These items were taken from the literature expressing potential improvements made to educational and training mandates for technicians, dating back to older calls and to the more recent aforementioned consensus gathering [16–18].

The third component of the survey to further assist in ascribing value to national certification included 13 items evaluated on five-point Likert-type scales of agreement asking respondents their opinions on various items such as the extent to which certification assists newer versus more experienced technicians, the extent that certification is associated with more greater employer commitment, whether certification should be required for advanced status, whether it helps prepare technicians for emerging roles (practice and organizational change), and whether certification is a determining factor in hiring decisions. These items were based upon findings from a previous nationwide survey of certified pharmacy technicians that examined descriptively pharmacy technicians' commitment levels and from previous studies of pharmacists who initially ascribed value to national certification based upon technicians' preparedness for entry-level practice at that time [27–29].

The fourth component of the survey asked responding pharmacists to rank eight potential characteristics or experiences of technicians as to their importance in that hiring decision. The items consisted of whether they were certified, previous work experience, anticipated job abilities, communication skills, emotional intelligence, and ability to adapt to practice change. As there were no previous studies on desired skills of technicians, these were adapted from a recent study of desire skills for pharmacists [31]. The fifth and final component of the survey solicited certain respondent demographic and practice setting characteristics.

2.2. Design and Sampling

The survey was constructed and disseminated using Qualtrics XM [32] and delivered via email to potential respondents. A list of pharmacists' email addresses was acquired from IQVIA, a company that among other things maintains a list of pharmacists who have agreed to be maintained on a list of theirs to potentially be contacted for research and other purposes. There was no formal sample size determination, as there were many potential variables upon which to base power. It was hoped to acquire at least 200 or more respondents, and the study's budget provided the purchase of 1800 emails from IQVIA.

The sampling frame was derived from four states: California, Florida, Tennessee, and Ohio. These states were selected in consultation with the study sponsor (PTCB) in identifying states that were geographically diverse with varied scopes of practice and licensure for pharmacy technicians. Concurrently, and even more importantly, these four states were without requirements for certification but still had relatively large proportions of technicians who were certified, thus yielding a greater likelihood that pharmacists would have had an opportunity to work with both certified and non-certified technicians, and particularly technicians who had been newly certified as to provide context and potential comparison for their answers to the survey. The states were sampled in relative proportion to the size of their technician population, but with some under sampling from California and some oversampling from Tennessee and Ohio to better assure a reasonable number of respondents from these states. The total number of participants contacted for participation was: 600 from California, 500 from Florida, 360 from Ohio, and 340 from Tennessee.

The procedures employed techniques recommended by Dillman et al. [33] to optimize survey response. An initial email notification of the upcoming survey was sent in early April 2019. Approximately one week later, an email with basic purpose and IRB approval (cover letter) was emailed with a link to the survey. Two reminders were sent via email to the entire sample (not knowing who had already responded) approximately one week apart, with the survey having been closed on 23 May 2019.

2.3. Analysis

Descriptive statistics were tabulated and reported here. There were no measures or other bases around which to frame any attempt to discern construct validity, as there were no attempts to create a summated scale score. However, internal consistency reliability was discerned among the various survey components by calculating Cronbach's alpha scores.

3. Results

3.1. Response Rate and Respondent Characteristics

Of the 1800 survey links disseminated, 110 were returned with undeliverable email addresses. There were valid responses from 326 respondents, resulting in a response rate of 19.3%. Response rates by U.S. state (assuming an equal proportion of undeliverable surveys for each) ranged from a low of 14.6% for Florida to a high of 21.3% for Tennessee. Just over 2/3 of respondents were White/Caucasian (see Table 1), and just over 1/8 indicated a preference not to answer. Nearly 3/4 of respondents worked the equivalent of full-time hours (i.e., greater than 39 h). Over half of the responding pharmacists came from the community pharmacy setting, with an approximately equal share among those from independent and chain settings, respectively. Just under 1/4 came from hospital/health-system settings. There were a considerable number (nearly 7%) who came from a compounding or other specialty practice, and several apiece representing various other practice settings. Staff pharmacists represented nearly 1/3 of respondents, while several respondents were in some sort of administrative or ownership position. Clinical pharmacists could have come from any of various settings, but many of the pharmacy managers likely came from community settings with administrative responsibilities in addition to staffing those pharmacies.

In comparison to the general population of pharmacists in the U.S., the Bureau of Labor Statistics only categorizes pharmacists into much broader work settings, with 26% working in hospital (compared with the current study's 23%) and 57% working in retail (compared with the current study's 54%), which is commensurate given that some of the current study respondents likely work in a hospital or retail setting but have a job title/responsibilities that might be more clinical or administrative [34]. A 2014 study of a national random sample of pharmacists also responding to a survey showed responses in their sample from 56% who were female and 44% male, compared with the current study of just over 52% female and just under 48% male [35].

3.2. Survey Results

Cronbach's alpha calculations for all subsets of items ranged from a low of 0.83 to a high of 0.97. Respondents' perceptions of the impact of certification on technician competence alone, or in combination with other types of education/training and with previous work experiences are described in Table 2. Certification alone was not deemed to have a very substantial impact on many of the general skills under question that generally transcend most, if not all practice settings. Some of the skills/items where certification alone was rated as having the least impact were billing/administrative functions, time management skills, leadership, and problem-solving. Although still under the median scale value ("3"), the areas in which certification alone was deemed to have greater impact were basic pharmacology/drug knowledge, math computation, medication order/prescription entry, and non-sterile compounding. Respondents were more positive about the impact of certification in combination with other types of education/training, with nearly all response means calculated to be at or above the median scale value (except for time management). In addition to time management, those items/areas where the impact of certification in combination with additional education/training was rated lowest included interpersonal communication, ethical decision making and managing organizational change. Those areas rated highest included mathematical computation and medication/prescription order entry, but also sterile compounding. Some of the larger incremental evaluations from combination of certification with education/training versus certification alone included medication/prescription preparation, sterile compounding, problem-solving, and billing/inventory management. Likewise, certification in combination with previous work experience as a technician was viewed to have a more positive impact, with positive mean values (above scale median) for all items except for ethical decision-making. Many of the mean values were similar to but in some cases perhaps somewhat greater than those of certification combined with other education/training. Higher mean values were seen with regard to tech-check-tech, emerging responsibilities (e.g., administering immunizations and assistance with medication therapy management), and a few others; however, these were not compared statistically.

Table 1. Demographic and work-setting characteristics of responding pharmacists (n = 326).

Characteristic	Number (%) *
U.S. State residing/practicing	
California	112 (34.5%)
Florida	83 (25.4%)
Ohio	63 (19.3%)
Tennessee	68 (20.9%)
Sex	
Female	170 (52.2%)
Male	156 (47.8%)
Race/ethnicity	
White/Caucasian	222 (68.1%)
Black/African-American	18 (5.6%)
Hispanic/Latino	24 (7.5%)
Asian/Pacific Islander	15 (4.6%)
Middle Eastern (e.g., Arabic, Persian, Palestinian)	5 (1.4%)
Prefer not to answer	42 (12.9%)
Hours worked per week	
Up to 20	42 (12.9%)
20–39	43 (13.2%)
Greater than 39	241 (73.9%)
Primary work setting	
Community independent	86 (26.3%)
Community chain	91 (27.9%)
Community health center (e.g., Federally Qualified Health Center)	2 (0.6%)
Hospital inpatient	49 (15.0%)
Hospital ambulatory care	12 (3.7%)
Hospital critical access	7 (2.1%)
Hospital other	6 (1.8%)
Compounding/other specialty	22 (6.7%)
Government state or local	9 (2.8%)
Government federal	7 (2.1%)
Government military	6 (1.8%)
Mail service	7 (2.1%)
Managed health care	12 (3.6%)
Pharmaceutical industry	4 (1.2%)
Other	6 (1.8%)
Job title	
Staff pharmacist	100 (30.7%)
Clinical pharmacist	71 (21.6%)
Pharmacy manager or supervisor	79 (24.2%)
District manager	2 (0.7%)
Chief pharmacist/Pharmacy Director/Assistant Director or Chief	28 (8.6%)
Pharmacy Owner	48 (14.7%)

* Percentages for each category may not summarily equal 100.0% due to rounding.

Table 3 provides mean ratings of items/factors contributing to making certification more impactful. Most items were evaluated quite highly on a three-point scale of importance, with all but one of them at or above the median scale value of "2". The factor rated below "2" was "more difficult examination". Items the respondents rated rather high on importance included better integration of the certification process with vocational training, more content on technical pharmacy knowledge/skills, more content on "soft skills", and more support for certification from employing organizations.

Table 2. Perceptions of the impact of certification on technician competence alone, in combination with other types of education/training, and in combination with previous work experience.

Skill/Behavior/Knowledge Item	Alone *	with Education *	with Work *
Medication order/prescription entry	2.38±1.24	3.54±1.42	3.65±1.35
Medication order/prescription preparation	2.15±1.07	3.46±1.49	3.62±1.18
Patient/customer service	1.92±1.17	3.15 ± 1.33	3.27 ± 1.37
Non-sterile compounding	2.35 ± 1.24	3.58 ± 1.42	3.65 ± 1.37
Sterile compounding	2.19 ± 1.00	3.54 ± 1.34	3.65 ± 1.36
Inventory management	1.92 ± 0.91	3.38 ± 1.42	3.46 ± 1.34
Billing and other administrative functions	1.73 ± 0.92	3.45 ± 1.30	3.53 ± 1.42
Interpersonal communication	1.65 ± 0.98	3.00 ± 1.36	3.02 ± 1.19
Time management/organization skills	1.73 ± 1.12	2.92 ± 1.47	3.04 ± 1.32
Ethical decision making	1.92 ± 1.22	3.04 ± 1.45	2.88 ± 1.40
Supervision of other technicians	2.19 ± 1.08	3.31 ± 1.40	3.42 ± 1.35
Tech-check-tech	2.31 ± 1.12	3.27 ± 1.31	3.46 ± 1.28
Quality assurance program activities	2.19 ± 1.15	3.38 ± 1.28	3.50 ± 1.24
Professionalism	2.12 ± 1.12	3.23 ± 1.37	3.27 ± 1.33
Problem-solving/innovativeness	1.88 ± 1.01	3.23 ± 1.29	3.37 ± 1.28
Accepting responsibility	1.88 ± 1.21	3.12 ± 1.28	3.15 ± 1.30
Leadership	1.77 ± 1.29	3.24 ± 1.37	3.38 ± 1.34
Emerging/new responsibilities (e.g., immunizations, assistance with MTM)	2.19 ± 1.28	3.48 ± 1.36	3.52 ± 1.33
Basic pharmacology/knowledge of drug names/OTCs	2.69 ± 1.34	3.58 ± 1.36	3.65 ± 1.31
Math computational skills	2.65 ± 1.20	3.65 ± 1.34	3.58 ± 1.28
Managing organizational change	2.08 ± 1.27	3.08 ± 1.28	3.12 ± 1.19

* Mean ± Standard deviation on a scale ranging from 1 = Not at all to 5 = Very much.

Table 3. Items/factors contributing to making certification more impactful.

Item/Factor	Mean ± S.D. *
More difficult examination	1.83 ± 0.69
More stringent criteria to sit, or be able to take the examination	2.00 ± 0.76
More specialty certifications (e.g., specifically in compounding, Inventory management)	2.00 ± 0.87
More process/logistical support from certification programs (PTCB, NHA)	2.05 ± 0.91
More support from your employing organization for certification	2.35 ± 0.74
More content on "soft skills" such as communication, leadership, and ethical decision-making	2.39 ± 0.65
More content on technical pharmacy knowledge and skills	2.45 ± 0.62
Better integrating the certification process with vocational training	2.50 ± 0.64

* Mean ± Standard Deviation on a three-point scale ranging from 1 = Not important to 3 = Very important.

Respondents' beliefs about various facets of the value of certification are shown in Table 4. Respondents slightly disagreed with the notion that certification is equally beneficial across different practice settings. There was also slight disagreement with mean scores toward neutral for items suggesting certified technicians make fewer mistakes, are more innovative in customer service, are better prepared to deal with organizational change, and are more committed to their employer. There was agreement with the idea that technicians with experience are able to leverage certification, are more committed to their occupation/profession, help to promote a stronger organizational culture, and are better prepared to accept new roles, as well as that hiring decisions are made at least in part on whether the technician is certified. There was strongest agreement with the idea that technician certification should be a requirement for advanced status and/or roles.

Table 4. Respondents' beliefs about various facets of the value of certification.

Item/Facet	Mean ± S.D. *
Certification imparts the same level of benefit to technicians regardless of setting	2.83 ± 1.51
Technicians with experience are able to leverage certification effectively	4.57 ± 1.24
Certification assists technicians who are new to this field of work	3.55 ± 1.57
I make (or would make) technician hiring decision at least in part upon whether or not they are certified	3.99 ± 1.75
Technician certification should be a requirement for advanced status/roles	4.84 ± 1.63
Technicians who are certified are better prepared to accept new roles and responsibilities	3.98 ± 1.84
Certified technicians make fewer mistakes/errors than non-certified ones	3.08 ± 1.56
Technicians who are certified are better prepared to deal with organizational change	3.25 ± 1.60
I feel more comfortable delegating to a technician who is certified	3.82 ± 1.80
Technicians who are certified help to promote a stronger organizational culture in my organization	3.77 ± 1.72
Technicians who are certified are more innovate in providing customer/client service	3.23 ± 1.60
Technicians who are certified are more committed to their employer	3.13 ± 1.68
Technicians who are certified are more committed to their occupation/profession	4.34 ± 1.75

* Mean ± standard deviation on a scale ranging from 1 = Strongly disagree to 6 = Strongly agree.

Table 5 provides the mean ranking of various factors responding pharmacists actually use or would use in hiring pharmacy technicians. Ranked highest (lowest mean) was the technician's demonstrated or anticipated job abilities. This was followed by their previous work history as a technician, their communication skills and moral integrity, whether or not they are certified, their ability to adapt to practice change, their emotional intelligence, and finally their acquisition of vocational school training.

Table 5. Mean ranking of factors in respondents' hiring or potential hiring decisions regarding pharmacy technicians.

Item/Factor	Mean ± S.D. *
Their demonstrated or anticipated job abilities	2.97 ± 1.78
Their previous work history as a technician	3.53 ± 1.37
Their communication skills	3.65 ± 1.64
Their professional/moral integrity	3.65 ± 1.79
Whether they are certified	4.54 ± 2.35
Their ability to adapt to practice change	5.61 ± 1.69
Their emotional intelligence	5.83 ± 2.14
Their acquisition of vocational school training	6.22 ± 1.97

* Mean ± standard deviation based on a ranking of each item/factor from 1 to 8.

4. Discussion

This study evaluated the opinions of pharmacists from four states regarding the value of and potential changes that might enhance the impact of pharmacy technician certification. In doing so, it updated previous assessments of certification undertaken over a decade ago after many changes in the pharmacy landscape and after continued calls for standardization in technician education and training. It also undertook this evaluation under the auspices of an organizational behavior framework, thus focusing more on general abilities that transcend practice setting while considering potential organization and further practice change.

Although approaching the topic from a different angle, namely with an organizational behavior framework, the study corroborates other research on pharmacist workforce, such as how technicians see themselves in regard to their own preparedness [29]. The results also align with a recent qualitative study of both pharmacists and technicians identifying a competency/preparedness for practice framework that identified six domains, including: communication in patient care, collaboration with other personnel, knowledge in pharmaceuticals, organization of care (including staffing and workflow issues), emerging leadership responsibilities, and personal development [36].

Pharmacists responding to the survey saw certification alone as having only a very modest impact on technician competence in various job responsibilities and behaviors. This is not surprising, given that certification involves a self-study process that does not include a didactic or experiential component and was basically designed to impart certain foundational knowledge concepts for test-takers [24]. As such, it also is not surprising that the competencies accorded the highest impact by certification were basic pharmacology and math computational skills. However, respondents saw certification as having a greater impact when it is combined with other types of education/training and with previous work experience. In comparison to certification alone, for certification in combination with other educational activities and/or work experience, the impact was evaluated much higher on competencies such as medication preparation, compounding, billing/administrative functions, problem-solving, and leadership. As such, the responding pharmacists likely recognize the importance of longitudinal and multiple types of exposure to more complex and cognitive functions administered or instructed in a variety of ways [37]. Likewise, there have been calls in Doctor of Pharmacy (PharmD) education to include various types of learning experiences for skills such as problem-solving, leadership, and managing change [38].

These results suggest that respondents see certification as an important component of a larger effort to promote technician competence and professionalization [39]. In fact, the action deemed most important by respondents in certification having an even greater impact was integration of the certification process with vocational training. This was echoed in the aforementioned stakeholder consensus conference and other calls for standardizing technician preparedness and entry into the field [18]. In the current study, pharmacists viewed technician vocational training as least impactful in potential hiring decisions, and this reflects concern pharmacists have expressed about the variation of quality in those vocational programs [40]. However, the pharmacists in the current study see certification's alignment with vocational programs as a potential way to further standardize and raise the quality of technician preparedness for practice. These phenomena warrant additional study.

Respondents reported nearly the same level of importance on content related to technical pharmacy skills and to the inclusion of "soft skills" such as leadership and ethical decision-making. Indeed, the evaluation of the impact of certification alone on items such as communication and leadership were relatively low. Previous research has found community pharmacists of the mindset that technicians are the "face" of the pharmacy [41] and have also expressed concern about technicians dealing with controlled substances (i.e., issues around ethical decision making) [42]. Thus, while it is unlikely that anyone expects a self-study examination process to fully prepare technicians for specific job competencies and soft skills, respondents did think it was an important component to add and perhaps integrate with other types of education and training. This is further amplified by a high importance rating given to the need for more support from employers, which likely also alludes to the need to increase technician salaries as well as to better leverage certification in their own in-house training. Previous qualitative research indicates pharmacist support for including more so-called soft skills [43]. Viewed as less than somewhat important in this study was the need to simply make the current certification examinations more difficult.

Respondents reiterated their perceptions of the importance of communication skills and professional judgment when these skills were rated rather highly in hiring decisions, only after previous work experience and expected overall abilities on the job. Certification was deemed to be relatively important, and alone, was deemed more important than vocational training as well as the technician's ability to adapt to practice change. Perhaps respondents believe that technicians' ability to adapt to change and their emotional intelligence will, or can be groomed by the employing organization. The results here would appear to corroborate recent explorations into the desired characteristics of pharmacists, as well. Alston et al. [31] found characteristics such as communication skills and moral integrity to be the most highly sought after among recent pharmacy graduates for new positions, and Wheeler et al. saw these types of competencies, as well as proven ability and experience, to be among the most frequent requirements listed in pharmacist job positions posted nationwide [44].

A composite view of certification was undertaken through the use of general items about various facets of the process. Respondents agreed that technicians with experience are able to leverage certification effectively, thus adding to perceptions of its importance but need for integration with experience, which would appear to be incumbent both on employers and certification boards. The responding pharmacists also agreed that certification should be required for designation into advanced status, as is becoming more common with career laddering options [45]. Respondents also agreed that technicians who are certified are more committed to their profession but slightly disagreed or were neutral in regard to employer commitment. Perhaps pharmacists are of the belief that having gained more marketability through certification might result in technicians being open to opportunities with other employers. The respondents also slightly disagreed or were neutral with the notion that certified technicians are more adept in customer service and commit fewer errors. Again, certification is not necessarily meant to improve skills that would be associated with reduced errors, but perhaps better integration and more emphasis on public health/safety and customer relations would be beneficial components to the certification process.

Taken together, the results suggest that pharmacists placed a good bit of value on technician certification but are aware that certification alone does not prepare technicians for greater competence in all facets of work and that the role it plays currently is in providing much needed background knowledge in certain areas. The results also suggest that respondents see certification as a needed component of technician education and particularly required for advancement into higher status/roles in the organization and helping to imbue greater commitment and professionalism through the self-study process while acknowledging that certification needs to be better synchronized and leveraged with other experiences and education. As such, these results call for action by employers, certification organizations, educators, and other leaders in the profession concurrently, thus echoing sentiments expressed for quite some time [46,47]. Even colleges/schools of pharmacy in the U.S. can consider interprofessional education options that include exposure of technicians to Doctor of Pharmacy curricula while providing Doctor of Pharmacy students an opportunity to gain greater appreciation for technician roles, which can ultimately assist as well in their supervision of technicians and thus technicians' competence [48]. Additionally, technician certification vendors (and educational organizations) might want to gear future education and assessment based more on the setting than on the particular task.

Study Limitations

Several study limitations are worth noting. The survey was administered to pharmacists in only four U.S. states. The response rate achieved was positive in light of evidence suggesting that surveys, particularly those executed through email, are otherwise quite low [49]. However, the response rate was low enough to preclude generalization of attitudes even to pharmacists in the four states comprising the sampling frame. The research involved the use of question items informed from previous research but without any sort of gold standard or an attempt to create an overall composite measure or index; thus, there was no basis by which to discern the construct or content validity of the measures used.

5. Conclusions

This study examined pharmacists' perceptions of the value of pharmacy technician certification within an organizational behavior framework. Pharmacists viewed certification as important for professionalization of technicians, suggested the need to include more soft skills training as part of the process, and implored leaders to better integrate certification with vocational training. Future research might attempt to replicate the current study with a more geographically diverse population and evaluate more specific strategies to integrate certification with other forms of training.

Even with many changes having taken place since initial evaluations of the value of certification, the results corroborate the importance of certification not only for specific skills but overall professionalism and commitment, yet recognizes the need for action by various stakeholders and leaders in pharmacy to better integrate certification with other educational components and past work experience to ensure a support workforce that has the competence needed to assist with the execution of effective patient care in a continuously changing health care environment.

Author Contributions: Research conceptualization by S.P.D.; methodology by S.P.D., K.C.M., and K.C.H.; validation by S.P.D., K.C.M., and K.C.H., data curation by S.P.D., K.C.M., and K.C.H.; writing—original draft preparation by S.P.D.; writing—review and editing by S.P.D., K.C.M., and K.C.H.; project administration, S.P.D., K.C.M., and K.C.H.; funding acquisition, S.P.D.

Funding: This research was funded by the Pharmacy Technician Certification Board (PTCB).

Acknowledgments: The authors would like to express their appreciation to the Pharmacy Technician Certification Board (PTCB) for their sponsorship and support of the study.

Conflicts of Interest: The authors declare no conflict of interest.

References

1. Schultz, K.M.; Jeter, C.K.; Keresztes, J.M.; Martin, N.M.; Mundi, T.K.; Van Cura, J.D. ASHP Statement on the Roles of Pharmacy Technicians. *Am. J. Health Syst. Pharm.* **2016**, *73*, 928–930. [CrossRef] [PubMed]
2. Lengel, M.; Kuhn, C.H.; Worley, M.; Wehr, A.M.; McAuley, J.W. Pharmacy technician involvement in community pharmacy medication therapy management. *J. Am. Pharm. Assoc.* **2018**, *58*, 179–185. [CrossRef] [PubMed]
3. Bryan, K. Optimizing the role of pharmacy technicians in patient care settings: First hand knowledge of the technician's value. *J. Am. Pharm. Assoc.* **2018**, *58*, 7–8. [CrossRef] [PubMed]
4. Mattingly, T.J. Optimizing the role of pharmacy technicians in patient care settings: Measuring pharmacy technician impact on desired outcomes. *J. Am. Pharm. Assoc.* **2018**, *58*, 8–9. [CrossRef] [PubMed]
5. Leong, A.Y.; Pederson, M. Optimizing workflow processes in an advanced medication dispensary. *Res. Soc. Adm. Pharm.* **2018**, *14*, 1072–1079. [CrossRef] [PubMed]
6. Mattingly, A.N.; Mattingly, T.J. Advancing the role of the pharmacy technician: A systematic review. *J. Am. Pharm. Assoc.* **2018**, *58*, 94–108. [CrossRef]
7. Gernant, S.A.; Nguyen, M.O.; Siddiqui, S.; Schneller, M. Use of pharmacy technicians in elements of medication therapy management delivery: A systematic review. *Res. Soc. Adm. Pharm.* **2018**, *14*, 883–890. [CrossRef]
8. Frost, T.P.; Adams, A.J. Expanded pharmacy technician roles: Accepting verbal prescriptions and communicating prescription transfers. *Res. Soc. Adm. Pharm.* **2017**, *13*, 1191–1195. [CrossRef]
9. McKeirnan, K.C.; Frazier, K.R.; Nguyen, M.; MacLean, L.G. Training pharmacy technicians to administer immunizations. *J. Am. Pharm. Assoc.* **2018**, *52*, 174–178. [CrossRef]
10. Mone, M.M. Optimizing the contributions of technicians in pharmacy practice—Moving the pharmacy profession forward. *Am. J. Health Syst. Pharm.* **2017**, *74*, 1333–1335. [CrossRef]
11. Desselle, S.P.; Hoh, R.; Rossing, C.; Holmes, E.R.; Gill, A.; Zamora, L. Work preferences and general abilities among U.S. pharmacy technicians and Danish pharmaconomists. *J. Pharm. Pract.* **2018**. [CrossRef] [PubMed]
12. Urick, B.Y.; Mattingly, T.J.; Mattingly, A.N. Relationship between regulatory burdens to entry and pharmacy technician wages. *Res. Soc. Adm. Pharm.* **2019**. [CrossRef] [PubMed]
13. Hohmeier, K.C.; Desselle, S.P. Exploring the implementation of a novel optimizing care model in the community pharmacy setting. *J. Am. Pharm. Assoc.* **2019**, *59*, 310–318. [CrossRef] [PubMed]
14. Schafheutle, E.I.; Jee, S.D.; Willis, S.C. Fitness of purpose for pharmacy technician education and training: The case of Great Britain. *Res. Soc. Adm. Pharm.* **2017**, *13*, 88–97. [CrossRef] [PubMed]
15. Abramowitz, P.W.; Cobaugh, D.J. Education and certification of technicians: A noble decision is long overdue. *Am. J. Health Syst. Pharm.* **2017**, *74*, 1303–1304. [CrossRef]
16. Pharmacy Technician Certification Board. Sesquicentennial stepping stone summits—Summit two: Pharmacy technicians. *J. Am. Pharm. Assoc.* **2003**, *43*, 84–92. Available online: https://www.pharmacist.com/sites/default/files/stepping_stone_summits_pharmacy_technicians.pdf (accessed on 1 November 2019).
17. Tice, L. White paper on pharmacy technicians 2002: Needed changes can no longer wait. *Am. J. Health Syst. Pharm.* **2003**, *60*, 37–51. Available online: https://www.japha.org/article/S1086-5802(15)30083-8/pdf (accessed on 1 November 2019). [CrossRef]
18. Zellmer, W.A.; Mcallister, E.B.; Silvester, J.A.; Vlasses, P.H. Toward uniform standards for pharmacy technicians: Summary of the 2017 Pharmacy Technician Stakeholder Consensus Conference. *Am. J. Health Syst. Pharm.* **2017**, *74*, 1321–1332. [CrossRef]

19. Mattingly, A.N. Entry-level practice requirements of pharmacy technicians across the United States: A review. *Am. J. Health Syst. Pharm.* **2018**, *75*, 1057–1063. [CrossRef]
20. The consensus of the Pharmacy Practice Model Summit. *Am. J. Health Syst. Pharm.* **2011**, *68*, 1148–1152. [CrossRef]
21. Justis, L.; Crain, J.; Marchetti, M.L.; Hohmeier, K.C. The effect of community pharmacy technicians on industry standard adherence performance measures after cognitive pharmaceutical services training. *J. Pharm. Technol.* **2016**, *32*, 230–233. [CrossRef]
22. California Board of Pharmacy 8/22/17 Meeting Materials. Available online: https://www.pharmacy.ca.gov/meetings/agendas/2017/17_aug_lic_mat.pdf (accessed on 15 May 2019).
23. Pharmacy Technician Career Guide. Washington Pharmacy Technician Requirements and Training Programs. Available online: https://v-tecs.org/washington-pharmacy-technician-requirements-and-training-programs.htm (accessed on 3 August 2019).
24. Pharmacy Technician Certification Board. Prepare for the Pharmacy Technician Certification Exam. Available online: https://ptcb.org/get-certified/prepare-for-the-ptce#.XNsFxdQrKY0 (accessed on 1 August 2019).
25. National Healthcareer Association. The ExCPT Exam: What to Expect and How to Prepare. Available online: https://info.nhanow.com/blog/the-excpt-exam-what-to-expect-and-how-to-prepare (accessed on 1 August 2019).
26. Desselle, S.P. An in-depth examination of pharmacy technician worklife through an organizational behavior framework. *Res. Soc. Adm. Pharm.* **2016**, *12*, 722–732. [CrossRef] [PubMed]
27. Schmitt, M.R.; Desselle, S.P. Pharmacists' perceptions of the value of certification. *J. Pharm. Technol.* **2010**, *26*, 340–351.
28. Schmitt, M.R.; Desselle, S.P. Pharmacists' attitudes toward technician certification: A qualitative study. *J. Pharm. Technol.* **2009**, *25*, 79–88. [CrossRef]
29. Desselle, S.P.; Holmes, E.R. Results of the 2015 National Certified Pharmacy Technician Workforce Survey. *Am. J. Health Syst. Pharm.* **2017**, *74*, 981–991. [CrossRef]
30. Roberts, A.S.; Benrimoj, S.I.; Chen, T.F.; Williams, K.A.; Hopp, T.R.; Aslani, P. Understanding practice change in community pharmacy: A qualitative study in Australia. *Res. Soc. Adm. Pharm.* **2005**, *1*, 546–564. [CrossRef]
31. Altson, G.L.; Marsh, W.; Castleberry, A.N.; Kelley, K.A.; Boyce, E.G. Pharmacists' opinions of the value of specific applicant attributes in hiring decisions for entry-level pharmacists. *Res. Soc. Adm. Pharm.* **2019**, *15*, 536–545.
32. Copyright 2015. Provo, Utah. Available online: www.qualtrics.com (accessed on 24 September 2019).
33. Dillman, D.A.; Smyth, J.D.; Christian, L.M. *Internet, Mail and Mixed-Mode Surveys: The Tailored Design Method*, 3rd ed.; John Wiley and Sons, Inc.: Hoboken, NJ, USA, 2009.
34. U.S. Bureau of Labor and Statistics. Pharmacists. Available online: https://www.bls.gov/ooh/healthcare/mobile/pharmacists.htm (accessed on 24 October 2019).
35. Mott, D.A.; Doucette, W.R.; Gaither, C.A.; Kreling, D.G.; Schommer, J.C. Trends in pharmacist participation in the workforce, 2009 to 2014. *J. Am. Pharm. Assoc.* **2016**, *54*, 433–440. [CrossRef]
36. Koehler, T.C.; Bok, H.; Westerman, M.; Jaarsma, D. Developing a competency framework for pharmacy technicians: Perspectives from the field. *Res. Soc. Adm. Pharm.* **2019**, *15*, 514–520. [CrossRef]
37. Vira, P.; Nazer, L.; Phung, O.; Jackevicius, J. A longitudinal evidence-based pharmacy curriculum and its impact on the attitudes and perceptions of pharmacy students. *Am. J. Pharm. Educ.* **2019**, *83*, 6510.
38. Accreditation Council for Pharmacy Education. Accreditation Standards and Key Elements for the Professional Program in Pharmacy Leading to the Doctor of Pharmacy Degree. Available online: https://www.acpe-accredit.org/pdf/Standards2016FINAL.pdf (accessed on 6 August 2019).
39. Gregory, P.A.M.; Austin, Z. Conflict in community pharmacy practice: The experience of pharmacists, technicians and assistants. *Can. Pharm. J.* **2016**, *150*, 32–41. [CrossRef] [PubMed]
40. Anderson, D.C.; Draime, J.A.; Anderson, T.S. Description and comparison of pharmacy technician training programs in the United States. *J. Am. Pharm. Assoc.* **2016**, *56*, 231–236. [CrossRef] [PubMed]
41. Kadia, N.K.; Schroeder, M.N. Community pharmacy-based adherence programs and the role of pharmacy technicians: A review. *J. Pharm. Technol.* **2015**, *31*, 51–57. [CrossRef]

42. Draime, J.A.; Anderson, D.C.; Anderson, T.S. Description and comparison of medication diversion in pharmacies by pharmacists, interns, and pharmacy technicians. *J. Am. Pharm. Assoc.* **2018**, *58*, 275–280. [CrossRef] [PubMed]
43. Desselle, S.P.; McKeirnan, K.C.; Hohmeier, K.C. A re-evaluation of the value of pharmacy technician certification. *Am. J. Health Syst. Pharm.* **2019**, in press.
44. Wheeler, J.S.; Ngo, T.; Cecil, J.; Borja-Hart, N. Exploring employer job requirements: An analysis of pharmacy job announcements. *J. Am. Pharm. Assoc.* **2017**, *57*, 723–728. [CrossRef]
45. Proposal for pharmacy technician education, training, practice, and career laddering: A proposal to advance pharmacy practice and promote patient safety. *Cali. J. Health Syst. Pharm.* **2015**, *27*, 29–40. Available online: https://cdn.ymaws.com/www.cshp.org/resource/resmgr/Files/Technician/Resources/CJHP_Pharm_Tech_Article_2015.pdf (accessed on 1 November 2019).
46. Wheeler, J.S.; Gray, J.A.; Gentry, C.K.; Farr, G.E. Advancing pharmacy technician training and practice models in the United States: Historical perspectives, workforce developments needs, and future opportunities. *Res. Soc. Adm. Pharm.* **2019**. [CrossRef]
47. Manasse, H.R.; Menighan, T.E. Single standard for education, training, and certification of pharmacy technicians. *Am. J. Health Syst. Pharm.* **2010**, *67*, 348–349. [CrossRef]
48. Mospan, C.M.; Bright, D.R.; Eid, D. Highlighting a gap in student pharmacist training: Intraprofessional education with pharmacy technicians. *Curr. Pharm. Teach. Learn.* **2018**, *10*, 1160–1164. [CrossRef]
49. Hardigan, P.C.; Popovici, I.; Carvajal, M.J. Response rate, response time, and economic costs of survey research: A randomized trial of practicing pharmacists. *Res. Soc. Adm. Pharm.* **2016**, *12*, 141–148. [CrossRef] [PubMed]

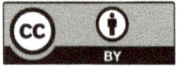

© 2019 by the authors. Licensee MDPI, Basel, Switzerland. This article is an open access article distributed under the terms and conditions of the Creative Commons Attribution (CC BY) license (http://creativecommons.org/licenses/by/4.0/).

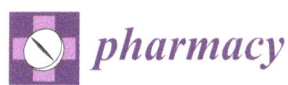

Article

Description of Position Ads for Pharmacy Technicians

Juanita A. Draime [1,*], Emily C. Wicker [2], Zachary J. Krauss [2], Joel L. Sweeney [2] and Douglas C. Anderson [1]

1. Department of Pharmacy Practice, Cedarville University School of Pharmacy, Cedarville, OH 45413, USA; andersond@cedarville.edu
2. Cedarville University School of Pharmacy, Cedarville, OH 45413, USA; ewicker217@cedarville.edu (E.C.W.); zacharykrauss@cedarville.edu (Z.J.K.); jsweeney@cedarville.edu (J.L.S.)
* Correspondence: juanitaadraime@cedarville.edu; Tel.: +(937)-766-7475

Received: 3 March 2020; Accepted: 21 May 2020; Published: 22 May 2020

Abstract: Pharmacy technician roles are evolving alongside the changing role of a pharmacist. There is currently no uniform definition of a pharmacy technician's role in the pharmacy workforce. The objective of this study was to look at the United States-based pharmacy technician advertisement database from Pharmacy Week to find patterns and commonalities in the duties and qualifications of pharmacy technicians. A retrospective analysis was performed on fourteen days of pharmacy technician job listings from Pharmacy Week from the year 2018. Information obtained from the listings included job title, location, setting, type of job, job duties, and job requirements. Job duties and requirements were coded by themes. Fourteen days of data resulted in 21,007 individual position listings. A majority of the job listings were for full-time positions (96.4%) and most were in the retail setting (96.78%). The most common requirements were registration with State Board, high school diploma, ability to perform tasks, communication, and physical. The most common job duties were general office etiquette, performing tasks under the direct supervision of the pharmacist, and professionalism. This study provides a description of the evolving role of pharmacy technicians through the broad variety in expectations for requirements of pharmacy technician applicants and the duties they perform when hired.

Keywords: pharmacy technician; technician duties; technician job requirements; technician role

1. Introduction

Over the last decade, pharmacy has seen a large shift in the role of both the pharmacist and pharmacy technician. For instance, pharmacists have increasingly focused on providing clinical care, and gradually fallen away from the traditional dispensing role [1]. Pharmacy technicians are personnel "working in a pharmacy who, under the supervision of the licensed pharmacist, assists in pharmacy activities that do not require the professional judgment of a pharmacist [1]." However, as pharmacists have decreased their focus on dispensing, pharmacy technicians have been given the opportunity to fill the traditional dispensing role in the pharmacist's place. These new changes have progressively become the normal pharmacy model, and many studies have shown the added value of this model in both improved quality of patient care and pharmacy efficiency [2–8]. This shift is a huge building block for the future, yet at the same time, it has resulted in the formation of unique and evolving roles for pharmacy technicians. These new roles are still in the development process, and research is beginning to roll out on the safety and efficacy of advanced pharmacy technician positions [9–12]. These changes, in due course, may be considerable innovations, but at the same time, they may pose poignant risks to patient safety. This study helps to define pharmacy technicians' new roles through the use of pharmacy technician job advertisements.

Understanding the way pharmacy technicians are recruited through job advertisements is helpful in defining the evolving role of pharmacy technicians. The recruitment process through job listings on social forums is an important and commonly-used tool by employers to convey job requirements and responsibilities. Additionally, job advertisements affect the number, type, and talent of possible hires. If effectively used, employers can use job advertisements to increase the quality and quantity of applicants by giving applicants a clear snapshot of future roles and responsibilities as well as the requirements for the job. While advertisements do not represent the formal contractual responsibilities and requirements of a technician, they do represent what the employer needs in a technician. Ultimately, looking at pharmacy technician advertisements can serve as an indicator of both the duties and qualifications desired for pharmacy technicians.

The roles and responsibilities of pharmacy technicians have been evolving from basic pharmacy organization and prescription assembly skills to complex dispensary, verification, immunization, education, and medication synchronization skills in the past decade [13]. Recently, the American Society of Health-System Pharmacists (ASHP) has defined the role of pharmacy technicians in three categories: entry-level, advanced, and specialized [13]. The listed skills needed for entry-level roles include pharmacology for technicians, pharmacy law and regulation, compounding including low- or medium-risk sterile compounding and non-sterile compounding, basic safe medication practices, pharmacy quality assurance, medication order entry and distribution, pharmacy inventory management, pharmacy billing and reimbursement, and medication-use system technology [13]. Interestingly, many of what the ASHP calls "entry-level skills" are what used to traditionally define the role of pharmacy technician [1]. However, as the pharmacy model has evolved, pharmacy technicians are now receiving new roles that are attained through additional education, training, and competency testing. These new advanced roles are supervised by pharmacists and/or approved by each state's Board of Pharmacy [1]. According to the ASHP, pharmacy technicians need to have certain skills to be included in this advanced category [13]. These skills include advanced medication systems including "tech-check-tech" programs, purchasing or fiscal management, management or supervision of other pharmacy technicians, medication history assistance, medication therapy management assistance, quality improvement, immunization assistance, hazardous drug handling, patient assistance programs, pharmacy technician education and training, community outreach, drug utilization evaluation and/or adverse-drug-event monitoring, industry, and informatics [13]. Furthermore, the ASHP says that some technicians receive even more specialized roles which are dependent upon each technician's individual situation [13]. They define these specialized roles as roles that require extra certification as specified by the Pharmacy Technician Certification Board (PTCB) [13]. These advanced and specialized roles contain many unique and innovative changes for pharmacy technicians which could ultimately improve patient care [13].

Despite the fact that these new technician roles may help alleviate a pharmacist's workload and allow for a more streamlined pharmacy, they may, at the same time, present safety and efficacy issues in patient care. For instance, many of these new roles are still in the research and development process and, therefore, require strict certification, regulation, and supervision by each state's Board of Pharmacy [9–12,14]. These innovative roles require exemptions as can be seen in the research studies done by Frost, Adams. McKeiran, Henriksen, and Bailey [9–12,14]. However, employers may knowingly or unknowingly try to utilize the added efficiency of these new roles in their pharmacies without receiving proper exemption status. Unfortunately, without the provided exemption, many of the strict protocols and regulations put into place by Boards of Pharmacy as safeguards may be ignored or improperly implemented. Without proper regulation, there is a higher chance of errors and mistakes. As a result, employers may run into legal issues, and, more importantly, patient safety and efficacy of care will be put at risk. A previous study on pharmacy technician training programs found that of 216 training programs, 29.6% were accredited and 46% had pharmacists as faculty of the program. It was concluded that there is little to no oversight of and consistency in pharmacy technician training [15].

While, this topic should be of great interest to employers, there is a lack of literature studying the hiring requirements and expectations of pharmacy technicians. A review of state regulations concerning entry-level pharmacy technicians in 2017 found that 86% of states required board registration or licensure. While only 16 states required any training programs for entry-level pharmacy technicians. This study reveals the legal requirements for the employment of pharmacy technicians, but did not study or discuss what employers actually look for in pharmacy technician candidates [16]. Therefore, the overall objective of this study was to look at the pharmacy technician advertisement database from the Pharmacy Week to find patterns and commonalities in the duties and qualifications of pharmacy technicians.

2. Materials and Methods

This study used a retrospective analysis study design to describe the current pharmacy technician job descriptions. Pharmacy technician job advertisements were obtained from Pharmacy Week for a 14 day period (26 November 2018–9 December 2018). PharmacyWeek.com was an online database of job advertisements for pharmacists, pharmacy technicians, and pharmacy interns started in 1990. Unfortunately, it is no longer maintained and can no longer be accessed. For all pharmacy technician job advertisements, the following items were obtained: (1) job title, (2) location of job (city and state), (3) what field of pharmacy job is in (hospital system, retail, [chain versus independent], long-term care, managed care, etc.), (4) position type (full or part time), (5) job duties, and (6) listed requirements for the position. Requirements within job advertisements were noted as being either required, preferred, not required, or not specified. Duties within job advertisements were noted as being either listed or not listed. Following data collection, related requirements and duties were combined into themes. These themes are detailed in Tables 1 and 2. The decision to code requirements and duties by themes verses individually was made by all researchers after listing were made of all the individual requirements and duties found in the position listing. The final themes agreed upon are depicted in the Tables 1 and 2.

Table 1. Job Requirements Themes.

	Job Requirements Themes
Ability to perform tasks	<ul><li>Data input</li><li>Intermediate calculations</li><li>Technical skills</li><li>Must be able to work in two specialty functions</li><li>Clerical skills</li></ul>
Technology	<ul><li>Windows product proficiency</li><li>Computer literacy</li><li>Epic experience</li><li>Use a 10-key pad</li></ul>
Communication	<ul><li>Language/communication (verbal, written, interpersonal)</li><li>English proficiency</li><li>Proficient in spoken Spanish</li><li>Bilingual</li></ul>
Knowledge	<ul><li>Knowledge of metric system</li><li>Special knowledge (drug names, Latin and chemical abbreviations, aseptic technique, storage of pharmaceuticals, determine drug's formulary status)</li><li>340B experience</li><li>Wholesale acquisition cost experience</li><li>Medical terminology</li></ul>

Table 1. *Cont.*

	Job Requirements Themes
Attributes	<ul><li>Reasoning/problem-solving skills</li><li>Team player/leadership</li><li>Customer service</li><li>Detail oriented</li><li>Time/work management (multitasking)</li><li>Friendly/courtesy</li><li>Flexibility</li><li>Punctuality</li><li>Professionalism</li><li>Attendance</li><li>Innovative</li><li>Enthusiasm</li><li>Salesman skills</li><li>Ability to listen and learn</li><li>Function in a normal work environment</li><li>Function with minimal supervision</li><li>Respect for confidentiality</li><li>Strong ethical standards</li></ul>
Legal requirements	<ul><li>No previous drug use or conviction</li><li>Subject to background and reference check</li><li>Basic life support certification</li><li>Have or get professional liability insurance</li><li>U.S. citizen</li><li>Driver's license</li><li>Selective service registration is required for males born after 12/31/1959</li><li>Up-to-date on vaccines</li></ul>
Physical	<ul><li>Physical demands (standing, lifting, bending)</li><li>Visual acuity</li><li>Auditory function</li></ul>
Age	<ul><li>18 years old or older</li><li>17 years old or older</li><li>16 years old or older</li></ul>
Previous experience	<ul><li>340B experience</li><li>Wholesale acquisition cost (WAC) experience</li></ul>
Transportation	<ul><li>Reliable transportation</li><li>Travel</li></ul>

Data were collected and entered into an Excel document. Data were de-identified prior to Excel entry. No information was recorded in a manner that could reveal the identity. Descriptive statistics were performed for all data in IBM© SPSS v 26.0 (Armonk, NY, USA). This included frequencies and percentages.

Table 2. Job Duties by Theme.

	Job Duties by Theme
Do things under the direct supervision of the pharmacist	• Do things under the direct supervision of the pharmacist • Obtain a final check from the pharmacist before releasing any prepared parenteral compounds, before packaging any medication, or dispensing any medication
Communication	• Triage requests and follow through with appropriate action(s) • Notifies pharmacist of relevant clinical information gathered during calls to provider or patient that may affect the patient's disease state or medication regimen • Contacting insurance companies • Provide information and assistance to pharmacies, members, and other callers regarding benefits, claims, and eligibility • Read, interpret, and write documents (store and third-party clerical) • Process faxes • Ask if patient wants "pharmacist counseling" • Refer any questions regarding prescriptions, drug information, or health matters to a pharmacist • Notify pharmacist to transfer prescriptions that can no longer be filled to appropriate pharmacy along with notifying the provider and the patient • Transcribe verbal prescriptions from doctors' offices at the discretion of the pharmacist on duty • Helping coordinate telehealth appointments
Perform pharmaceutical calculations	• Calculate figures (mathematics) • Calculate drug volumes to deliver correct dosages
Fill prescription orders	• Receiving written prescription or refill requests and verify that information is complete and accurate • Receives refill requests from patients and obtains authorization for refills from physicians' offices • Decipher and accurately enter orders for new prescriptions • Billing/coding • Identify and complete prior authorizations • Prepare and distribute non-sterile medications • Medication delivery (to home, pyxis...) • Prescription counting, processing, filling, and labeling • Maintain pharmacy records • Pulling hard copy scripts to return to patient with an appropriate letter if pharmacy is unable to fill the order • Ensure that patients receive the correct medication in a safe and timely manner
Fill IV medication orders	• Prepare and distribute sterile medications • Handles all home infusion functions as needed, including pump programming
Fill chemotherapy medication orders	• Preparation of chemotherapy • Demonstrates advanced knowledge of hazards of cytotoxic chemotherapeutic agents, including but not limited to the dangers posed to those who prepare, deliver, administer and/or receive treatment with these agents
Provider oversight of other employees	• Oversight of other technicians • Administrative task and staff support • Coordinate technician activities (unit dose (UD) distribution, intravenous admixture, compounding, purchasing, controlled substances, OR drug preparation, pharmacy automation, investigational drug services, and inventory control) • Assists in the supervision, scheduling, payroll maintenance, administration of disciplinary action, and evaluation of technical personnel • Participates in recruitment activities and decisions to hire or terminate • Provide and coordinate training
General office etiquette	• Maintain clean work area • Provide customer service • Follow organization policies and procedures

Table 2. Cont.

	Job Duties by Theme
Professionalism	<ul><li>Maintain personal appearance</li><li>Work in a team (w/ other medical professionals)</li><li>Participate in and successfully completes mandatory education</li><li>Possess strong ethical standards</li><li>Travel/attend meetings and conferences</li></ul>
Quality assurance/improvement	<ul><li>Develop and implement new systems and procedures</li><li>Practice preventive maintenance by properly inspecting equipment and notify appropriate department or store manager of any items in need of repair</li><li>Perform daily quality assurance monitoring/performance improvement activities</li><li>Follow HIPPA standards for confidentiality</li><li>Work with the pharmacist to ensure that the pharmacy functions and keeps within federal and state requirements</li><li>Report medication diversions</li><li>Report regulatory deficiencies (medication and billing errors)</li><li>Notify the pharmacist when agents from any regulatory agency or law officers contact/visit the pharmacy.</li><li>Assist with audits/work with auditing software</li><li>Understand and adhere to guidelines on accepting and tendering vendor coupons, company limits on cash shortages and shrink guidelines.</li><li>Participate in safety initiatives</li><li>Follow United States Pharmacopeia (USP) standards (cleaning, PPE...)</li><li>Inspect storage and maintain the safety of medications</li><li>Assist in medication formulary management and compliance</li></ul>
Use of technology	<ul><li>Operate automated pharmacy technology systems</li><li>Cash register operations</li><li>Use computer system to credit unused doses back to patient accounts</li><li>Use tools like a fork lift, hand tools, etc.</li><li>Proficient in the use and application of new medications and technology</li><li>Test client system</li></ul>
Inventory maintenance	<ul><li>Maintain/order inventory and supplies</li><li>Manage the schedule for patient deliveries, manage inventory, create and maintain supply templates in the pharmacy computer database</li></ul>
Clinical tasks	<ul><li>Discusses with patients life issues affecting medication adherence and provide advice on improving drug regimen compliance</li><li>Assist the pharmacist in medication reconciliation</li><li>Reviews medication regimen for disease state and provide summaries and guidance on future medication plans. Advice may include alternate drug therapies, stopping a medication and/or lower cost alternative</li><li>Help patients in over-the-counter (OTC) medication aisle</li><li>Gather patient medication history</li><li>Provide patient-oriented clinical pharmacy services to patients</li><li>Provide care appropriate to the population served</li><li>First line screening for medication order errors, drug or allergy contraindications, and processing non-formulary drug requests</li><li>Checking for possible interactions</li><li>Assist patients in solving issues and problems related to acquired immunodeficiency syndrome (AIDS)</li></ul>
Maintain workflow in a high-volume pharmacy	
HIV knowledgeable	
Maintain narcotic coordination and investigational drug therapy	
Perform duties of a technician	
Business configuration duties	
Provides PAP assistance	

Table 2. *Cont.*

	Job Duties by Theme
Promotion of services	• Set up and maintain pharmacy display cases • Be aware of competitor services and effectiveness • Promote company services to obtain new customers
Prepare, distribute, and maintain records for investigational drug products ensuring that you understand study protocols needed to accurately fulfill orders	
Research how the pharmacy can acquire contracts for certain state Medicaid's/Adaps/Networks, depending on the needs at the moment	
Pick-up orders, requisitions, and medications when on delivery rounds	
Subject matter expert of delivery services and leader of delivery initiatives	
Opening, counting, barcoding, and profiling incoming mail	
Manages difficult or emotional patient situations	
Other duties as assigned to include	• This job description is not intended, nor should it be construed to be an exhaustive list of all responsibilities, skills, efforts or working conditions associated with the job. It is intended to indicate the general nature and level of work performed by employees within this classification. • Other duties as assigned

3. Results

Fourteen days of data resulted in 21,007 individual position listings, with 96.78% of those being in a retail setting. These technician position listings included positions from all 50 states, Puerto Rico, and the District of Columbia. A little over one-third (37.5%) of the positions were from California, Florida, Illinois, New York, or Texas (N = 1983, 9%; N = 1889, 9%; N = 1242, 6%; N = 1188, 5.7%; and N = 1568, 7.5%, respectively). A majority of the job listings were for full-time positions (96.4%). Settings for these positions included hospital systems, retail pharmacies, and managed care companies (Figure 1).

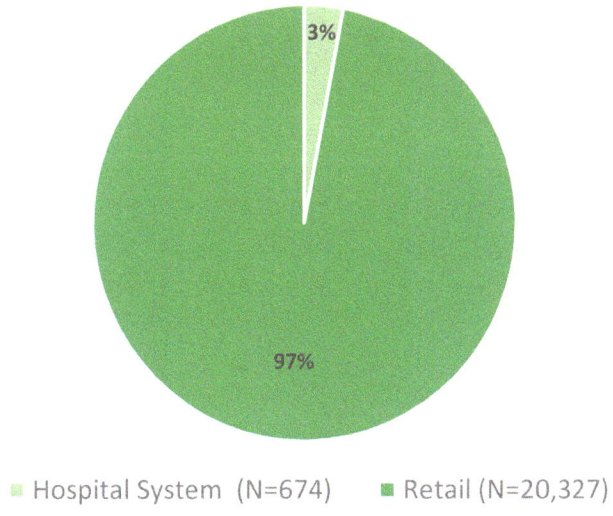

Figure 1. Pharmacy technician job listings by setting.

Pharmacy technician job listing in the managed care setting are not reflected in Figure 1 due to sample size of 6.

The requirements included in the listings are displayed in Table 3. The most common requirements were registration with State Board, high school diploma, ability to perform tasks, communication, and physical (N = 18,261 86.9%, N = 17,325 82.5%, N = 16,861 80.3%, N = 16,436 78.2%, and N = 15,908 75.7%, respectively).

Table 3. Pharmacy Technician Job Requirements.

Requirement	Required Number (%)	Preferred Number (%)	Not Required Number (%)	Not Specified Number (%)
Registration with State Board	18,261 (86.9%)	16 (0.1%)	102 (0.5%)	2628 (12.5%)
High school diploma	17,325 (82.5%)	69 (0.3%)	116 (0.6%)	3497 (16.6%)
Ability to perform tasks	16,861 (80.3%)	-	-	4146 (19.7%)
Communication	16,436 (78.2%)	-	-	4571 (21.8%)
Physical	15,908 (75.7%)	-	-	5099 (24.3%)
Technology	10,132 (48.2%)	-	-	10,875 (51.8%)
Attributes	6478 (30.8%)	-	-	14,529 (69.2%)
PTCB or exCPT certification	2583 (12.3%)	17,114 (81.5%)	4 (0%)	1306 (6.2%)

PTCP = Pharmacy Technician Certification Board; exCPT = Exam for the Certification of Pharmacy Technicians.

Additional information collected but not reported in Table 3 include that 9.1% (N = 1904) required some form of technician program coursework and almost 1% of listings required or preferred at least an associate's degree level of education (required N = 131, 0.6%; preferred N = 56, 0.3%).

The job duties included in the listings are displayed in Table 4. The most common job duties were general office etiquette, performing tasks under the direct supervision of the pharmacist, and professionalism (19,961 95%, 18,043 85.9%, and 10,560 50.3%, respectively).

Table 4. Pharmacy Technician Job Duties.

Duty	Listed Number (%)	Not Listed Number (%)
General office etiquette	19,961 (95%)	1046 (5%)
Do things under the direct supervision of the pharmacist	18,043 (85.9%)	2964 (14.1%)
Professionalism	10,560 (50.3%)	10,447 (49.7%)
Fill prescription orders	10,079 (48%)	10,928 (52%)
Quality assurance and improvement	8870 (42.2%)	12,137 (57.8%)

Additional information collected related to duties worth noting include 10 listings that required pharmacy technicians to have experience in patient assistance programs (0.0%, N = 10), HIV knowledge (0.0%, N = 3), maintaining narcotic coordination and investigational drug therapy (0.8%, N = 167), calculations (0.4%, N = 76), and managing difficult or emotional patient situations (0.0%, N = 2).

In Figures 2 and 3, the pharmacy technician position ad requirements and duties are indicated by job setting.

Of note in the pharmacy requirements as separated by setting, 11.7% (N = 79) of included hospital advertisements included a legal piece of some sort, whereas less than 1 % (0.3%, N = 55) of retail and 0 in managed care did.

Some individual technician ads listed unique and unheard of duties and requirements for applicants. One example of this would be a job duty listed as "be HIV knowledgeable" without further context; the same ad listed that technicians were expected to assist patients in "solving issues and problems related to AIDS." Another example was a pharmacy technician position that expected the applicant to be able to operate a forklift and hand tools. One technician position examined included requirements that technicians be willing to travel for meetings, conferences, and "field support" in order to "support and grow key customer relationships."

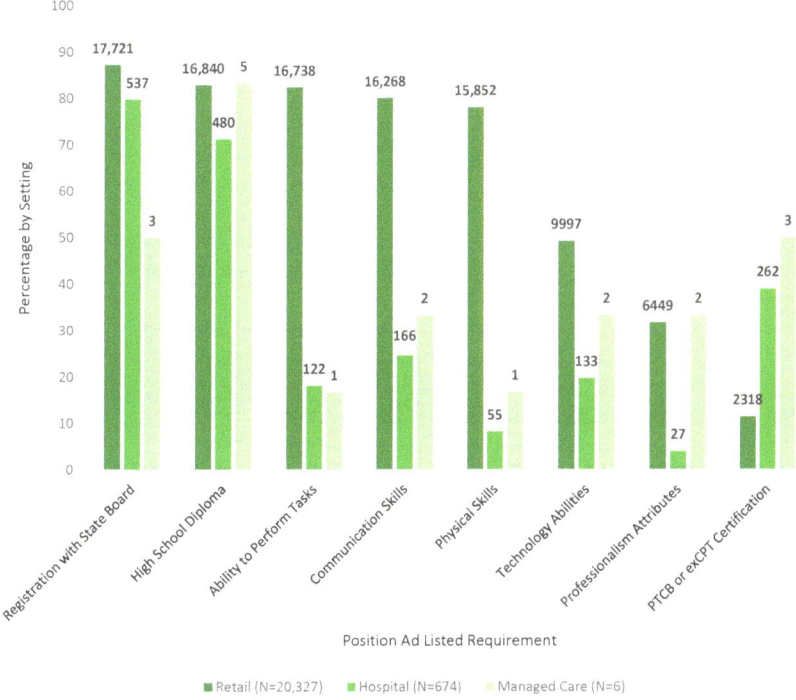

Figure 2. Pharmacy technician position ad requirements by setting.

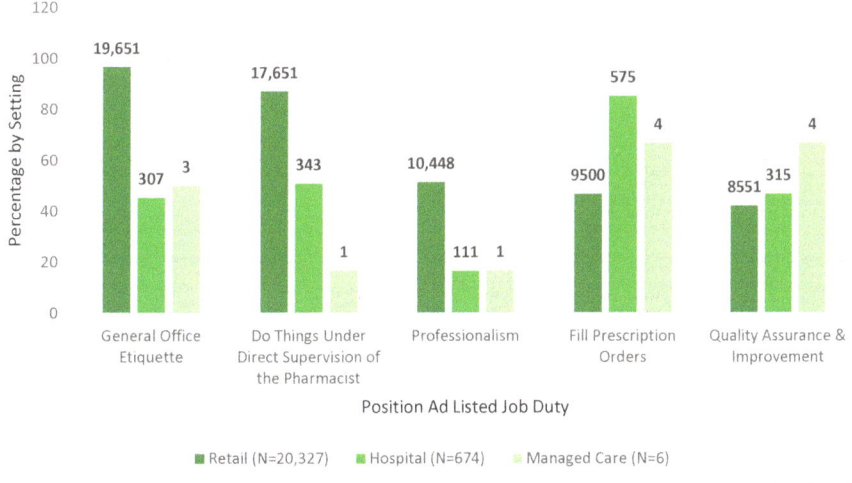

Figure 3. Pharmacy technician position ad job duties by setting.

4. Discussion

A review of job postings for pharmacy technicians provided a rich description of the different roles and skills currently needed across pharmacy settings. Technicians remain in many traditional settings, such as retail/community pharmacy. This is consistent with other descriptions that place technicians in supportive roles at community pharmacies and health-system pharmacies [1]. In these settings, technicians often assist with technical pharmacy functions and interact with patients. However, this can expand to other roles, such as providing support for medication therapy management (MTM) services and other clinical services [1]. Interestingly, there are emerging areas that are hiring technicians, such as managed care. As pharmacists in managed care continue to expand their opportunities to provide clinical services and chronic care management, technicians may have increasing roles to support data collection and documentation [15].

The data show that 12.3% (N = 2583) of pharmacy technicians are required to have standard certifications in pharmacy technician work such as PTCB and exCPT. Many states have a requirement that pharmacy technicians get certified either through these routes or through a standardized exam with similar content within a year of hiring, but there is little standardization across the board for these exams [17,18]. On multiple occasions, calls for standard national training and certification processes have been made, and it is clear that multiple organizations find it crucial to have this kind of a standard for certified pharmacy technicians [19,20]. While 81.5% (N = 17,114) did prefer a certified technician, it is surprising that more employers do not share the same national desire.

To fill these roles in a variety of settings, pharmacy technicians appear to need a variety of skills—many of which lie in the affective domain, i.e., professionalism and communication. Given the customer/patient service role many technicians provide, it is essential that they exhibit professionalism and can communicate appropriately in both written and verbal formats [2]. Further, analysis of the ads underscored the importance of technicians in quality assurance. Given their role in the dispensing process, inventory management, and other aspects of the pharmacy, technicians play a vital role in fostering an environment that promotes safe and effective medication use. For example, Odukoya, Schleiden, and Chui (2015), found that pharmacy technicians play a vital role in preventing e-prescribing errors by catching errors before the prescription is sent to the pharmacist to verify [16].

Expanding the roles of certified pharmacy technicians continues to be a discussion in the literature and the profession of pharmacy. States continue to explore tech-check-tech programs to free up pharmacist time to focus on clinical activities [9]. Some recent research also has explored the use of pharmacy technicians to extend medication management to the home setting, performing medication reconciliation and reiterating key counseling points from the pharmacist using motivational interviewing and the teach-back method [14]. Others have explored creating a clinical pharmacy technician to expand patient medication education [17]. While the job postings do not necessarily reflect these expansions, it would be important to continue to monitor ads to determine if the roles of pharmacists and particularly, certified pharmacy technicians, are altering and expanding to allow pharmacists to focus on clinical activities.

As noted in the results, a small portion of the data included advertisements that required the technicians to be knowledgeable in HIV-related patient care. While this was not a substantial portion of the data, it is interesting to note that it is an area of potential growth for pharmacy technicians in the US. An article from 2013 found that a pharmacy technician-centered medication reconciliation for ART therapy of patients in the hospital was successful in assisting with the prevention of drug-drug interactions, as well as other medication errors. The program showed that ART and OI prophylaxis in HIV/AIDS patients was improved by the utilization of pharmacy technicians [21]. Similar data were collected related to a pharmacy technician-centered medication reconciliation unit at a mental health location in 2014 [22]. These articles and pieces of literature show that there is potential for pharmacy technician-led integration of prevention of med errors even in disease-specific areas of healthcare.

In order to continue integrating pharmacy technicians into the practice of pharmacy, it is important for those pharmacy technicians to be highly skilled to enhance the clinical reach of the pharmacist.

Projected pharmacy technician skills that could potentially be sought out by progressive employers include skills such as managing certain aspects of clinical tasks such as medication management and medication reconciliation, reiterating counseling points to reinforce statements made by the pharmacist, exceptional skills in communication and professionalism, as well as being able to quickly and accurately review information regarding patients' prescriptions during data collection and order entry. One systematic review found that pharmacy technicians are often utilized to support MTM through medication reconciliation and that adherence and medication utility can be improved. However, standardization for administration utilization and educational training in this setting is necessary [23].

Another study found that the implementation of pharmacy technicians into a nursing team in an acute admissions unit in a hospital setting allowed for the prevention of omitted doses and helped all members of the team make better use of their time [24]. Another similar study showed that pharmacy technicians working in hospital wards in order to improve medication management and to prevent the utilization of expired or misplaced medications caused significant cost savings, as well as per-patient time savings for the nurses also working in the wards [25]. These and other studies like it allow us to see the benefit of utilizing pharmacy technicians in expanded definitions of the traditional pharmacy tech role. These articles and trials of expanding the role of pharmacy technicians have given insight into ways to continue utilizing pharmacy technicians well. Due to the vast amount of pharmacy technician positions in the US, and the variety in settings that pharmacy technicians can explore, it is expected that these potentially beneficial positions will continue to develop in the United States as pharmacy practice continues to move forward.

In addition to defining potential expansion of the role for technicians, the literature also emphasizes the importance of education and training in order to standardize patient care and to ensure best practice is being followed. Pharmacy technicians must be competent, able to communicate, and behave in a professional manner. Given their integral role in the profession of pharmacy, providing opportunities for pharmacy technicians to develop professionally is vital. Multiple professional organizations have provided outlines of competencies and training/education to assist pharmacy settings in providing these opportunities [1,13]. Opportunities also remain for technicians to become certified, and some jobs preferred or required this additional training [1,13]. However, the benefits of completing additional training for technicians may not yet be balanced with the costs of obtaining it [18].

Limitations

This study, though novel, was limited in several ways. First, the available data were only taken from one source, Pharmacy Week. While Pharmacy Week does have a variety of job listings that encompass the entire United States, there are other sources of advertisements that are used to hire pharmacy technicians. The short data collection window only provides a brief snapshot of what jobs were being advertised during that time frame. While the sample size is robust for 14 days, it only reflects the needs at that specific time. Further, data collection was performed by four different researchers. While they all received training on the research protocol and data collection tools, no assessment for interrater reliability was performed.

5. Conclusions

This study represents a unique view of the state of pharmacy technician practice in the United States. Data showed demand for a broad variety of duties ranging from traditional to clinical to managerial. This represents an increased demand for skills and training requirements for pharmacy technicians. Further, due to the lack of standardization in certification and training for pharmacy technicians, it is important to research the future potential of policy, practice, and educational innovation in order to ensure safety and proper utilization of the pharmacy technician workforce.

Author Contributions: Conceptualization, D.C.A. and J.A.D.; methodology, J.A.D.; formal analysis, E.C.W.; data curation, E.C.W., Z.J.K., and J.L.S.; writing—original draft preparation, J.A.D., E.C.W., Z.J.K.; writing—review and editing, J.A.D., E.C.W., Z.J.K., and D.C.A.; visualization, E.C.W. and Z.J.K.; supervision, J.A.D. and D.C.A.; project administration, D.C.A. All authors have read and agreed to the published version of the manuscript.

Funding: This research received no external funding.

Acknowledgments: Thank you to Philip White for his coding assistance. Thank you to Kevin Mero and Pharmacy Week for allowing us to have access to their job database. Thank you to Seth Campbell and Zach Bevins for their assistance with data entry.

Conflicts of Interest: The authors declare no conflict of interest.

References

1. Albanese, N.P.; Rouse, M.J.; Schlaifer, M.; Pharmacy, C.O.C.I. Scope of contemporary pharmacy practice: Roles, responsibilities, and functions of pharmacists and pharmacy technicians. *J. Am. Pharm. Assoc.* **2010**, *50*, e35–e69. [CrossRef] [PubMed]
2. Bluml, B.M. Definition of medication therapy management: Development of professionwide consensus. *J. Am. Pharm. Assoc.* **2005**, *45*, 566–572. [CrossRef] [PubMed]
3. Brummel, A.; Lustig, A.; Westrich, K.; Evans, M.A.; Plank, G.S.; Penso, J.; Dubois, R.W. Best practices: Improving patient outcomes and costs in an ACO through comprehensive medication therapy management. *J. Manag. Care Speéc. Pharm.* **2014**, *20*, 1152–1158. [CrossRef] [PubMed]
4. Isetts, B.J.; Schondelmeyer, S.W.; Artz, M.B.; Lenarz, L.A.; Heaton, A.H.; Wadd, W.B.; Brown, L.M.; Cipolle, R.J. Clinical and economic outcomes of medication therapy management services: The Minnesota experience. *J. Am. Pharm. Assoc.* **2008**, *48*, 203–214. [CrossRef] [PubMed]
5. Moore, J.M.; Shartle, D.; Faudskar, L.; Matlin, O.S.; Brennan, T.A. Impact of a patient-centered pharmacy program and intervention in a high-risk group. *J. Manag. Care Pharm.* **2013**, *19*, 228–236. [CrossRef] [PubMed]
6. Touchette, D.R.; Masica, A.L.; Dolor, R.; Schumock, G.T.; Choi, Y.K.; Kim, Y.; Smith, S.R. Safety-focused medication therapy management: A randomized controlled trial. *J. Am. Pharm. Assoc.* **2012**, *52*, 603–612. [CrossRef] [PubMed]
7. Viswanathan, M.; Kahwati, L.C.; Golin, C.E.; Blalock, S.J.; Coker-Schwimmer, E.; Posey, R.; Lohr, K.N. Medication therapy management interventions in outpatient settings: A systematic review and meta-analysis. *JAMA Intern. Med.* **2015**, *175*, 76. [CrossRef]
8. Wittayanukorn, S.; Westrick, S.C.; Hansen, R.; Billor, N.; Braxton-Lloyd, K.; Fox, B.I.; Garza, K.B. Evaluation of medication therapy management services for patients with cardiovascular disease in a self-insured employer health plan. *J. Manag. Care Pharm.* **2013**, *19*, 385–395. [CrossRef]
9. Frost, T.P.; Adams, A.J. Pharmacist and technician perceptions of tech-check-tech in community pharmacy practice settings. *J. Pharm. Pract.* **2017**, *31*, 190–194. [CrossRef]
10. Adams, A.J.; Martin, S.J.; Stolpe, S.F. "Tech-check-tech": A review of the evidence on its safety and benefits. *Am. J. Health-Syst. Pharm.* **2011**, *68*, 1824–1833. [CrossRef]
11. McKeirnan, K.C.; Frazier, K.R.; Nguyen, M.; MacLean, L.G. Training pharmacy technicians to administer immunizations. *J. Am. Pharm. Assoc.* **2018**, *58*, 174–178. [CrossRef] [PubMed]
12. Henriksen, J.P.; Noerregaard, S.; Buck, T.C.; Aagaard, L. Medication histories by pharmacy technicians and physicians in an emergency department. *Int. J. Clin. Pharm.* **2015**, *37*, 1121–1127. [CrossRef] [PubMed]
13. Schultz, J.M.; Jeter, C.K.; Keresztes, J.M.; Martin, N.M.; Mundy, T.K.; Reichard, J.S.; Van Cura, J.D. ASHP statement on the roles of pharmacy technicians. *Am. J. Health-Syst. Pharm.* **2016**, *73*, 928–930. [CrossRef] [PubMed]
14. Bailey, J.E.; Surbhi, S.; Bell, P.C.; Jones, A.M.; Rashed, S.; Ugwueke, M.O. SafeMed: Using pharmacy technicians in a novel role as community health workers to improve transitions of care. *J. Am. Pharm. Assoc.* **2016**, *56*, 73–81. [CrossRef]
15. Anderson, D.C.; Draime, J.; Anderson, T.S. Description and comparison of pharmacy technician training programs in the United States. *J. Am. Pharm. Assoc.* **2016**, *56*, 231–236. [CrossRef]
16. Mattingly, A.N. Entry-level practice requirements of pharmacy technicians across the United States: A review. *Am. J. Health-Syst. Pharm.* **2018**, *75*, 1057–1063. [CrossRef]

17. Mattingly, A.N.; Boyle, C.J. Salary and entry-level requirements for pharmacy technicians compared with other health technologist and technician occupations in Maryland. *J. Am. Pharm. Assoc.* **2019**, *60*, 17–21. [CrossRef]
18. Urick, B.Y.; Mattingly, T.J.; Mattingly, A.N. Relationship between regulatory barriers to entry and pharmacy technician wages. *Res. Soc. Adm. Pharm.* **2020**, *16*, 190–194. [CrossRef]
19. Smith, M.A.M.; Boyle, C.J.; Keresztes, J.M.; Liles, J.; MacLean, L.G.; McAllister, E.B.; Silvester, J.; Williams, N.T.; Bradley-Baker, L.R. Report of the 2013–2014 Professional Affairs Standing Committee: Advancing the pharmacy profession together through pharmacy technician and pharmacy education partnerships. *Am. J. Pharm. Educ.* **2014**, *78*, S22. [CrossRef]
20. Manasse, H.R.; Menighan, T.E. Pharmacy technician education, training, and certification: Call for a single national standard and public accountability. *J. Am. Pharm. Assoc.* **2011**, *51*, 326–327. [CrossRef]
21. Siemianowski, L.A.; Sen, S.; George, J.M. Impact of pharmacy technician-centered medication reconciliation on optimization of antiretroviral therapy and opportunistic infection prophylaxis in hospitalized patients with HIV/AIDS. *J. Pharm. Pract.* **2013**, *26*, 428–433. [CrossRef] [PubMed]
22. Brownlie, K.; Schneider, C.R.; Culliford, R.; Fox, C.; Boukouvalas, A.; Willan, C.; Maidment, I. Medication reconciliation by a pharmacy technician in a mental health assessment unit. *Int. J. Clin. Pharm.* **2013**, *36*, 303–309. [CrossRef] [PubMed]
23. Gernant, S.A.; Nguyen, M.-O.; Siddiqui, S.; Schneller, M. Use of pharmacy technicians in elements of medication therapy management delivery: A systematic review. *Res. Soc. Adm. Pharm.* **2017**, *14*, 883–890. [CrossRef]
24. El-Fahimi, N.; Dube, M.; Savage, K.; Elsender, P.; Costello, C.; Rojas, W.; Calleja, M.A. The impact of implementing a pharmacy technician role as part of a nursing team in an acute admissions unit. *Eur. J. Hosp. Pharm.* **2019**, *27*, 114–116. [CrossRef] [PubMed]
25. Lynch, E.; O'Flynn, J.; O'Riordan, C.; Bogue, C.; Lynch, D.; McCarthy, S.; Murphy, K.D. The impact of a ward-based pharmacy technician service in an Irish hospital. *Pharmacoepidemiol. Drug Saf.* **2019**, *28*, 3–16. [CrossRef]

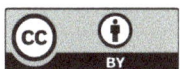

© 2020 by the authors. Licensee MDPI, Basel, Switzerland. This article is an open access article distributed under the terms and conditions of the Creative Commons Attribution (CC BY) license (http://creativecommons.org/licenses/by/4.0/).

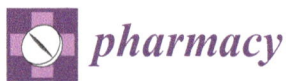

Article

Wage Premiums as a Means to Evaluate the Labor Market for Pharmacy Technicians in the United States: 1997–2018

David P. Zgarrick [1],*, Tatiana Bujnoch [2] and Shane P. Desselle [3]

1. Department of Pharmacy and Health Systems Sciences, School of Pharmacy, Bouvé College of Health Sciences, Northeastern University, Boston, MA 02115, USA
2. Division of Pharmacy, Memorial Hermann Health System, Houston, TX 77024, USA; Tatiana.bujnoch@memorialhermann.org
3. Department of Social, Behavioral & Administrative Sciences, College of Pharmacy, Touro University California, Vallejo, CA 94592, USA; shane.desselle@tu.edu
* Correspondence: d.zgarrick@northeastern.edu; Tel.: +1-617-373-4664

Received: 2 March 2020; Accepted: 15 March 2020; Published: 17 March 2020

Abstract: Pharmacy technicians are integral members of the health care team, assisting pharmacists and other health professionals in assuring safe and effective medication use. To date, evaluation of the labor market for pharmacy technicians has been limited, and relatively little has been evaluated regarding trends in wages. The objective of this research is to use US Bureau of Labor Statistics (US BLS) data to evaluate changes in pharmacy technician wages in the United States from 1997 to 2018 relative to changes in the US consumer price index (CPI). Median hourly wages for pharmacy technicians were collected from US BLS data from 1997 to 2018. Median hourly wages were compared to expected hourly wages, with the difference, a wage premium, indicative of imbalances in the supply and demand of labor. Both positive and negative wage premiums were observed, with most positive wage premiums occurring prior to 2007 and most negative wage premiums observed after 2008. Differences in wage premiums were also observed between technicians working in various practice settings. Given the median length of employment of pharmacy technicians, it is likely that the majority of technicians working in US pharmacies have not experienced increases in their wages relative to what would be expected by changes in the CPI. This has occurred at a time when pharmacies and pharmacists are asking more of their pharmacy technicians. Researchers and pharmacy managers must continue to evaluate the pharmacy technician labor market to assure that technician wage and compensation levels attract an adequate supply of sufficiently skilled workers.

Keywords: pharmacy technicians; labor market; wages

1. Introduction

The labor markets for health care workers are important to monitor and evaluate, as these workers are still the driving force behind the delivery of goods and services that improve the health of individuals and entire populations. This is particularly important in the profession of pharmacy, where the increased reliance on medications as a form of treatment requires trained personnel to ensure that medications deliver desired outcomes and avoid undesired outcomes.

Some degree of attention has been paid over the years to the labor markets for health care professionals, such as those for physicians, pharmacists, nurses and others who are educated and trained to play specific roles in serving our health needs [1–3]. As health care has become more specialized and complex, health professionals have increasingly relied on para-professional workers to support their clinical roles and provide administrative assistance. In pharmacy, the role of the pharmacist has been increasingly supported by the pharmacy technician. Pharmacy technicians support pharmacists in dispensing medications, performing clinical functions needed to improve the outcomes of mediation use [4–6], and to perform a number of administrative functions which assist in the operations of a pharmacy [7]. Pharmacy technicians have been asked to increasingly take on roles that had previously been exclusively performed by pharmacists, including reviewing medications and checking the work of other technicians prior to dispensing [8,9], taking medication histories [10], managing warfarin therapy within a clinical pharmacy anticoagulation service [11] and immunization delivery [12]. Pharmacists depend upon a stable labor market of pharmacy technicians to support them in optimizing patient health outcomes. The ability to delegate and empower others is demonstrative of a pharmacist practicing at the top of their license [13].

The number of pharmacy technicians working in the United States has grown from 165,400 in 1997 to 420,400 in 2018 [14]. The number of pharmacy technicians in the US now surpasses the number of pharmacists (314,300). The United States Bureau of Labor Statistics (US BLS) projects that the job market for pharmacy technicians will grow by 7% between 2018–2028, adding 31,500 positions [15]. At the same time that the US BLS is not projecting any net growth in the number of pharmacist positions needed in the US [16].

The supply and demand of health care professionals has been the subject of considerable research. The labor market for pharmacists in the United States has been evaluated by means of the aggregate demand index (ADI) [17], and later by the pharmacist demand indicator (PDI) [18]. Pharmacist demographics, working conditions and other trends in pharmacist practice in the US are examined in the National Pharmacist Workforce Survey, which has been conducted every five years since 2000 [19]. Our understanding of the supply and demand of pharmacy technicians in the US and their working conditions are more limited. Desselle and Holmes conducted a National Certified Pharmacy Technician Workforce Survey in 2015 which described various aspects of their working conditions, including a finding that over one in four certified pharmacy technicians (26.6%) were "highly dissatisfied" with their wages [20]. Urick and colleagues noted that while many US states adopted additional barriers to entry to working as a pharmacy technician between 1997 and 2017, such as registration with a state entity and national certification requirements, these barriers were not associated with any changes in pharmacy technician wages [21]. Mattingly and Mattingly also found that that were no significant differences in pharmacy technician wages in 2016 based on the degree of regulation of pharmacy technician practice in that state or the cost of living in a state as measured by the salary housing index [22]. Mattingly and Mattingly also concluded in their systematic review of literature regarding the roles of pharmacy technicians that while evidence supports technicians performing roles which advance pharmacy practice and improve patient outcomes, the benefits to technicians in performing these roles have been limited to increases in their job satisfaction and work schedules, and not in their levels of wages or other forms of financial compensation [23]. They further concluded that if pharmacy technicians are to take on more roles in the future, they may need to be offered more tangible forms of benefits, particularly if these roles require completion of formalized education and training programs.

Limitations of much of the previous research on pharmacy technician labor is that it is cross sectional and only describes labor market conditions at a particular point in time. Little research has been done to evaluate how pharmacy technician wages have changed over time, and how that in turn this has been reflected by changes in the number of technicians leaving or entering the labor market. Even more scarce is research evaluating trends in various sectors of the labor market for pharmacy technicians, sectors which can be defined by the setting in which the work takes place (e.g., chain and independent pharmacies, grocery store pharmacies, mass merchandise store pharmacies, hospitals, government agencies).

Since 1997, the US BLS has collected data annually on over 800 occupational groups, including pharmacists and pharmacy technicians. Among the data collected by the BLS for each occupational group are the mean and median annual salary and hourly wage levels, as well as the number employed in that group. US BLS occupational group data can be further analyzed by workplace setting. The objective of this research is to use US BLS data to evaluate changes in pharmacy technician wages in the United States from 1997 to 2018 relative to changes in the US consumer price index (CPI) over that time. The underlying hypothesis for this comparison is that if the supply and demand for labor are in balance, changes in wages for that occupation will match changes in the CPI. If differences between an occupation's wages from what would be predicted by changes in CPI are noted, that would be a signal that the supply and demand are not in balance. For example, increases in real wages over those predicted by CPI could be explained by both shortages of labor, and/or increased demand for that service. Decreases in real wages relative to CPI may be indicative of just the opposite; a combination of oversupplies of labor in that market and/or decreased demand for that particular type of labor.

2. Methods

Each May since 1998 the US BLS has released occupational employment statistics (OES) for over 800 occupational groups, reflecting information collected in May of the preceding year [24]. From this OES data the median hourly wage for pharmacy technicians (US BLS OES code 29-2052) was collected for each year from May 1997 through May 2018 [25]. In addition to collecting median hourly wages for all pharmacy technicians, median hourly wages were also collected each year for pharmacy technicians employed in industry sectors, including chain and independent pharmacies, grocery store pharmacies, mass merchandise pharmacy, hospitals, and government agencies. The percentage change in the US consumer price index (CPI) from May to May of each year from 1997 through 2018 was also gathered from US BLS [26].

Beginning with 1997, the actual median pharmacy technician hourly wage was multiplied by the percentage change in CPI over the next year to determine the expected median pharmacy technician hourly wage for the following year. This expected median hourly wage was then multiplied by the CPI for each subsequent year to determine the median hourly wage that would have been expected for each year from the base year through May 2018. The actual median pharmacy technician hourly wage for each following year was then compared to the expected median pharmacy technician hourly wage for that year as calculated above. This is demonstrated in Figure 1, in which, beginning with the actual median pharmacy technician hourly wage in 1997, expected median hourly wages for future years were calculated, and then comparisons were made to the actual median hourly wage pharmacy technicians had each year. The primary research hypothesis is that when these comparisons are made the difference will be $0, reflecting a balance in compensation paid to these employees and their ability and willingness to accept these wages in the market. Any differences found between the actual median hourly wage and the expected median hourly wage for any particular year is defined as a wage premium (wage premium = actual median hourly wage − expected median hourly wage). Wage premiums which occurred prior to 2018 were adjusted to reflect 2018 net present values. The adjusted wage premiums were then summed from the base year through 2018, and then divided by the number of years being analyzed to determine the mean wage premium experienced by pharmacy technicians for each year over the term being considered. In the example described in Figure 1, pharmacy technicians in the United States experienced a mean adjusted wage premium of $1.99/hour between 1997 and 2018, meaning that the median hourly wage for pharmacy technicians who worked between these years was, on average, $1.99/hour higher than would had been expected had their wages increased by the CPI each year.

Figure 2 describes changes in the median hourly wages from 2009 to 2018. Pharmacy technician median hourly wages in the United States decreased by an average of $0.35/hour relative to what would have been expected had their median hourly wage increased by the CPI over that time.

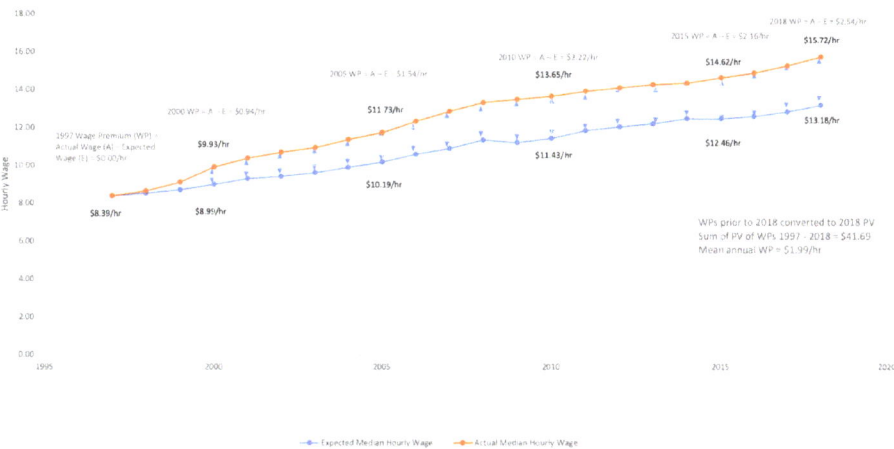

Figure 1. Calculation of the Mean Annual Hourly Wage Premium for Pharmacy Technicians from Base-year 1997 to 2018.

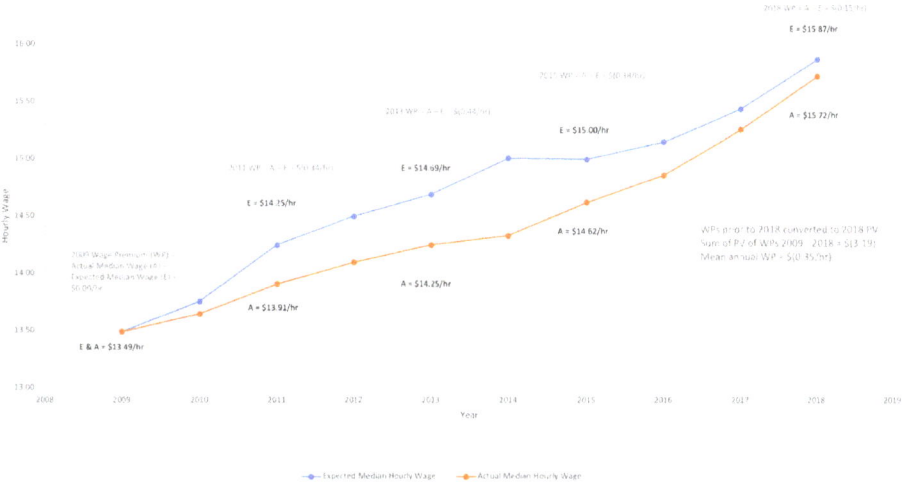

Figure 2. Calculation of the Mean Annual Hourly Wage Premium for Pharmacy Technicians from Base-year 2009 to 2018.

This analysis was repeated for all base years from 1997 to 2017, resulting in ranges from one year (2017 to 2018) to twenty-one years (1997 to 2018). This analysis was also performed on subsets of data for pharmacy technicians working in chain and independent pharmacies, grocery store pharmacies, mass merchandise store pharmacies, hospitals, and for government agencies. An analysis was also performed to evaluate the presence of wage premiums across all workers in all occupational groups in the United States.

3. Results

Figure 3 represents trends in the median hourly wages received by pharmacy technicians between 1997 and 2018. Median hourly wages across all pharmacy technicians have increased from $8.39/hour in 1997 (which, adjusting based on changes in the US CPI is the equivalent to $13.18/hour in 2018) to $15.72/hour in 2018. Variation in median hourly wages is noted between the settings where pharmacy technicians work. Median hourly wages for pharmacy technicians in 2018 ranged from $14.65/hour in chain and independent pharmacies and $14.73/hour in food store pharmacies to $17.97/hour in hospitals and $21.10/hour in government settings. It should also be noted that the median hourly wage in the United States in May 2018 for all workers across all occupations was $18.58/hour [24].

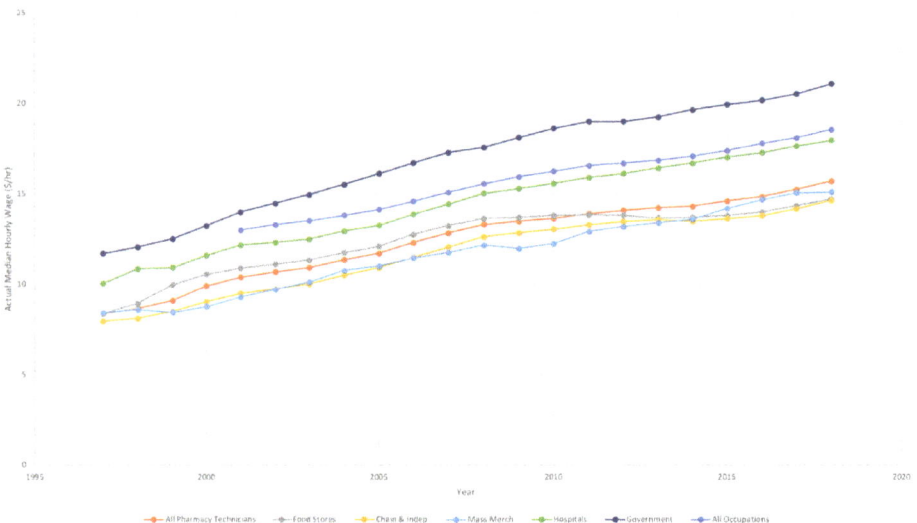

Figure 3. Median Hourly Wages for Pharmacy Technicians, by work setting, from 1997 to 2018.

Figure 4 represents the trends in wage premiums in pharmacy technician hourly wages which occurred between 1997 and 2018. Pharmacy technician median hourly wages consistently experienced positive wage premiums from base years prior to 2007, meaning that the median hourly earnings of technicians from the base year to 2018 were higher than would had been expected had their hourly wages increased by the CPI. Since 2007, pharmacy technicians in the United States have been much less likely to experience positive wage premiums. In the 2009 and 2010 base years, median hourly wages for pharmacy technicians were $0.35/hour and $0.25/hour less than what would had been expected than if their wages had kept up with the CPI over that time. The wage premiums experienced by pharmacy technicians since 2006 have been very similar to those experienced by all workers in all occupations in the US over that time.

The presence and absence of wage premiums also varied between sectors of the US pharmacy technician workforce. Pharmacy technicians in grocery store settings have been experiencing negative wage premiums since 2000, some earning over $1.00/hour less than would have been expected given changes in CPI. On the other hand, pharmacy technicians in mass merchandiser settings experienced higher wages than would have been expected by changes in CPI for all years up to 2016.

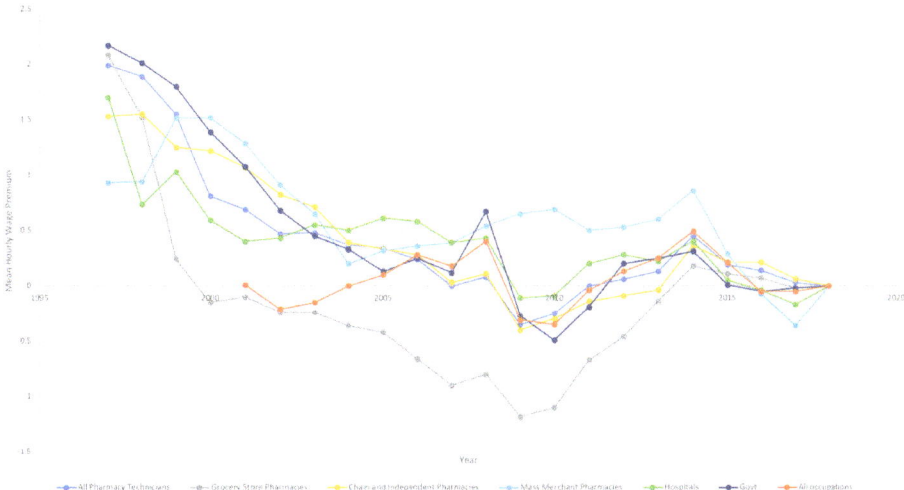

Figure 4. Mean Annual Hourly Wage Premiums for Pharmacy Technicians, from 1997 to 2018, and All Occupations, from 2001 to 2018.

4. Discussion

While pharmacy technicians in the United States who began their work between 1997 and 2006 have likely experienced modest positive wage premiums over time, pharmacy technicians who begun their work after 2007 have likely not experienced any positive wage premiums, with some earning less than what would have been expected had their wages kept up with the CPI. It should be noted that pharmacy technicians who have been working in this role since the late 1990s and early 2000s likely account for a very small portion of the pharmacy technician workforce in the United States. According to data from Desselle and colleagues, the median length of employment as a pharmacy technician in the US is approximately 9–10 years [27] compared to a median length of employment of approximately 22 years for pharmacists [28]. The majority of pharmacy technicians in the US have entered the workforce since 2006, and as such have not experienced much in the way of positive wage premiums, and may have even experienced negative wage premiums. Pharmacy technicians who have entered the work force since 2006 may have benefitted indirectly from hourly wage levels that were higher in CPI-adjusted dollars than if had they started in the field earlier. Since 2006 wage premiums for pharmacy technicians in the US have fluctuated in a manner and to a degree similar to those experienced by the median of "all occupations" in the US economy. Yet, what has been asked of pharmacy technicians in terms of expanded job roles [4–12] and regulatory requirements [21–23] has increased over this time. While one would expect to see positive wage premiums as a result of these increases in job roles and requirements, this was not observed in our analysis, and is consistent with the findings of other researchers [21,22]. Pharmacy technicians in the United States also have not experienced wage changes in the manner of those experienced by pharmacists, who experienced relatively large positive wage premiums in the late 1990s through the late 2000s [29].

Pharmacy technicians employed in community pharmacy settings in the United States (grocery stores, chain and independent pharmacies, mass merchandise stores) have generally experienced lower hourly wages and have been more likely to experience negative wage premiums than pharmacy technicians in hospitals and government settings. Community pharmacy technicians have been described as "the face of the community pharmacy", which translates into them being a critical source of patient loyalty, satisfaction and engagement. Their expanded job scope has resulted in higher levels of job stress [30]. As pharmacy technicians are essential to community pharmacy in the midst of their practice becoming more patient-centric model, community pharmacies must compensate their technicians at levels in line with the responsibilities they are increasingly being asked to take on, or risk losing them to other practice settings (such as hospitals and government, which has consistently paid pharmacy technicians higher hourly wages) or to other jobs outside of pharmacy entirely. Mattingly and Boyle have found that pharmacy technicians were the lowest compensated of 14 health technologist occupations in the U.S. state of Maryland, despite having education, training, and regulatory requirements similar to those other occupations [31]. Chui and colleagues stated that community pharmacies must redesign technician jobs, deploy them more effectively, and provide the training and compensation commensurate with these jobs so as to re-engineer practice with greater patient safety in mind [32]. In a 2005 study, Desselle found that as little as a $0.75/hour difference in hourly wages (approximately $1.00/hour when converted to 2018 levels) explained a significant portion of a pharmacy technician's intention to remain with their current employer or seek other employment [33].

This study has limitations that are important to recognize. The US Bureau of Labor Statistics Occupational Employment Statistics are exclusively collected in the United States and its territories. The results described here are limited to pharmacy technicians in the United States. The manner in which the US BLS provides its data (it is over one year old at the time it first becomes available), and the subsequent use of this data to calculate the presence of positive or negative wage premiums means that the findings reported here are a trailing indicator of the state of the labor market in the past. This study of US BLS data precludes any ability to discern from pharmacy hiring managers and other stakeholders the realities of the hiring market at the present time. While this analysis enables identification of past incongruities in the labor market (e.g., groups who have experienced either positive or negative wage premiums), the analysis does not allow us to separate to the extent to which wage premiums (or lack thereof) can be explained by changes in the supply of labor willing to work at these wage levels, or changes in the demand for services provided by pharmacy technicians. There is ample evidence that the demand for the services of pharmacy technicians in the United States has been high during this time period. The fact that significant positive wage premiums have not been observed, particularly since 2006, may be due a variety of factors. These include increases in the supply of pharmacy technician labor that kept up with the changes in demand. The lack of wage premiums may also be explained by other factors, including the role that technology has played in automating various dispensing and administrative roles that had previously been performed by pharmacy technicians, as well as negative pressures on pharmacy revenues generated by dispensing, which are needed to pay employee wages and other expenses.

5. Conclusions

The period from 1997 to the present has been one of transition for pharmacy across all settings in the United States, with increased demands for patient safety, access to safe and effective medication therapy, and value for what payers obtain from medications. Pharmacy technicians have been an essential component of these transitions, with pharmacies and pharmacists increasingly depending on them to support the delivery of high-quality patient care. This study provides evidence that compensation levels for the majority of pharmacy technicians in the United States have not increased in line with changes in the US consumer price index, nor have they increased in line with their increased responsibilities. It is important that the compensation, and particularly the hourly wage levels, of pharmacy technicians continue to be evaluated. This evaluation is essential to maintaining and supporting this important segment of the pharmacy workforce.

Author Contributions: Conceptualization, D.P.Z. and T.B.; methodology, D.P.Z.; validation, D.P.Z. and T.B.; formal analysis, D.P.Z.; writing—original draft preparation, D.P.Z.; writing—review and editing, D.P.Z., T.B. and S.P.D.; project administration, D.P.Z.; All authors have read and agreed to the published version of the manuscript.

Acknowledgments: Portions of this manuscript were previously presented at the 2018 American Pharmacists Association Annual Meeting, Nashville, TN (USA). Portions were also presented in research seminars at

Northeastern University, University of Minnesota, South University, Auburn University, and the University of Mississippi. The authors would like to thank everyone who provided input in these sessions.

Conflicts of Interest: The authors declare no conflict of interest.

References

1. Zhang, X.; Lin, D.; Pforsich, H.; Lin, V.W. Physician workforce in the United States of America: Forecasting nationwide shortages. *Hum. Resour. Health* **2020**, *18*, 8. [CrossRef]
2. Watanabe, J.H. Examining the Pharmacist Labor Supply in the United States: Increasing Medication Use, Aging Society, and Evolution of Pharmacy Practice. *Pharmacy* **2019**, *7*, 137. [CrossRef]
3. Benson, A. Labor market trends among registered nurses: 2008–2011. *Policy Politics Nurs. Pract.* **2012**, *13*, 205–213. [CrossRef] [PubMed]
4. Gernant, S.A.; Nguyen, M.O.; Siddiqui, S.; Schneller, M. Use of pharmacy technicians in elements of medication therapy management delivery: A systematic review. *Res. Soc. Adm. Pharm.* **2018**, *14*, 883–890. [CrossRef] [PubMed]
5. Hill, H.R.; Cardosi, L.; Desselle, S.P. Evaluating Advanced Pharmacy Technician Roles in the Provision of Point-of-Care Testing. *J. Am. Pharm. Assoc.* **2020**. [CrossRef]
6. Borchert, J.S.; Phillips, J.; Thompson Bastin, M.L.; Livingood, A.; Andersen, R.; Brasher, C.; Bright, D.; Fahmi-Armanious, B.; Leary, M.-H.; Lee, J.C. Best practices: Incorporating pharmacy technicians and other support personnel into the clinical pharmacist's process of care. *J. Am. Coll. Clin. Pharm.* **2019**, *2*, 74–81. [CrossRef]
7. Schultz, J.M.; Jeter, C.K.; Martin, N.M.; Mundy, T.K.; Reichard, J.S.; Van Cura, J.D. ASHP Statement on the Roles of Pharmacy Technicians. *Am. J. Health Syst. Pharm.* **2016**, *73*, 928–930. [CrossRef]
8. Adams, A.J.; Martin, S.J.; Stolpe, S.F. "Tech-check-tech": A review of the evidence on its safety and benefits. *Am. J. Health Syst. Pharm.* **2011**, *68*, 1824–1833. [CrossRef]
9. Napier, P.; Norris, P.; Braund, R. Introducing a checking technician allows pharmacists to spend more time on patient-focused activities. *Res. Soc. Adm. Pharm.* **2018**, *14*, 382–386. [CrossRef]
10. Davidson, T.R.; Hobbins, M.A.; Blubaugh, C.M. Development and Implementation of a Pharmacy Technician Medication History Program. *J. Pharm. Pract.* **2019**. [CrossRef]
11. Hawkins, K.L.; King, J.; Delate, T.; Martinez, K.; McCool, K.; Clark, N.P. Pharmacy Technician Management of Stable, In-Range INRs Within a Clinical Pharmacy Anticoagulation Service. *J. Manag. Care Spec. Pharm.* **2018**, *24*, 1130–1137. [CrossRef] [PubMed]
12. Adams, A.J.; Desselle, S.P.; McKeirnan, K.C. Pharmacy Technician-Administered Vaccines: On Perceptions and Practice Reality. *Pharmacy* **2018**, *6*, 124. [CrossRef] [PubMed]
13. Lau, G.; Alwan, L.; Chi, M.; Lentz, M.; Hone, K.; Segal, E. Expanding pharmacy practice through the use of pharmacy technicians as process navigators to facilitate patient access of oral anticancer agents. *J. Am. Pharm. Assoc.* **2019**, *59*, 586–592. [CrossRef] [PubMed]
14. US Bureau of Labor Statistics. Occupational Employment Statistics. Occupational Employment and Wages, May 2018, 29-2052 Pharmacy Technicians. Available online: https://www.bls.gov/oes/current/oes292052.htm (accessed on 28 February 2020).
15. US Bureau of Labor Statistics. Occupational Outlook Handbook. Pharmacy Technicians. Available online: https://www.bls.gov/ooh/healthcare/pharmacy-technicians.htm#:~{}:text= (accessed on 28 February 2020).
16. US Bureau of Labor Statistics. Occupational Outlook Handbook. Pharmacists. Available online: https://www.bls.gov/ooh/healthcare/pharmacists.htm#:~{}:text= (accessed on 28 February 2020).
17. Knapp, K.K.; Livesey, J.C. The Aggregate Demand Index: Measuring the balance between pharmacist supply and demand, 1999–2001. *J. Am. Pharm. Assoc.* **2002**, *42*, 391–398. [CrossRef]
18. Pharmacist Demand Indicator. Available online: https://pharmacymanpower.com/ (accessed on 28 February 2020).
19. Mott, D.A.; Cline, R.R.; Kreling, D.H.; Pedersen, C.A.; Doucette, W.R.; Gaither, C.A.; Schommer, J.C. Exploring trends and determinants of pharmacist wage rates: Evidence from the 2000 and 2004 National Pharmacist Workforce Survey. *J. Am. Pharm. Assoc.* **2008**, *48*, 586–597. [CrossRef]
20. Desselle, S.P.; Holmes, E.R. Results of the 2015 National Certified Pharmacy Technician Workforce Survey. *Am. J. Health Syst. Pharm.* **2017**, *74*, 981–991. [CrossRef]

21. Urick, B.Y.; Mattingly, T.J., 2nd; Mattingly, A.N. Relationship between regulatory barriers to entry and pharmacy technician wages. *Res. Soc. Adm. Pharm.* **2020**, *16*, 190–194. [CrossRef]
22. Mattingly, A.N.; Mattingly, T.J., 2nd. Regulatory burden and salary for pharmacy technicians in the United States. *Res. Soc. Adm. Pharm.* **2019**, *15*, 623–626. [CrossRef]
23. Mattingly, A.N.; Mattingly, T.J., 2nd. Advancing the role of the pharmacy technician: A systematic review. *J. Am. Pharm. Assoc.* **2018**, *58*, 94–108. [CrossRef]
24. US Bureau of Labor Statistics. Occupational Employment Statistics. May 2018 National Occupational Employment and Wage Estimates: United States. Available online: https://www.bls.gov/oes/current/oes_nat.htm (accessed on 28 February 2020).
25. US Bureau of Labor Statistics. Occupational Employment Statistics. OES Data. Available online: https://www.bls.gov/oes/tables.htm (accessed on 28 February 2020).
26. US Bureau of Labor Statistics. CPI Inflation Calculator. Available online: https://data.bls.gov/cgi-bin/cpicalc.pl (accessed on 28 February 2020).
27. Desselle, S.P.; Hoh, R.; Rossing, C.; Holmes, E.R.; Gill, A.; Zamora, L. Work Preferences and General Abilities Among US Pharmacy Technicians and Danish Pharmaconomists. *J. Pharm. Pract.* **2018**. [CrossRef]
28. Mott, D.A.; Doucette, W.R.; Gaither, C.A.; Kreling, D.H.; Schommer, J.C. Trends in pharmacist participation in the workforce, 2009 to 2014. *J. Am. Pharm. Assoc.* **2016**, *56*, 433–440. [CrossRef] [PubMed]
29. Zgarrick, D.; Bujnoch, T. Examination of Premiums in Pharmacists' Median Annual Salaries between 1997 and 2016. *J. Am. Pharm. Assoc.* **2018**, *58*, e1–e201. [CrossRef]
30. Desselle, S.P. An in-depth examination into pharmacy technician worklife through an organizational behavior framework. *Res. Soc. Adm. Pharm.* **2016**, *12*, 722–732. [CrossRef] [PubMed]
31. Mattingly, A.N.; Boyle, C.J. Salary and entry-level requirements for pharmacy technicians compared with other health technologist and technician occupations in Maryland. *J. Am. Pharm. Assoc.* **2020**, *60*, 17–21. [CrossRef] [PubMed]
32. Chui, M.A.; Mott, D.A.; Maxwell, L. A qualitative assessment of a community pharmacy cognitive pharmaceutical services program, using a work system approach. *Res. Soc. Adm. Pharm.* **2012**, *8*, 206–216. [CrossRef] [PubMed]
33. Desselle, S.P. Job turnover intentions among Certified Pharmacy Technicians. *J. Am. Pharm. Assoc.* **2005**, *45*, 676–683. [CrossRef]

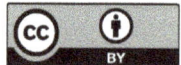

© 2020 by the authors. Licensee MDPI, Basel, Switzerland. This article is an open access article distributed under the terms and conditions of the Creative Commons Attribution (CC BY) license (http://creativecommons.org/licenses/by/4.0/).

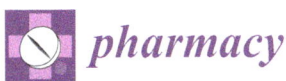

Opinion

Embracing the Evolution of Pharmacy Practice by Empowering Pharmacy Technicians

Ryan Burke

Pharmacy Technician Certification Board, Washington, DC 20037, USA; rburke@ptcb.org

Received: 16 March 2020; Accepted: 14 April 2020; Published: 15 April 2020

Abstract: While pharmacy technician roles in some practice settings are expanding beyond the traditional dispensing activities to include advanced or specialized tasks such as immunization administration, medication history collection, and final product verification, these practices are not yet widespread. There are apparent barriers to expanding the role of pharmacy technicians, including inconsistency in the education, training, and certification requirements across the United States, and regulations that have not kept pace with the evolving role of pharmacy technicians. Every corner of the profession has an opportunity, and responsibility, to elevate pharmacy technicians in an effort to advance safety and better serve patients. Regulators can expand the responsibilities that may be delegated to technicians, professional organizations can bring pharmacy technicians into the fold, employers can build career ladders to allow for advancement, and individual pharmacists and pharmacy technicians can advocate and engage.

Keywords: pharmacy technicians; pharmacy workforce; certification; education; regulations; board of pharmacy

---

Pharmacy technicians are the backbone of pharmacies across the globe. In the United States (U.S.), there are more than 420,000 pharmacy technicians in the workforce and the occupation is expected to grow by 7% during the next 10 years. Pharmacy technicians work under the supervision of pharmacists and are typically responsible for tasks such as data entry, medication dispensing, inventory management, insurance claims processing, and customer service [1]. While technicians' roles in some practice settings are expanding beyond the traditional activities to include advanced or specialized tasks such as immunization administration, medication history collection, and final product verification, these practices are not yet widespread. The pharmacy profession has an opportunity to embrace the evolution of practice and determine how to best position pharmacy technicians to meet the public's health care needs and enable pharmacists to fully utilize their clinical knowledge and skills. Achieving this in a comprehensive way requires all stakeholders, from regulators and professional associations to individual pharmacy technicians and pharmacists, to engage and take action.

Research supports the safety and efficacy of advanced pharmacy technician roles. Studies have demonstrated that the implementation of technician product verification in institutional and community pharmacy settings is a safe and effective way to allow pharmacists to focus on direct patient care. Frost and Adams summarized the findings of four community, pharmacy-focused studies that revealed trained pharmacy technicians perform product verification as accurately as pharmacists [2]. In another study by Hohmeier and colleagues, implementation of a practice model in which pharmacy technicians were responsible for product verification resulted in pharmacists spending significantly more time delivering patient care services [3].

Similarly, studies focused on medication history collection have found that pharmacy technicians are accurate and time efficient and, in some cases, may also decrease costs [4,5]. In terms of immunization administration, McKeirnan and Sarchet have affirmed that appropriately trained pharmacy technicians improve access to vaccination care, thereby having the potential to increase the number of immunizations given and reduce the number of deaths from vaccine-preventable diseases [6].

There are two apparent barriers to expanding the role of pharmacy technicians: inconsistency in the education, training, and certification requirements across the U.S., and regulations that have not kept pace with the evolving roles of pharmacy technicians.

Notably, there is stark disparity between consumers' high expectations for technician training and the reality of pharmacy practice, suggesting public support for more consistent requirements for technician education and credentialing to advance safety. A 2016 public perception survey revealed that U.S. consumers view pharmacy technician education, training, and certification requirements as critically important. In fact, 94% said their trust in pharmacy would increase with standardized certification for pharmacy technicians; 88% say it is very important for people who compound or mix custom medications to be specially trained and certified; 77% of respondents said states should require all pharmacy technicians to be trained and certified, and 76% said they would seek out a different pharmacy if they knew technicians working in their current pharmacy were not certified [7].

The reality is that state regulations for education, training, and certification vary widely, thus creating a barrier to advancing technician roles. There are 45 states that require pharmacy technicians to be registered or licensed by the state's board of pharmacy, and while 22 states require technicians to obtain national certification, only nine of those states require them to maintain certification throughout their careers.

There are inherent benefits to national pharmacy technician certification. Wheeler and colleagues recently compared the viewpoints of certified and noncertified technicians and explored the perceived value of certification in the areas of medication safety, skills and abilities, experience, career engagement and satisfaction, and productivity. They found that certified technicians have a stronger commitment to their careers and employers, a perceived lower rate of medication errors, and a stronger desire to take on new roles than technicians who are not certified [8]. In recent focus groups, Desselle and colleagues concluded that national certification has a positive impact on technician maturation, professional socialization, and career commitment [9].

In some states, national certification enables pharmacy technicians to perform certain tasks that noncertified technicians are prohibited from performing. For example, in Ohio, certified pharmacy technicians may accept verbal prescription orders, transfer prescriptions, and perform sterile compounding while those without certification may not [10].

In terms of pharmacy technician education and training, there are two accreditation standards: one created jointly by the American Society of Health-System Pharmacists and the Accreditation Council for Pharmacy Education (ASHP/ACPE) [11], and the other created by the Accrediting Bureau for Health Education Schools (ABHES) [12]. Aside from these accrediting organizations, both national pharmacy technician certification organizations require completion of an education and training program or work experience as part of their certification program's eligibility criteria [13,14]. To date, only two states, North Dakota and Louisiana, have adopted accredited education and training as the entry-level requirement for all pharmacy technicians in the state. Illinois and Virginia are pursuing legislative and regulatory changes to implement similar requirements in their respective states.

The second primary barrier to expanding technician roles is that, despite the evidence, many states' current regulations do not enable pharmacy technicians to take on advanced or specialized tasks. This must change if the profession is to fully realize the benefits of a trained, certified, and committed pharmacy technician workforce. There has been some progress on this front. Two states, California and New Hampshire, are aiming to create an advanced pharmacy technician license category that would have different requirements and privileges than a standard technician registration or license [15,16]. In other places, like Idaho, the board of pharmacy has taken a less prescriptive approach by allowing pharmacists to use their professional judgment to determine which tasks to delegate to pharmacy technicians [17].

Today, 18 states allow technician product verification in some form, though in some cases it is limited to specific processes in the institutional setting (e.g., filling or replenishing an automated dispensing cabinet). While only three states currently allow technicians to administer immunizations, several states are actively exploring this task, and it is reasonable to expect more states to follow suit in the coming years.

While research and regulatory changes are important, pharmacy technicians also need to be engaged and prepare for new roles. This may come in the form of professional development through their employers or by seeking advanced or specialized training and credentials. Likewise, both pharmacy technicians and pharmacists have a responsibility to advocate for change through state or national professional associations and by voicing their opinion at state board of pharmacy meetings.

Twelve states have taken the positive step of appointing pharmacy technicians to serve on the state board of pharmacy. Other states should consider this approach to ensure pharmacy technicians have a voice in the critical regulatory process.

While some professional associations, such as ASHP, have a robust pharmacy technician membership focused on issues of importance to those professionals, many do not [18]. Anecdotally, some pharmacy technicians question the value in organizations that seek to represent them but have a name that implies exclusivity (i.e., "pharmacists"). Professional organizations should consider how their governance structures, membership models, messaging, and policy positions can be changed to better include and represent pharmacy technician viewpoints.

The pharmacy profession is evolving at a rapid pace. Every corner of the profession has an opportunity, and responsibility, to elevate pharmacy technicians in an effort to advance safety and better serve patients. Regulators can expand the responsibilities that may be delegated to technicians, professional organizations can bring pharmacy technicians into the fold, employers can build careers ladders to allow for advancement, and individual pharmacists and pharmacy technicians should advocate and engage.

Funding: This research received no external funding.

Conflicts of Interest: The authors declare no conflict of interest.

References

1. Bureau of Labor Statistics. Available online: https://www.bls.gov/ooh/healthcare/pharmacy-technicians.htm (accessed on 4 March 2020).
2. Frost, T.P.; Adams, A.J. Tech-Check-Tech in Community Pharmacy Practice Settings. *J. Pharm. Technol.* **2017**, *33*, 47–52. [CrossRef]
3. Hohmeier, K.C.; Garst, A. The Optimizing Care Model: A novel community pharmacy approach to enhance patient care delivery by leveraging the technician workforce through technician product verification. *JAPhA* **2019**, *59*, 880–885. [CrossRef] [PubMed]
4. Johnston, R.; Saulnier, L. Best Possible Medication History in the Emergency Department: Comparing Pharmacy Technicians and Pharmacists. *Can. J. Hosp. Pharm.* **2010**, *63*, 359–365. Available online: https://www.ncbi.nlm.nih.gov/pmc/articles/PMC2999367/ (accessed on 4 March 2020). [CrossRef] [PubMed]
5. Jobin, J.; Irwin, A.N. Accuracy of Medication Histories Collected by Pharmacy Technicians during Hospital Admission. *Res. Soc. Adm. Pharm.* **2018**, *14*, 695–699. [CrossRef] [PubMed]
6. McKeirnan, K.; Sarchet, G. Implementing Immunizing Pharmacy Technicians in a Federal Healthcare Facility. *Pharmacy* **2019**, *7*, 152. [CrossRef] [PubMed]
7. Pharmacy Technician Certification Board (PTCB). Available online: https://www.ptcb.org/news/survey-shows-three-quarters-of-americans-would-seek-out-a-pharmacy-where-pharmacy-technicians-are-certified (accessed on 4 March 2020).
8. Wheeler, J.S.; Renfro, C.P. Assessing Pharmacy Technician Certification: A National Survey Comparing Certified and Noncertified Pharmacy Technicians. *JAPhA* **2019**, *59*, 369–374. [CrossRef] [PubMed]
9. Desselle, S.P.; McKeirnan, K.C. Pharmacists Ascribing Value of Technician Certification Using an Organizational Behavior Framework. *AJHP* **2020**, *77*, 457–465. [CrossRef] [PubMed]

10. State of Ohio Board of Pharmacy. Available online: https://www.pharmacy.ohio.gov/Documents/Licensing/PTech/General/Pharmacy%20Technician%20Registration%20-%20Frequently%20Asked%20Questions.pdf (accessed on 12 April 2020).
11. American Society of Health-System Pharmacists (ASHP). Available online: https://www.ashp.org/-/media/assets/professional-development/technician-program-accreditation/docs/ashp-acpe-pharmacy-technician-accreditation-standard-2018 (accessed on 4 March 2020).
12. Accrediting Bureau of Health Education Schools (ABHES) Accreditation Manual. Available online: https://www.abhes.org/wp-content/uploads/2020/01/18th-Edition-Accreditation-Manual-Effective-12020.pdf (accessed on 4 March 2020).
13. Pharmacy Technician Certification Board (PTCB). Available online: https://www.ptcb.org/guidebook/ (accessed on 6 March 2020).
14. National Healthcareer Association (NHA). Available online: https://www.nhanow.com/docs/default-source/pdfs/handbooks/candidate_handbook.pdf (accessed on 6 March 2020).
15. California State Board of Pharmacy. Available online: https://www.pharmacy.ca.gov/meetings/agendas/2019/19_dec_lic_mat.pdf (accessed on 6 March 2020).
16. The General Court of New Hampshire. Available online: http://gencourt.state.nh.us/bill_status/billText.aspx?sy=2019&id=465&txtFormat=html (accessed on 6 March 2020).
17. Idaho State Board of Pharmacy. Available online: https://bop.idaho.gov/wp-content/uploads/sites/99/2019/07/2019_Law_Book.pdf (accessed on 6 March 2020).
18. American Society of Health-System Pharmacists. Available online: https://www.ashp.org/Pharmacy-Technician/Pharmacy-Technician-Forum (accessed on 6 March 2020).

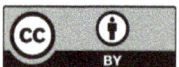

© 2020 by the author. Licensee MDPI, Basel, Switzerland. This article is an open access article distributed under the terms and conditions of the Creative Commons Attribution (CC BY) license (http://creativecommons.org/licenses/by/4.0/).

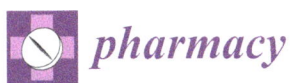

Commentary

Practice, Skill Mix, and Education: The Evolving Role of Pharmacy Technicians in Great Britain

Melanie Boughen [1,*] and Tess Fenn [2]

1. School of Pharmacy, University of East Anglia, Norwich NR4 7TJ, UK
2. European Association of Pharmacy Technicians, 2500 Valby, Denmark; eaptsecretary@outlook.com
* Correspondence: m.boughen@uea.ac.uk

Received: 6 March 2020; Accepted: 24 March 2020; Published: 26 March 2020

Abstract: Pharmacy technicians' roles are rapidly evolving in Great Britain (GB) as they undertake more extended activities with increased autonomy across the different pharmacy sectors. This paper compares the GB pharmacy regulator initial education and training standards recently introduced (2017) with the qualifications currently used in practice and discusses whether future qualifications will be 'fit for purpose'. In this context, knowledge, skills, and competence are reviewed to assess whether they will meet the expectations and underpin the evolving pharmacy technician role as integral to healthcare provision. Based on drivers, policy change, and the changing GB healthcare landscape, effectiveness of skill mix is analysed to establish whether this is being optimised to support person-centred pharmacy in response to the challenges and pressures faced within the NHS. On this basis and given there is a limited evidence base, this review has highlighted a need for larger scale research to reassure the pharmacy and wider healthcare professions, and the public, that the evolving pharmacy technician role presents no increased risk to patient safety and contributes significantly to releasing pharmacists time for person-centred clinical activities.

Keywords: pharmacy technician; education; skill mix; extended roles; patient safety; medicines reconciliation

1. Introduction

Pharmacy technicians in Great Britain were first accepted onto the General Pharmaceutical Council (GPhC) register, the pharmacy regulator, in 2011 and practice to the same GPhC professional standards as pharmacists [1]. Since registration, they have gained increased recognition for their contribution to the healthcare agenda as their roles, scope of practice, and autonomy increase. This is partly due to the realisation that many 'traditional' pharmacists' roles have become increasingly technical due to the introduction of automation and enhancement of information technology as well as the changing focus of practice to become person/patient-centred.

As a result, particularly in the hospital sector, with specific training, these extended roles have evolved from traditional pharmacy technician activities such as dispensing and stock management, to final accuracy checking (in the UK this is a nonclinical check for accuracy of prescribed and dispensed medicines, as opposed to the clinical check conducted by a pharmacist for clinical appropriateness for a patient), medicines optimisation skills* (see Table 1), and pharmacy management. All of these roles have previously been traditional pharmacists' roles. However, although the UK government vision for the community pharmacist role has significantly changed from the supply of medicines to the clinical provision of patient care—and this gives opportunities for pharmacy technician role development—this has been slower to evolve in community pharmacy. Currently, pharmacy legislation relating to the 'supervision' of the preparation, assembly, sale, and supply, including dispensing, of medicines from GPhC-registered pharmacies prevents pharmacists from leaving the pharmacy for significant periods of time [2]. Therefore, pharmacy technicians have not been able to assume responsibility for all activity within the dispensary in the same manner as that seen in the hospital setting.

Albeit, at a varying pace across the different sectors and settings, the pharmacy technician landscape is changing, and in addition to the traditional settings of community and hospital, pharmacy technicians are now increasingly located within care homes and GP Practices (doctors surgeries and health centres) performing very much a clinical role as part of medicines optimisation* teams.

In recent years, there has been some growth in the body of literature on extended/advance roles and although these are generally limited to small local studies, they do provide insight into pharmacy technician role development [3–7]. The literature also highlights the positive contribution that pharmacy technicians, with specific training, can make to pharmacy services and patient care, with the general theme that the extended roles release pharmacists for more patient-facing clinical activity and further developing their clinical skills and knowledge to train as nonmedical prescribers. On a more global scale, it should be noted that releasing pharmacists time is not always the reason that pharmacy technicians scope and autonomy has increased—there are countries with rural and remote environments and populations where with little infrastructure and few pharmacists, pharmacy technicians and other support staff operate autonomously out of necessity [8].

Table 1. Medicines optimisation definition and activities undertaken by pharmacy technicians.

*Medicines Optimisation **Definition** Medicines optimisation is an approach that seeks to maximise the beneficial clinical outcomes for patients from medicines with an emphasis on safety, governance, professional collaboration, and patient engagement [9]. **Pharmacy Technician activities supporting patient safety include the following:** • Communicating with patients, patients' representatives, and the public providing advice about their medicines. • Shared decision making with patients about taking their medicines. • Providing patients with compliance aids when required and demonstrating their use. • Supplying medicines for individual patients. • Assessing appropriateness of medicine forms for patients. • Referring complex clinical inventions to pharmacist or prescriber. • Providing advice about repeat supplies and storage of medicines. • Analysing quantities of medicines to reduce waste and safe disposal. • Assessing patients' own medicines for use ensuring they are fit for purpose. • Taking a history of a patient's medication use. • Reconciling a patient's medicines from one setting to another. • Communication with the multidisciplinary team to streamline patient care.

To better understand the evolving role in GB, in this article we will look at the main drivers for change of the pharmacy technician role, how the role has evolved in response to this, what needs to change to support the transition (education), and finally, how the role may evolve further in the future.

2. Drivers and Responding to Change in Great Britain

In pharmacy, as well as all other sectors of healthcare, there never seems a point when the workforce is not under extreme pressure to deliver services. This has led to several NHS 'White Paper' publications including The Interim NHS People Plan [10] and the Interim NHS People Plan: the future pharmacy workforce [11], which state the importance of pharmacy involvement in patient and public care and identifying the support that pharmacy technicians can provide across different sectors, practicing to the 'top of their licence'. The NHS England (NHSE) review on secondary care productivity in NHS Hospitals [12] (commonly known as the Carter Review) and most recently in 2020, the NHS England Update to the GP Contract [13], formally recognise pharmacy technicians alongside pharmacists as part of the skill mix needed to deliver person-centred care. It is through this formal recognition that pharmacy technicians as healthcare professionals can progress further alongside other healthcare professions.

For changes to be successful, understanding skill mix efficiency (ensuring the right people, with the right skills, are in the right place at the right time) and what can be achieved by maximising skill mix is critical. Poorly managed skill mix to just 'get a job done' could be counterproductive and a risk to patient safety. McIntosh and Sheppy highlighted that productivity and safety can be enhanced simultaneously by greater use of the skills and experiences of all staff and could enhance outcomes both clinically and economically [14].

Arguably, in the UK, there still remains some confusion as to pharmacy technicians' scope of practice, role boundaries, and accountability. This is more prevalent in the community sector, where there is often a blurring of pharmacy technician and pharmacy/dispensing assistant roles. One activity that does separate pharmacy technicians from pharmacy assistants is final accuracy checking, and a major training and development-funded initiative was introduced in 2016 by NHS England (Pharmacy Integration Fund) [15]. The intention of this ongoing initiative is to drive the greater use of pharmacists and pharmacy technicians in new, integrated local care models. Part of this initiative is to broaden the skills of pharmacy technicians working in the community sector by funding final accuracy checking—however, as this is still ongoing, no evaluation of its success is available.

In comparison, in the UK, the pharmacy assistant is an essential member of the pharmacy team and assists pharmacists and pharmacy technicians in both community and hospital pharmacy settings. In the secondary care setting, there is more variety and clarity of the role, whereas in community the role generally focuses on stock maintenance and the assembly aspect of the dispensing process but with less demarcation of responsibilities within the pharmacy team. On-the-job training, equivalent to UK level 2, is provided to meet the GPhC education requirements, however the pharmacy assistant is not a registrant.

Another contributing factor in community pharmacy is the use of locum pharmacists who may not be familiar with the team, and therefore be less forthcoming or possibly less confident in delegating tasks when they are the 'Responsible Pharmacist' [16]. However, this is not always the reason, and sometimes it is time pressures on management that prevent implementation of skill mix strategy or staff that recognise greater use of extended roles and responsibilities [17] but may not feel empowered to influence any change. Although this is occurring less, it remains a barrier and can restrict flow of patient services. According to West [18], organisational skill mix reviews are key to ascertain what activities need to be carried out, who has the minimum level of skills to undertake them, and if new roles need to be created to fulfil optimisation. Pharmacists spending time on 'traditional' roles do not optimise their skills as they do not need to final-accuracy-check prescriptions, manage the day-to-day supervision of staff, or prepare staff rotas—which are technical duties. With effective communication, robust procedures, and clear understanding of boundaries and lines of responsibility, the majority of pharmacy technicians have the knowledge and skills or the potential to undertake these activities. As many pharmacists are managers, another aspect for making skill mix work is recognising the needs of the pharmacist—pharmacists need developed skills in delegation and managing teams, which some see as their own development requirements [19].

With further regard to skill mix, emerging evidence does not suggest that pharmacy technicians are less safe when taking on extended roles. Rather, it suggests that because they are trained for the specific role, they are likely to have fewer competing demands and have been found to have a higher level of accuracy than pharmacists and other healthcare professionals [20–22]. However, this evidence is still very limited with small scale studies and wider, larger scale research needs to be undertaken to reassure pharmacists and wider healthcare teams that from these roles there is no worsening risk to patient safety or systems.

3. Education

In light of the changing roles of pharmacy technicians, education is pivotal, and a key point of interest is the level of the baseline pharmacy technician qualifications, which vary considerably from country to country.

In 2017, the European Association of Pharmacy Technicians (EAPT) undertook a European-wide survey of education and training programmes [23]. The results highlighted the variation in pharmacy technician education in Europe with levels of study required for practice, licensing, or registration ranging from post-secondary diplomas to bachelor's degrees. Interestingly, comparison between the level of initial education requirements and the role undertaken by community pharmacy technicians in the EAPT 2017 European Survey [23] shows a correlation between countries with higher level education requirements and pharmacy practice activities. The volume and complexity of the dispensing activities carried out and the application of problem-solving skills are specifically enhanced in Denmark and Portugal, where bachelor's degrees are in place as the baseline education. Interestingly, comparing the academic credits of these bachelor's degrees using the European Credit Transfer and Accumulation System (ECTS) shows a further differential between the countries, with Denmark accruing 180 ECTS credits and Portugal 240.

In Great Britain, trainee pharmacy technicians are known as preregistration trainee pharmacy technicians (PTPTs) and undertake their training over a two-year period. Trainees are employed, therefore much of their learning and competence is gained in the workplace as they complete a competence-based qualification. They are also required to complete an academic (theoretical knowledge) qualification, which is delivered either as study days away from the workplace or distance learning. The qualification standards set by the GB pharmacy regulator are currently the Level 3 Diploma in Pharmacy Service Skills (work-based) and Level 3 Diploma in Pharmaceutical Science (theory) [24] which predate mandatory registration of 2011. These standards are still in use up until August 2020.

As the pharmacy technician role has developed, the underpinning education model in GB has failed to keep up with the practice, which has caused considerable confusion for pharmacists and employers as pharmacy technician roles, boundaries, and accountability have been difficult to define [25,26].

Role definition is also a challenge across the globe as both the EAPT survey 7 and the International Pharmaceutical Federation (FIP) 2017 [8] introductory global descriptive survey blend the pharmacy technician role with that of 'pharmacy support workforce cadres' who work with pharmacists. Vast global variation compounds the barriers to understanding the pharmacy technician role, the education and competencies needed to underpin their work, and ultimately the autotomy of their professional practice.

Across the USA and Australia, current rules and regulations concerning the education and training of pharmacy technicians varies from state to state, and applying a national certified educational programme is a source of much debate. In comparison however, mirroring GB, Canada's national model for the regulation of pharmacy technicians exists across 90% of its provinces, and the pharmacy technician title is restricted to those who meet the qualification requirements and are registered with their provincial regulatory body [27].

Acknowledging the changing healthcare landscape and the need to upskill the pharmacy technician workforce, in October 2017, the GB pharmacy regulator published the new Initial Education and Training Standards (IETS) [28]. The outcome-based standards now being introduced (2020) incorporate the shift in knowledge and skills required for patient/person-centred practice. This involves four domains of study: 1. Person-centred care; 2. Professionalism; 3. Professional knowledge and skills; 4. Collaboration. Using Miller's Pyramid (1990) [29] theory of assessment and competence, the new standards will require building from fundamental knowledge level of 'knows', to the application level of 'knows how', to measuring competence at the 'does' level and having to achieve and exceed at the lower level before moving on.

Whilst providing a broad base of knowledge and skills for work in a range of pharmacy settings across GB, the IETS have a strong emphasis on effective communication to support the clinical, operational, and scientific practices, procedures, and professionalism required of the registered pharmacy technician. Requiring a qualification of a minimum Level 3 (broadly equating to the UK subject advanced level qualifications—A level), Figures 1 and 2 illustrate the comparison of activities from the previous qualification to the new IETS and measures these along a continuum of pharmacy skills.

Figure 1 illustrates the mandatory skills required for the 2010 GB qualification at day one of practice and extended skills along a continuum of skill complexity and autonomy. It shows inclusion of the traditional skills of dispensing, receiving prescriptions, and managing the stock of the pharmacy. Another inclusion is extemporaneous dispensing skills, sometimes referred to as compounding. In the UK, this skill has become all but non-existent with community pharmacies in particular due to the high risk involved in the preparation, with pharmacies opting to outsource these requests to organisations specifically set up for this type of production. The communication skills required for these standards are at a basic or routine level for handing out prescriptions, giving mainly noncomplex instructions and dealing with routine queries and customer service issues. Figure 1 also illustrates the addition of final accuracy checking. This was the first extended skill to be undertaken by pharmacy technicians approximately 20 years ago, originally in hospital pharmacy but now also widely practiced in community pharmacy. Medicines reconciliation (an activity that is integral to medicines optimisation*) was the second extended role introduced in acute hospitals following the publication of guidance by the National Institute for Health and Care Excellence in 2007 [30] (then called the National Institute for Clinical Excellence). Originally a role for pharmacists, this became a delegated activity and pharmacy technicians have been training to undertake medicines reconciliation over the last 10 years. This activity has increased and is now accepted as part of the pharmacy technicians' progression and practiced across all settings where there is patients' transfer of care.

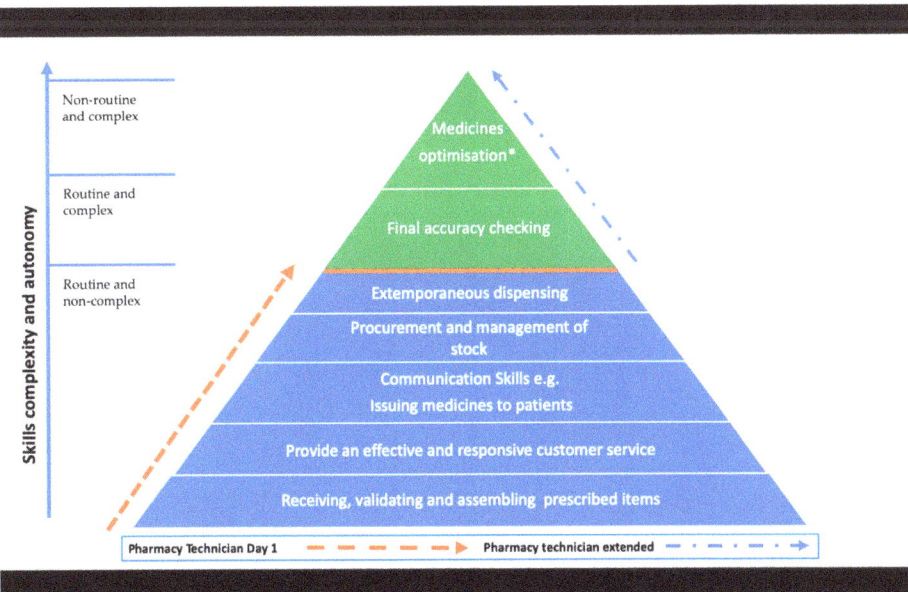

Figure 1. Great Britain (GB)-registered pharmacy technician role and skills—2010 General Pharmaceutical Council (GPhC) education standards.

In comparison, the first three levels of Figure 2 show that the core skill of dispensing—in its broadest definition of receiving prescriptions, validating, assembling medicines, and issuing medicine to a named person—remains. The next four levels then illustrate the mandatory activities newly introduced in the 2017 IETs, with extemporaneous dispensing removed from the standards completely as it was considered an obsolete activity. In addition to Medicines Optimisation* and Accuracy Checking, previously widely recognised as extended, advanced communication and leadership skills have been introduced. These changes and additions reflect the expectations of pharmacy technician practice by the GB regulator as well as working within the regulatory Standards for Pharmacy Professionals [1]. The mandatory inclusion of medicines optimisation* and accuracy checking activities which are delivered through person-centred care, commands taking responsibility for the legal, safe, and efficient supply of medicines together with using professional judgement and strategies for continuous quality improvement. The additional skills required to support this competence are now intrinsically embedded within new IETS [26] learning outcomes along with the required leadership and advanced communication skills. Although skills such as procurement and stock management have been removed from the IETS at the 'does' level, they have not been removed entirely and PTPTs will need to learn and be assessed at the 'knows how' level of the Miller's pyramid.

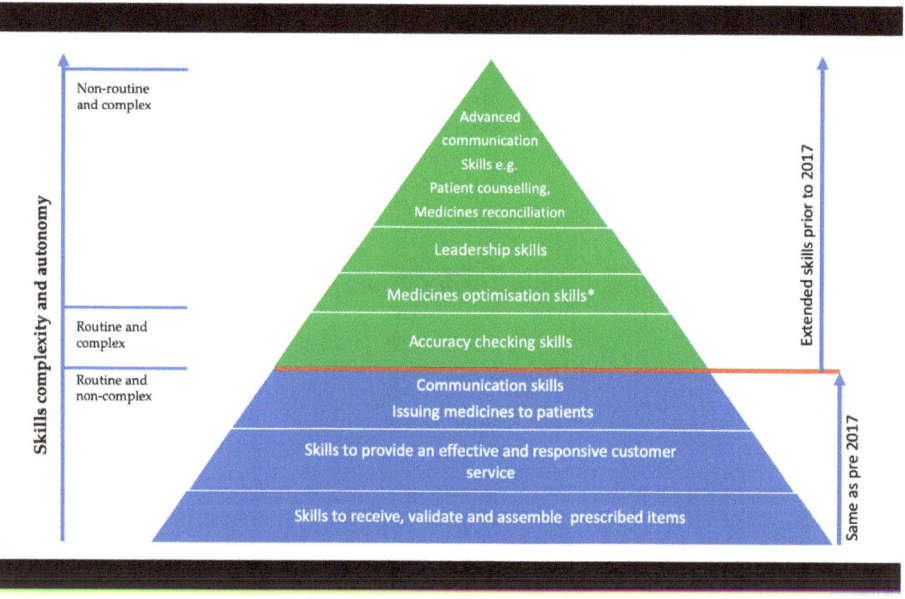

Figure 2. GB-registered pharmacy technician role and skills—2017 GPhC standards.

Recognising that the regulatory purpose of the IETS [28] is to ensure that newly registered pharmacy technicians are competent to practise safely and effectively, it is important to acknowledge that competence is much broader than skills alone. Whereas skills are specific to a task or activity, to perform these competently to an acceptable level of ability requires the appropriate depth and breadth of underpinning knowledge and understanding. Thus, professional pharmacy technicians need to be able to identify the required knowledge that underpins their job role and must be able to apply it in practice.

Given that competence is said to build on a foundation of clinical skills, scientific knowledge, and professional development, it also begs the question as to what extent of knowledge is required to combine both the knowledge and competency elements of the evolving job role.

Accepting that Miller's Pyramid requires achieving and exceeding the preceding level [29], and the regulators expectation that the newly registered pharmacy technician will be acting autonomously and consistently in complex situations [27], albeit defined situations, it can be argued that the level of knowledge required is considerable.

As the GB pharmacy regulatory Professional Standards [1] are very much reflected in the new IETs [28] and these include the complexity of ethical and effective decision making, identifying and responding to errors, and raising concerns, this arguably raises the level and expectations from day 1 of practice and that of a qualification fit for purpose.

4. Conclusions

Responding to the pressures of the NHS in delivering patient care, every healthcare profession in the UK has been called upon to maximise their outputs in the most efficient and cost-effective way. The expectations of UK healthcare policy and the integrated care model are already being transposed into new pharmacy services and managing skill mix efficiency will be a major contribution to its success.

The introduction of a new 'NHS Discharge Medicines Service' [30] in addition to the 'NHS Community Pharmacist Consultation Service' (already part of the Community Pharmacy Contractual Framework [31]) adds to the expanse of the pharmaceutical care provision, providing development opportunities for community pharmacy technicians. A pharmacy technician qualifying with the new IETs should have the fundamental education and competence to support pharmacists in these services and allow scope for ongoing development. However, the legacy workforce would need additional training to ensure they did not present any risk to patient safety. With this in mind, alongside the expanding role of primary care and news that pharmacy technicians have been added to the list of healthcare professions in the evolving NHSE primary care network structure, undeniably, the primary care pharmacy technician role will also continue to evolve. Thus, there is clearly a significant correlation between progression of pharmacy services, workforce capacity, and utilising pharmacy technicians aligned with their professional knowledge and skills.

There is no doubt that the intention of the new IETS is to embed what was previously seen as extended roles for GB pharmacy technicians into standard practice and develop the profession further. This is indeed required to empower both pharmacists and pharmacy technicians to deliver the aspirations of the NHS England's Long-term plan [31]. Delivering person-centred care to help patients optimise their medicines and support shared decision-making depends on skilful and proficient communication and skills. Of course, the content of the new qualification must be sound to transfer the acquired behaviours, knowledge, and skills into professional practice. Only time will tell whether the minimum level 3 adequately supports this new, complex role and if two years is sufficient for the trainee to achieve the outcomes and full potential as a healthcare professional. An in-depth evaluation will need to be undertaken once the first trainees come through to explore these aspects.

Moving forward, with the paucity of literature available, larger scale research would provide further insight to reassure the pharmacy and wider healthcare professions, and the public, that the evolving pharmacy technician role presents no increased risk to patient safety and contributes significantly to releasing pharmacists' time for person-centred clinical activities.

Author Contributions: Conceptualization, M.B., T.F.; resources, M.B.; writing—original draft preparation, M.B., T.F.; writing—review and editing, M.B., T.F.; visualization, M.B., T.F.; project administration, M.B.; All authors have read and agreed to the published version of the manuscript.

Funding: This research received no external funding.

Acknowledgments: The authors would like to acknowledge the advice provided by David Wright in the writing of this article.

Conflicts of Interest: There are no conflicts of interest.

References

1. General Pharmaceutical Council. Standards for Pharmacy Professionals. 2017. Available online: www.pharmacyregulation.org/sites/default/files/standards_pharmacy_professionals_may-2017_f.pdf (accessed on 15 February 2020).
2. Gov.UK. Rebalancing Medicines Legislation and Pharmacy Regulation Programme Board. Available online: https://www.gov.uk/government/groups/pharmacy-regulation-programme-board (accessed on 20 March 2020).
3. Wanbon, R.; Lyder, C.; Villeneuve, E.; Shalansky, S.; Manuel, L.; Harding, M. Medication reconciliation practices in Canadian emergency departments: A national survey. *Can. J. Hosp. Pharm.* **2015**, *68*, 202–209. [CrossRef] [PubMed]
4. Pevnick, J.M.; Nguyen, C.; Jackevicius, C.A.; Palmer, K.A.; Shane, R.; Cook-Wiens, G.; Rogatko, A.; Bear, M.; Rosen, O.; Seki, D.; et al. Improving admission medication reconciliation with pharmacists or pharmacy technicians in the emergency department: A randomised controlled trial. *BMJ Qual. Saf.* **2018**, *27*, 512–520. [CrossRef] [PubMed]
5. Kraus, S.K.; Sen, S.; Murphy, M.; Pontiggia, L. Impact of a pharmacy technician-centered medication reconciliation program on medication discrepancies and implementation of recommendations. *Pharm. Pract.* **2017**, *15*. [CrossRef]
6. Newby, B. Expanding the role of pharmacy technicians to facilitate a proactive pharmacist practice. *Am. J. Health Syst. Pharm.* **2019**, *76*, 398–402. [CrossRef] [PubMed]
7. Boughen, M.; Sutton, J.; Fenn, T.; Wright, D. Defining the Role of the Pharmacy Technician and Identifying Their Future Role in Medicines Optimisation. *Pharmacy* **2017**, *5*, 40. [CrossRef] [PubMed]
8. Koehler, T.; Brown, A. Documenting the evolution of the relationship between the pharmacy support workforce and pharmacists to support patient care. *Res. Soc. Adm. Pharm.* **2017**, *13*, 280–285. [CrossRef] [PubMed]
9. UK Medicines Information. Medicines Optimisation in England: A Consultation. Available online: https://www.ukmi.nhs.uk/filestore/ukmiuu/ukmi_meds_opt_consultation_final_11sept12.pdf (accessed on 4 March 2020).
10. NHS England. Interim People Plan. 2019. Available online: https://www.longtermplan.nhs.uk/publication/interim-nhs-people-plan/ (accessed on 27 February 2020).
11. NHS England. Interim People Plan—The Future Pharmacy Workforce. Available online: https://www.longtermplan.nhs.uk/wp-content/uploads/2019/06/ipp-p-future-workforce.pdf (accessed on 27 February 2020).
12. Department of Health. Operational Productivity and Performance in English NHS Acute Hospitals: Unwarranted Variations. 2016. Available online: https://www.gov.uk/government/publications/productivity-in-nhs-hospitals (accessed on 23 February 2020).
13. NHS England. Update to the GP Contract Agreement 2020/21—2023/24. Available online: https://www.england.nhs.uk/publication/investment-and-evolution-update-to-the-gp-contract-agreement-20-21-23-24/ (accessed on 20 February 2020).
14. McLntosh, B.; Sheppy, B. Skill maximisation: The future of healthcare. *Br. J. Healthc. Manag.* **2013**, *19*, 118–122. [CrossRef]
15. NHS England. Pharmacy Integration Fund. Available online: https://www.england.nhs.uk/primary-care/pharmacy/pharmacy-integration-fund/ (accessed on 22 March 2020).
16. Bradley, F.; Schafheutle, E.I.; Willis, S.C.; Noyce, P.R. 'Supervision in Community Pharmacy' Pharmacy Research UK. 2013. Available online: http://pharmacyresearchuk.org/wp-content/uploads/2014/01/Supervision-in-Community-Pharmacy-Full-Report-070114.pdf (accessed on 19 February 2020).
17. Barnes, E.; Bullock, A.; Allan, M.; Hodson, K. Community pharmacists' opinions on skill-mix and delegation in England. *Int. J. Pharm. Pract.* **2018**, *26*, 398–406. [CrossRef] [PubMed]
18. West, M.A. *Effective Teamwork: Practical Lessons from Organizational Research*, 3rd ed.; John Wiley & Sons: Chichester, West Sussex, 2012; p. 53.
19. Hickman, L.; Poole, S.G.; Hopkins, R.E.; Walters, D.; Dooley, M.J. Comparing the accuracy of medication order verification between pharmacists and a tech check tech model: A prospective randomised observational study. *Res. Soc. Adm. Pharm.* **2018**, *14*, 931–935. [CrossRef] [PubMed]

20. Jobin, J.; Irwin, A.N.; Pimentel, J.; Tanner, M.C. Accuracy of medication histories collected by pharmacy technicians during hospital admission. *Res. Soc. Adm. Pharm.* **2018**, *14*, 695–699. [CrossRef] [PubMed]
21. Snoswell, C.L. A meta-analysis of pharmacists and pharmacy technicians' accuracy checking proficiency. *Res. Soc. Adm. Pharm.* **2019**. [CrossRef]
22. European Association of Pharmacy Technicians. Education and Training Programmes of Pharmacy Technicians: European Survey. Available online: https://www.eapt.info/pharmacy-technician-in-europe/ (accessed on 16 February 2020).
23. General Pharmaceutical Council. Approved Pharmacy Technician Courses. Available online: https://www.pharmacyregulation.org/education/pharmacy-technician/accredited-courses (accessed on 12 February 2020).
24. Health Education England. Advancing Pharmacy Education and Training: A Review. 2019. Available online: https://www.hee.nhs.uk/sites/default/files/documents/Advancing%20Pharmacy%20Education%20and%20Training%20Review.pdf (accessed on 2 March 2020).
25. International Pharmaceutical Federation. Technicians and Pharmacy Support Workforce Cadres Working with Pharmacists: An. *Introductory Global Descriptive Study*. 2017. Available online: https://www.fip.org/www/streamfile.php?filename=fip/publications/2017-02-Technicians-Pharmacy-Support-Worforce-Cadres.pdf (accessed on 24 February 2020).
26. General Pharmaceutical Council. Standards for the Initial Education and Training of Pharmacy Technicians. 2017. Available online: https://www.pharmacyregulation.org/sites/default/files/standards_for_the_initial_education_and_training_of_pharmacy_technicians_october_2017.pdf (accessed on 15 February 2020).
27. Gp-training.net. The Miller Pyramid and Prism. Available online: https://www.gp-training.net/training/educational_theory/adult_learning/miller.htm (accessed on 4 March 2020).
28. National Institute for Health and Care Excellence. Medicines Optimisation. 2016. Available online: https://www.nice.org.uk/guidance/qs120 (accessed on 15 February 2020).
29. Pharmaceutical Services Negotiating Committee. Discharge Medicines Service. Available online: https://psnc.org.uk/services-commissioning/essential-services/discharge-medicines-service/ (accessed on 27 February 2020).
30. Gov.UK. Community Pharmacy Contractual Framework. 2019–2024. Available online: https://www.gov.uk/government/publications/community-pharmacy-contractual-framework-2019-to-2024 (accessed on 3 March 2020).
31. NHS England. NHS Long Term Plan. Available online: https://www.longtermplan.nhs.uk (accessed on 20 February 2020).

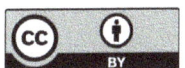

© 2020 by the authors. Licensee MDPI, Basel, Switzerland. This article is an open access article distributed under the terms and conditions of the Creative Commons Attribution (CC BY) license (http://creativecommons.org/licenses/by/4.0/).

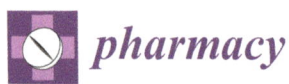

Review

Impact of Up-Scheduling Medicines on Pharmacy Personnel, Using Codeine as an Example, with Possible Adaption to Complementary Medicines: A Scoping Review

Kristenbella AYR Lee [1], Joanna E. Harnett [1], Carolina Oi Lam Ung [2] and Betty Chaar [1,*]

[1] School of Pharmacy, The University of Sydney School of Pharmacy, Sydney 2006, Australia; klee7377@uni.sydney.edu.au (K.A.L.); joanna.harnett@sydney.edu.au (J.E.H.)
[2] State Key Laboratory of Quality Research in Chinese Medicine, Institute of Chinese Medical Sciences, University of Macau, Macau SAR, Macau 999078, China; carolinaung@um.edu.mo
* Correspondence: betty.chaar@sydney.edu.au; Tel.: +61-02-9036-7101

Received: 21 March 2020; Accepted: 13 April 2020; Published: 15 April 2020

Abstract: Within Australia, vitamins, minerals, nutritional supplements, essential oils, and homoeopathic and herbal preparations are collectively termed and regulated as Complementary Medicines (CMs) by the Australian Therapeutic Goods Administration (TGA). CMs are predominantly self-selected through a pharmacy, providing pharmacy personnel an opportunity to engage with the public about their CM use. CMs are currently non-scheduled products in Australia. This review aimed to summarize the literature reporting the potential effect on pharmacies if scheduling of CMs was adopted, using codeine as an example. A scoping review methodology was employed. Seven databases were searched to identify four key concepts, including: CMs, scheduling and rescheduling, codeine, and pharmacists. Seven studies were included for analysis. The majority of the literature has explored qualitative studies on the perception and opinion of pharmacists in relation to the up-scheduling of codeine. The case of codeine illustrates the possible impact of up-scheduling. If CMs were to be up-scheduled, the accessibility of CMs would be limited to the pharmacy providing a role for pharmacy personnel, including both pharmacists and pharmacy technicians, to counsel on CM use. However, careful collaboration and consideration on how such a regulatory change would impact other key-stakeholders, including CM practitioners, requires both a strategic and collaborative approach.

Keywords: scheduling; complementary medicines; dietary supplements; regulation

1. Introduction

Within Australia, vitamins, minerals, nutritional supplements, essential oils, and homoeopathic and herbal preparations are collectively termed and regulated as Complementary Medicines (CMs) by the Australian Therapeutic Goods Administration (TGA) [1]. The prevalent use of CMs has steadily increased over the last two decades [2,3]. An estimated 53% of CMs are self-selected and mainly accessed through pharmacy outlets, providing pharmacists, technicians, and sales assistants an opportunity to engage with the public about their CM use [4,5]. CMs are currently non-scheduled products in Australia. However, as they are provided from within pharmacy premises. According to the principles of professional ethics clearly articulated in the Code of Ethics for Pharmacists [6], pharmacists and pharmacy personnel are expected to counsel patients and provide sufficient information to ensure safe and appropriate use, and pharmacists are expected to adopt an engaged professional role in relation to CMs provision [4,5]. This is particularly important in light of the growing body of evidence reporting potential side effects and drug-CM interactions that can impact patient safety and clinical outcomes of therapy. A well-established drug-herb interaction is *Hypericum perforatum* (St John's Wort, or SJW) [7], which is used in the management of mild to moderate depression [7]. In Australia, St John's Wort is easily accessed over-the-counter (OTC). Hyperforin, an active constituent of John's Wort, is known to induce the cytochrome P-3A4 (CYP3A4) enzyme and the drug transporter p-glycoprotein, which are involved in the metabolism of many medications [8,9]. Concurrent use of SJW with these CYP3A4-metabolized medicines is well documented as resulting in significant interactions associated with patient harm [10].

Despite this, there are reports that barriers exist in the pharmacy environment which prevent pharmacists and pharmacy personnel from adopting professional standards regarding CMs. These barriers appear to be: time constraints, limited resources within the pharmacy, and a lack of knowledge about CMs [11]. Some pharmacists report that CMs were secondary to their primary concerns in patient care. They considered these products as being mostly "retail" products, available through a range of retail outlets in addition to pharmacies, indicating the uncertainty about whether they should assume professional responsibility for ensuring the appropriate and safe use of widely available CMs [11]. Consumers' lack of respect towards the potential safety issues with the use of CMs was suggested to be yet another challenge experienced by pharmacists when trying to provide professional care related to CMs. To some consumers, as reflected by some pharmacists, having the CMs available at different retail outlets might indicate an "assurance of safe"; thus, pharmacists' advice or intervention was not needed [11]. Whilst there appears to be consensus among pharmacists and associated stakeholders about the responsibility of the pharmacist to actively supervise provision of CMs, as is legally required in the case of 'Pharmacist-Only' (Schedule 3 in Australia) and 'Prescription-Only' (Schedule 4 in Australia) medicines [5], as well as clearly mentioned in the Code of Ethics for Pharmacists, it is unclear whether such professional responsibility could be extended to CMs in their current status; or should up-scheduling be considered?

Scheduling of medicines is one of the global key pillars of the pharmacy practice business model, with decisions to reschedule or up-schedule medicines made in an attempt to improve medicine use at a population level [12]. In Australia, the scheduling of medications is assigned according to the appropriate level of safety and control over the accessibility and availability of medicines. The aim of rescheduling is to safeguard the health and safety of the public. There are several schedules within the Australian classification system. Schedule 2 medications, also known as "Pharmacy Medicines", are restricted to pharmacies and can be managed by non-pharmacist staff within the pharmacy. Provision of Schedule 3 medications ("Pharmacist-only Medicines") require a pharmacist to engage in a consultation session with the patient to ascertain if there is a therapeutic need for the medication and to advise on its use [12]. Provision of "Prescription-only" medicines are classified under Schedule 4 and require a prescriber to fill a prescription for it to be dispensed by the pharmacist.

One example of the complexities and impact of rescheduling was the rescheduling in Australia of codeine-containing products (CCPs) in 2010, which was a very controversial topic at the time. Some low dose CCPs were previously scheduled at Schedule 2 or over-the-counter (OTC). However, with intense scrutiny of the misuse of opioid-containing medicines, and the rising incidence of addiction on these medicines in Australia, on the 1 May 2010, regulatory changes were made to minimize access and misuse, and all low dose CCPs were up-scheduled from Schedule 2 to Schedule 3 [13]. In Australia, patients could therefore no longer self-select CCPs, and the pharmacist was required to have some level of consultation with the patient before supply of the product. Being a Pharmacist-Only Medicine implied that the pharmacist had all professional and legal responsibilities for the supply of the Schedule 3 medicine, and as such, up-scheduling impacted on the practice of community pharmacists all around Australia [13]. Inadvertently, however, pharmacists became involved in the supply and identification of misuse of CCPs. Thus, despite the rescheduling in 2010, the rate of misuse did not decline with heightened pharmacists' involvement. According to Cairns et al., even after the change in drug scheduling, phone calls made to New South Wales Poisons Information Centre (NSWPIC), coded under codeine-misuse, continued to rise [14]. Therefore, in December 2016, the TGA announced that CCPs were to undergo another round of up-scheduling to make them unavailable OTC or pharmacist-only, due to the safety issues of codeine. Accordingly, codeine was up-scheduled to Schedule 4 (prescription only) by the TGA on 1 February 2018, in an effort to address the increasing use and/or misuse of pharmaceutical opioids, particularly in relation to codeine abuse. The action of regulatory up-scheduling was therefore undertaken in the interest of patient safety and to minimize the risks of drug dependence and toxicity [14].

While the safety and implications of most CMs is incomparable to CCPs, the role of scheduling in relation to the accessibility of products and professionalism of pharmacists is worthy of discussion. To date, the scheduling of CMs has not even been considered or explored. Despite rising consumption and current safety concerns around some CMs, CMs remain unscheduled. And while CMs are clearly not drugs of abuse, there is an increasing demand from professional organizations, and within the literature, advocating for pharmacists and pharmacy personnel to adopt heightened professional duties as related to the supply of CMs [15]. According to the position statement issued by the Pharmaceutical Society of Australia, *"pharmacists are recommended to assume the responsibility of providing sound evidence-based advice to assist consumers in making informed decisions regarding CMs"* [16]. In the United States of America, where CMs are also over the counter, the position statement published by the American Society of Health System Pharmacists also urged pharmacists to integrate awareness of patients' use of dietary supplements into everyday practice and to increase efforts to prevention of interactions between these products and prescriptions medicines [17]. This responsibility may be aided by community workforce personnel, such as pharmacy assistants, who, if trained appropriately, may direct requests for CMs to the pharmacist in charge, where necessary.

The Australian Industry and Skills Committee published a report on community pharmacy in April 2020 [18], stating the following: *"The Community Pharmacy sector plays an important role in the Health Care sector through the supply to the general public of prescription-based medicine, non-prescription-based medicine when permitted, and a range of information and health care services ... As a result, the community pharmacy sector is pivotal in reducing the demand and burden on primary health care facilities ... The Community Pharmacy sector includes a workforce of 41,400 pharmacy sales assistants and generated $18.4 billion in revenue in the 2018-19 period, up from $16.3 billion in 2016-17."* And according to Australian government statistics, approximately 59% of the community pharmacy workforce is comprised of pharmacy assistants, many of whom undergo specific training to enable them to undertake tasks allocated to them in pharmacy [19]. As most requests for CMs come from the OTC areas (or shelves) within a typical community pharmacy, usually allocated to oversight of pharmacy assistants, there may be an important role for pharmacy personnel, such as pharmacy assistants, to support the pharmacist with streamlining of requests for CMs in a community pharmacy. This role would be particularly effective if CMs were to be scheduled in Australia.

We hypothesize that the scheduling of CMs to enable holding pharmacists and pharmacy personnel responsible for oversight of the supply of CMs could, theoretically at least, be a reasonable approach to enhance safe and appropriate use of self-selected CMs [11]. It would therefore follow that we seek to explore the literature for evidence of the impact of re-scheduling of other medicines in Australia. Hence, this is an exploratory study aimed to investigate the potential effect on pharmacy practice if scheduling of CMs was adopted, using the case of up-scheduling of codeine in Australia as an example.

2. Methodology

Arksey and O'Malley's scoping review framework was adopted in our literature review [20]. The scoping review methodology involves five different stages: (i) identifying a research question, (ii) identifying relevant studies, (iii) the selection of the studies, (iv) charting of data, and (v) summarizing and reporting of the results.

This scoping review was conducted in accordance to the Preferred Reporting Items for Systematic Reviews and Meta-Analyses (PRISMA) statement [21]. A PRISMA chart was constructed (Figure A1). The databases used in the literature search were: Cumulative Index to Nursing and Allied Health

Literature (CINAHL), Embase, Medline, PubMed, Scopus, Google Scholar and Web of Science. Our search strategy can also be found in Figure A2.

Studies that revolved around four concepts: (i) CMs, (ii) Scheduling and rescheduling, (iii) Codeine and (iv) Pharmacist, which were published in the English language between 10 March 2014 and 10 March 2019, were included. A timeframe of five years was selected due to the increasing trend of the use of CMs by consumers over this period [22]. Terminologies used in the search strategy for the four respective concepts are shown below:

- CMs: Complementary medicines, natural medicines, dietary supplements, vitamins, minerals, herbal supplements, homeopathic medicines, complementary therapy, CMs, and aromatherapy oils.
- Scheduling and rescheduling: regulations, up-schedule.
- Codeine.
- Pharmacist: Pharmacist, retail pharmacy, community pharmacy, pharmacy management and pharmacist autonomy.

Research articles that did not follow IMRAD (Introduction, Methods, Results, and Discussion) format were excluded from the study. Letters, editorials, and commentaries were also excluded. Search term criteria and terminologies were agreed upon among the four authors, and one author performed the literature search. The same author who conducted the literature search completed the title and abstract screening of the yield, along with the removal of duplicates. The review of full text articles was performed by four authors.

3. Results

From the initial literature search, a total of 2748 articles were identified across 7 databases (Figure A1). Following the removal of duplicate articles, titles and abstracts were screened for our key concepts, resulting in 21 articles being selected for full text assessment and a final 7 selected for inclusion. No studies were identified in our search when (1) and (5), and (4) and (5) were combined (Figure A2). There were no CMs' scheduling studies identified in the search conducted. All studies focused on the impact of scheduling codeine products, and this was judged as relevant to understanding more broadly what needs to be considered in the scheduling of any medicines, including CMs.

Four of the studies examined the perceptions and perspectives of pharmacists in relation to the up-scheduling of codeine. Two quantitative studies examined retrospective data from the Poison Information Centres, in Australia and Ireland. One study explored the characterization of Schedule 2, Schedule 3, and unscheduled medicines. As presented in Table 1, five themes were identified related to the purpose, attitudes, and implications.

4. Discussion

To our knowledge, this is the first study to explore the effects of regulatory scheduling of medicines and its impact on pharmacists' in terms of workload or professional behaviors. This review has illustrated the impact of up-scheduling medicines, using codeine as an example, and it was conducted with a view for theoretically extrapolating to other medicines, specifically to CMs. The findings of this study suggested there was a lack of quantitative data to provide specific outcomes relating to the schedule change. The majority of the literature was comprised of exploratory qualitative studies on the perceptions and opinions of pharmacists in relation to codeine.

Table 1. Systematic review of the selected studies.

	Theme	Sub-themes	Key Findings	Reference
1	Purpose		To address codeine misuse	[23]
2	Attitudes	2.1 Positive	Pharmacists were proactive in prompting discussions with patients	[23]
			Pharmacists recommended patients with appropriate medicines management	[23]
			Less addiction and toxicity were reported due to restrictions	[24]
			General Practitioners were in support of scheduling changes	[24]
			Up scheduling positively impacted the practice of community pharmacists in Australia	[13]
			Improvements to practice behaviors	[13]
		2.2 Negative	Did not solve misuse as patient shifted from "pharmacist-shopping" to "doctor-shopping"	[23]
			Some pharmacists felt that it might have possibly lead to escalation of stronger medications	[23]
			Limited pharmacists' capacity in offering pain management	[23]
			Some pharmacies viewed up scheduling of codeine as increasing GP's burden	[23]
			Opposition to the scheduling by pharmacists and users	
			Had a negative impacts on consumers' health, finances and pain management	
3	Potential impact on practice	3.1 Treatment options	Concerns raised around treatment options and support for pain management after the restriction	[23]
			Establishing therapeutic needs, inconsistent supplying issue between pharmacies and intervening with codeine-dependent individuals	[13]
		3.2 Challenges	Impact on business and environmental factors	[23]
		3.3 Funding models of payment	Implications to pharmacies income	[23]
4	Experiences of impact	4.1 Positive	Resulted in a decrease in the reported poison cases involving non-prescription codeine products in 2011	[24]
			Pharmacists required to monitor supply and identify more cases of misuse	[25]
		4.2 Insignificant	Rate of codeine poisoning remained stable and at a lower level	[26]
		4.3 Negative	Had no impact on misuse; Possible reason to why Schedule 3 failed to make an impact: People misusing codeine did not necessarily fit the 'addict' stereotype	[14]
			Pharmacists were not confident discussing possible codeine dependence with patients	[26]
5	Related issues	5.1 Marketing and advertising	Misleading patients to think that codeine is an effective treatment for pain	[12]
		5.2 Compliance with legislation and professional guidelines	Greater staff involvement for scheduled medicines	[12]

The intent of up-scheduling codeine was to minimize codeine misuse. When codeine was up-scheduled from Schedule 2 to Schedule 3, a pharmacist's involvement in the supply of codeine-containing medicines became a legal requirement. Pharmacists had a legal obligation and professional responsibility to ensure that codeine use was therapeutically appropriate for a patient before permitting sale. In such circumstances, pharmacists uphold an important role as a "gatekeeper" by counseling and, if required, intervening in OTC CCP misuse. In the qualitative study by Hamer et al., it was reported that there was an increase in the workload on pharmacists due to these new legal obligations [25]. Pharmacists also noted that they became more aware about misuse as a result of the increase in patients requesting codeine [25]. Some pharmacists felt that it gave them confidence to discuss with patients any codeine-related problems [25]. Some pharmacists would attempt to address a patient's concerns and recommend alternatives to minimize codeine use [13,23]. Other pharmacists felt that rescheduling to Schedule 3 prompted them to upskill in the area of pain management [23]. Following the second up-scheduling to Schedule 4 for any product containing codeine, it was reported that the up-scheduling actually created an opportunity for patients to openly discuss their pain issues with the pharmacist and seek non-codeine strategies to manage their pain [23,24].

Whilst CMs and codeine (which has potential for misuse) are very different classes of medicines, we propose that the fundamental principles that prompted changes to the up-scheduling of codeine are the same, i.e., pharmacists' responsibility to engage in patient care that ensures the appropriate and safe use of medicines. Currently, CMs are categorized as unscheduled medicines, and, as such, there is no legal implications for pharmacists if they do not directly engage in the supply of CMs. However, there is growing evidence of adverse reactions between certain medicines and some CMs, which potentially have serious effects on patient safety [27,28]. Therefore, there is a gap between the regulation of supply of CM products and pharmacy personnel's, including pharmacists', professional responsibilities. To date, up-scheduling of CMs has not been discussed in the literature.

Shifting CMs to Schedule 2 could theoretically increase pharmacy personnel's involvement in supply. When codeine was up-scheduled to "Pharmacist-only medicine", Hamer et al. reported that pharmacists' awareness about patients' request for codeine increased, which prompted for identification of codeine misuse and changes in pharmacists' practices with regard to supplying of CCPs [25]. Again, while CMs are overall a lower risk than CCPs, they are not without risk.

Therefore, we hypothesize that, by having an established legal framework, subjecting CMs to up-scheduling to at least Schedule 2, and educating pharmacy assistants, technicians, and pharmacists in the handling of CMs will enable closer monitoring [11] of CM use and identification of drug–herb interactions. With heightened regulation, pharmacy personnel would be required by law to interact and engage with the patients during the sale of CMs. This will create an opportunity for patients to make more informed decisions about the CMs of interest and encourage appropriate and safe use. At the same time, having CMs available exclusively through the pharmacy could be a strong message to consumers to be aware of and comply with advice offered with respect to the safety of CMs, as they would have with other medicines or prescription medicines. Consumers' perceived need to consult with pharmacy personnel when deciding on the use of CMs would, therefore, also be prompted. As indicated by a consumer advocacy group representative, *"it would be ideal to have pharmacists to deal with consumers' use of CMs"*. Initiating the regulatory scheduling of CMs might be the remedial policy needed to correct consumers' belief systems about the safety of CMs.

Furthermore, in a study conducted by Emmerton in 2003, it was noted that Schedule 3 medicines have higher rates of in-store interventions and pharmacist engagement, as compared to unscheduled medicines [8]. A probable conclusion drawn from this study could be that medicines assigned with higher risk value would be prioritized by pharmacy staff [13]. While CMs are commonly perceived by the public to be safe medicines [5], adverse reactions, drug-herb interactions and serious toxicities, if used inappropriately have been reported [27,28]. Increased risk of drug and CMs interaction is present in physiologically-compromised individuals and the elderly that are on polypharmacy [29,30]. Up-scheduling of CMs can encourage more patient-pharmacist/pharmacist technician interactions on the use of CMs. This may also potentially increase the reporting of drug-herb interactions and raise awareness among CM users and pharmacy personnel about interactions and, even more importantly, add to building the evidence-base about CM safety.

Another significant finding of this study was that one of the major challenges reported by pharmacists with the scheduling of codeine to Schedule 3 was having to establish a "therapeutic need" as required by law. Due to time constraints in real-time pharmacy practice, pharmacists felt that they were unable to perform a detailed consultation session with patients to determine a therapeutic need [13]. Based on the codeine example, we might be able to extrapolate that pharmacists might see it as a challenge to conduct a comprehensive consultation with their patients on their conventional medications and CMs, with time being the limiting factor. This provides an opportunity for pharmacy assistants/technicians to extend their role and be trained in CMs counseling. Doucette reported that pharmacy technicians were willing to perform new tasks that are needed to support emerging patient care services within community pharmacies [31]. The need for pharmacist assistants' or technicians' roles to evolve through appropriate education and collaborative working relations with pharmacists has been suggested [32]. Such an evolution would be suited to filling the current gap in the provision of professional care related to CMs use.

Despite legal obligations for the supply of Schedule 3 codeine, there was a reported lack of conformity between Australian pharmacies [13]. Inconsistencies in pharmacists' practices were found in different pharmacies, which can also become a potential barrier between patient and pharmacist. Some patients reported that pharmacists were not able to provide the information about CMs' they needed and therefore decided not to ask the pharmacist's assistance in making a decisions about CMs again [11]. Other patients may become confused and interpret the behavior of pharmacists exercising a duty of care as being unnecessarily prohibitive in comparison to other pharmacists who do not exercise professional behaviors related the provision of CM products [13]. With that in view, if CMs were to be up-scheduled, we might also be faced with varying pharmacy practices in the supply of CMs. Perhaps some of this inconsistency would be reduced if Schedule 2 was applied to CMs and well-trained pharmacy assistants and technicians could 'absorb' the professional responsibility of the counseling session and refer to the pharmacist only when necessary.

In addition, it was reported that when codeine was regulated to Schedule 3, some pharmacists were concerned about their clinical competence not being sufficient to help patients with pain management without the aid of over-the-counter CCPs [24]. It was consistent in most of the studies that the up-scheduling of codeine required additional educational training for pharmacists in the area of pain management, counseling skills, and the handling of drug misuse [13,23,24]. This could imply that, if a change in CMs scheduling were to eventuate, pharmacists, pharmacy assistants, and pharmacy technicians would need to undertake professional training in the area of CMs to build on their evidence-based CMs knowledge. In the study by Ung et al., education is identified as one of the solutions to facilitate the integration of CMs into pharmacy practice [33].

We suggest that up-scheduling of CMs should be based on an evidence-based model and conducted in a step-up approach. Suggestions include up-scheduling CMs that are associated with high interactions-risk and used as a therapeutic agent. Some Australian CMs companies have attempted to promote practitioner-only CMs. Yet little is known about the impact on improving pharmacy personnel engagement with consumers who are buying these products. With that in mind, scheduling of medicines should be explored in depth in relation to the possible implications for other healthcare professionals, retail outlets owners, and, more specifically, CMs practitioners. The aim of such research would be to promote a coordinated approach to supporting the appropriate and safe use of CMs across different sectors.

This study does have some limitations. As this is a newly emerging topic, there is limited research to date and lack of sufficient opportunity to compare with previous studies. Hence, it may not be an adequately comprehensive study to fully inform readers and policy makers on the impact of rescheduling. However, the findings of our study have clearly flagged several suggested initiatives that are worthy of consideration.

As codeine is a drug of addiction, we also need to be mindful that the purpose and effects of up-scheduling could be different to the case of CMs; although patient safety is of the essence of the approach taken and clearly has become applicable to CMs. Further research to inform enhancement of the role of pharmacy personnel engagement in the sale of CMs in view of the position statement from PSA may be required.

5. Conclusions

The case of codeine illustrates the possible impact of regulatory up-scheduling of medicines in community pharmacy. If CMs were to be up-scheduled to a rigorous pharmacy-specific regulatory level, such as Pharmacy-only (Schedule 2), the accessibility of CMs would be restricted to the community pharmacy setting, providing more opportunities for pharmacists and pharmacy personnel to engage with a patient's request for CMs and counsel on CM use, thereby contributing substantially to the appropriate and safe use of CMs. An added benefit would be enhancing patient or consumer awareness of any potential risks or interactions of CMs, rather than the current common belief that CMs are 'natural' products with no risks associated to their intake, regardless of patient history or conditions. However, careful collaboration and consideration about how such a regulatory change would impact other key-stakeholders, including other types of retailers providing these products and CM practitioners, requires a strategic and collaborative approach.

Author Contributions: B.C., C.O.L.U. and J.E.H. conceptualized the review and developed the search strategy. K.A.L. conducted the search and initial screening of papers. K.A.L., B.C. and J.E.H. reviewed the papers. K.A.L. and B.C. conducted the coding. J.E.H., B.C. and K.A.L. conducted the thematic analysis. K.A.L. drafted the manuscript that was reviewed by B.C. and J.E.H. C.O.L.U. conducted a critical review. All authors have read and agreed to the published version of the manuscript.

Funding: This research received no external funding.

Conflicts of Interest: The authors declare no conflict of interest relevant to this study.

Appendix A

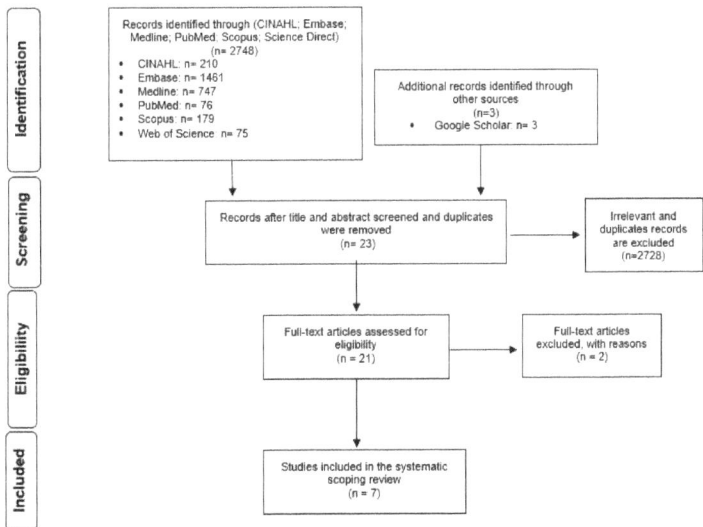

Figure A1. Preferred Reporting Items for Systematic Reviews and Meta-Analyses (PRISMA) model.

```
Database: Ovid MEDLINE(R) ALL <1946 to August 13, 2019>
Search Strategy:
--------------------------------------------------------------------------------
1     ("Impact of scheduling and rescheduling" or "scheduling and rescheduling" or
"regulations" or "up schedule").mp. [mp=title, abstract, original title, name of
substance word, subject heading word, floating sub-heading word, keyword heading
word, organism supplementary concept word, protocol supplementary concept word,
rare disease supplementary concept word, unique identifier, synonyms] (42203)
2     ("Pharmacist" or "retail pharmacy" or "community pharmacy" or "pharmacy
management" or "pharmacist autonomy").mp. [mp=title, abstract, original title, name
of substance word, subject heading word, floating sub-heading word, keyword
heading word, organism supplementary concept word, protocol supplementary
concept word, rare disease supplementary concept word, unique identifier,
synonyms] (18616)
3     codeine.mp. (6755)
4     ("regulation" or "reschedul*").mp. [mp=title, abstract, original title, name of
substance word, subject heading word, floating sub-heading word, keyword heading
word, organism supplementary concept word, protocol supplementary concept word,
rare disease supplementary concept word, unique identifier, synonyms] (1356723)
5     ("Complementary medicine*" or "natural medicines" or "dietary supplements" or
"vitamins" or "minerals" or "herbal supplements" or "homeopathic medicines" or
"complementary therapy" or "CM" or "aromatherapy oils").mp. [mp=title, abstract,
original title, name of substance word, subject heading word, floating sub-heading
word, keyword heading word, organism supplementary concept word, protocol
supplementary concept word, rare disease supplementary concept word, unique
identifier, synonyms] (490700)
6     1 and 2 and 3 and 5 (0)
7     1 and 3 (25)
8     3 and 4 (92)
9     1 and 2 and 5 (3)
10    1 and 5 (652)
11    4 and 5 (11602)
12    2 and 4 and 5 (7)

*****************************
```

Figure A2. Sample of search strategy (Medline).

References

1. Therapeutic Goods Administration. *Complementary Medicines*; Therapeutic Goods Administration: Canberra, Australia, 2019. Available online: https://www.tga.gov.au/complementary-medicines (accessed on 2 March 2020).
2. Xue, C.; Zhang, A.; Lin, V.; Da Costa, C.; Story, D. Complementary and alternative medicine use in Australia: A national population-based survey. *J. Altern. Complement. Med.* **2007**, *13*, 643–650. [CrossRef]
3. Steel, A.; McIntyre, E.; Harnett, J.; Foley, H.; Adams, J.; Sibbritt, D.; Wardle, J.; Frawley, J. Complementary medicine use in the Australian population: Results of a nationally-representative cross-sectional survey. *Sci. Rep.* **2018**, *8*, 17325. [CrossRef]
4. Cramer, H.; Shaw, A.; Wye, L.; Weiss, M. Over-the-counter advice seeking about complementary and alternative medicines (CAM) in community pharmacies and health shops: An ethnographic study. *Health Soc. Care Community* **2010**, *18*, 41–50. [CrossRef]
5. Ung, C.O.L.; Harnett, J.; Hu, H. Community pharmacist's responsibilities with regards to traditional medicine/complementary medicine products: A systematic literature review. *Res. Soc. Adm. Pharm.* **2017**, *13*, 686–716. [CrossRef]
6. Pharmaceutical Society of Australia. *Pharmacuetical Society of Australia Code of Ethics for Pharmacists*; Pharmaceutical Society of Australia: Canberra, Australia, 2017. Available online: https://www.psa.org.au/membership/ethics/ (accessed on 13 April 2020).

7. Soleymani, S.; Bahramsoltani, R.; Rahimi, R.; Abdollahi, M. Clinical risks of St John's Wort (Hypericum perforatum) co-administration. *Expert Opin. Drug Metab. Toxicol.* **2017**, *13*, 1047–1062. [CrossRef]
8. Chrubasik-Hausmann, S.; Vlachojannis, J.; McLachlan, A.J. Understanding drug interactions with St John's wort (Hypericum perforatum L.): Impact of hyperforin content. *J. Pharm. Pharmacol.* **2019**, *71*, 129–138. [CrossRef]
9. Hennessy, M.; Kelleher, D.; Spiers, J.; Barry, M.; Kavanagh, P.; Back, D.; Mulcahy, F.; Feely, J. St John's wort increases expression of P-glycoprotein: Implications for drug interactions. *Br. J. Clin. Pharmacol.* **2002**, *53*, 75–82. [CrossRef]
10. Biffignandi, P.M.; Bilia, A.R. The growing knowledge of St. John's wort (Hypericum perforatum L) drug interactions and their clinical significance. *Curr. Ther. Res.* **2000**, *61*, 389–394. [CrossRef]
11. Ung, C.O.L.; Harnett, J.; Hu, H. Key stakeholder perspectives on the barriers and solutions to pharmacy practice towards complementary medicines: An Australian experience. *BMC Complement. Altern. Med.* **2017**, *17*, 394. [CrossRef]
12. Pharmacy Board of Australia. *Guidelines on Practice-Specific Issues*; Australian Government Australia: Canberra, Australia, 2015. Available online: http://www.pharmacyboard.gov.au (accessed on 13 April 2020).
13. Emmerton, L. The 'third class' of medications: Sales and purchasing behavior are associated with pharmacist only and pharmacy medicine classifications in Australia. *J. Am. Pharm. Assoc.* **2009**, *49*, 31–37. [CrossRef]
14. Cairns, R.; Brown, J.A.; Buckley, N.A. The impact of codeine re-scheduling on misuse: A retrospective review of calls to Australia's largest poisons centre. *Addiction* **2016**, *111*, 1848–1853. [CrossRef]
15. Harnett, J.E.; Ung, C.O.L.; Hu, H.; Sultani, M.; Desselle, S.P. Advancing the pharmacist's role in promoting the appropriate and safe use of dietary supplements. *Complement. Ther. Med.* **2019**, *44*, 174–181. [CrossRef]
16. Pharmaceutical Society of Australia. Complementary Medicines Position Statement. 2015. Available online: http://www.psa.org.au/downloads/ent/uploads/filebase/policies/position-statement-complementary-medicines.pdf (accessed on 13 April 2020).
17. American Society of Health-System Pharmacists. Statement on the use of dietary supplements. *Am. J. Health-SystPharm.* **2004**, *61*, 1707–1711.
18. The Australian Government Department of Education: The Australian Industry and Skills Committee. Community Pharmacy. The Australian Government. 2020. Available online: https://nationalindustryinsights.aisc.net.au/industries/retail-and-wholesale/community-pharmacy (accessed on 13 April 2020).
19. The Australian Government Department of Health and Ageing Australia. *Pharmacy Guild of Australia*; Australian Government the Pharmacy Workforce Planning Study: Canberra Australia, 2020; Chapter 3, p. 14, Table 3.
20. Arksey, H.; O'Malley, L. Scoping studies: Towards a methodological framework. *Int. J. Soc. Res. Methodol.* **2005**, *8*, 19–32. [CrossRef]
21. Shamseer, L.; Moher, D.; Clarke, M.; Ghersi, D.; Liberati, A.; Petticrew, M.; Shekelle, P.; Stewart, L.A. Preferred reporting items for systematic review and meta-analysis protocols (PRISMA-P) 2015: Elaboration and explanation. *BMJ* **2015**, *349*. [CrossRef]
22. Harnett, J.E.; McIntyre, E.; Steel, A.; Foley, H.; Sibbritt, D.; Adams, J. Use of complementary medicine products: A nationally representative cross-sectional survey of 2019 Australian adults. *BMJ Open* **2019**, *9*, 024198. [CrossRef]
23. Carney, T.; Wells, J.; Bergin, M.; Dada, S.; Foley, M.; McGuiness, P.; Rapca, A.; Rich, E.; Van Hout, M.C. A Comparative exploration of community pharmacists' views on the nature and management of over-the-counter (OTC) and prescription codeine misuse in three regulatory regimes: Ireland, South Africa and the United Kingdom. *Int. J. Ment. Health Addict.* **2016**, *14*, 351–369. [CrossRef]
24. Kennedy, C.; Duggan, E.; Bennett, K.; Williams, D.J. Rates of reported codeine-related poisonings and codeine prescribing following new national guidance in Ireland. *Pharmacoepidemiol. Drug Saf.* **2019**, *28*, 106–111. [CrossRef]
25. Hamer, A.M.; Spark, M.J.; Wood, P.J.; Roberts, E. The upscheduling of combination analgesics containing codeine: The impact on the practice of pharmacists. *Res. Soc. Adm. Pharm.* **2014**, *10*, 669–678. [CrossRef]
26. Mishriky, J.; Stupans, I.; Chan, V. Pharmacists' views on the upscheduling of codeine-containing analgesics to 'prescription only' medicines in Australia. *Int. J. Clin. Pharm.* **2019**, *41*, 538–545. [CrossRef]
27. Izzo, A.A.; Hoon-Kim, S.; Radhakrishnan, R.; Williamson, E.M. A critical approach to evaluating clinical efficacy, adverse events and drug interactions of herbal remedies. *Phytother. Res.* **2016**, *30*, 691–700. [CrossRef]

28. Posadzki, P.; Watson, L.; Ernst, E. Herb-drug interactions: An overview of systematic reviews. *Br. J. Clin. Pharmacol.* **2013**, *75*, 603–618. [CrossRef]
29. De Souza Silva, J.E.; Souza, C.A.S.; da Silva, T.B.; Gomes, I.A.; de Carvalho Brito, G.; de Souza Araújo, A.A.; de Lyra-Júnior, D.P.; da Silva, W.B.; da Silva, F.A. Use of herbal medicines by elderly patients: A systematic review. *Arch. Gerontol. Geriatr.* **2014**, *59*, 227–233. [CrossRef] [PubMed]
30. Tachjian, A.; Maria, V.; Jahangir, A. Use of herbal products and potential interactions in patients with cardiovascular diseases. *J. Am. College Cardiol.* **2010**, *55*, 515–525. [CrossRef] [PubMed]
31. Doucette, W.R.; Schommer, J.C. Pharmacy technicians' willingness to perform emerging tasks in community practice. *Pharmacy* **2018**, *6*, 113. [CrossRef]
32. Desselle, S.P.; Hoh, R.; Holmes, E.R.; Gill, A.; Zamora, L. Pharmacy technician self-efficacies: Insight to aid future education, staff development, and workforce planning. *Res. Soc. Adm. Pharm.* **2018**, *14*, 581–588. [CrossRef] [PubMed]
33. Ung, C.O.L.; Harnett, J.E.; Hu, H.; Desselle, S. Barriers to US pharmacists adopting professional responsibilities that support the appropriate and safe use of natural products by Americans—Key stakeholders perspectives. *Am. J. Hosp. Pharm.* **2019**, *76*, 980–990.

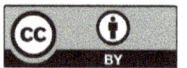

© 2020 by the authors. Licensee MDPI, Basel, Switzerland. This article is an open access article distributed under the terms and conditions of the Creative Commons Attribution (CC BY) license (http://creativecommons.org/licenses/by/4.0/).

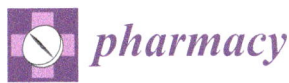

Article

Pharmacy Technicians' Contribution to Counselling at Community Pharmacies in Denmark

Mira El-Souri [1,*], Rikke Nørgaard Hansen [1], Ann Moon Raagaard [2], Birthe Søndergaard [3] and Charlotte Rossing [1,*]

[1] Department of Research and Development, Pharmakon, Danish College of Pharmacy Practice, 3400 Hilleroed, Denmark; rnh@pharmakon.dk
[2] Danish Association of Pharmacy Technicians, 2500 Valby, Denmark; amr@farmakonom.dk
[3] Association of Danish Pharmacies, 1260 Copenhagen, Denmark; bis@apotekerforeningen.dk
* Correspondence: mso@pharmakon.dk (M.E.-S.); cr@pharmakon.dk (C.R.)

Received: 25 February 2020; Accepted: 19 March 2020; Published: 23 March 2020

Abstract: (1) **Background:** pharmacy technicians are the largest group of staff at Danish community pharmacies and play a vital role in counselling customers on prescription medication, over-the-counter (OTC) medication and non-medical products. This is the first study carried out to specifically analyse how they contribute to counselling and identification of drug-related problems (DRPs) at Danish community pharmacies. (2) **Methods:** seventy-six pharmacy technicians from 38 community pharmacies registered data on all of their customer visits for five days, over a four-week period, between January and March 2019. Data were analysed in SPSS version 24. (3) **Results:** 58.9% of all registered customers (n = 10,417) received counselling. They identified DRPs for 15.8% of all registered customers (n = 2800). Counselling by pharmacy technicians solved, or partially solved, problems for 70.4% of customers with DRPs. Pharmacy technicians estimated that 25.2% of customers receiving counselling (n = 2621) were saved a visit to the general practitioner (GP). (4) **Conclusions:** as community pharmacists get more involved in complex services, it would be necessary to expand the roles of pharmacy technicians. Pharmacy technicians contribute to medication safety via counselling, and identifying and handling DRPs for all customers. This study documents the role of pharmacy technicians in customer counselling at Danish community pharmacies. It provides evidence to researchers and policy makers to support discussions on the future role of pharmacy technicians at community pharmacies.

Keywords: pharmacy technicians; counselling; drug-related problems; community pharmacy; OTC medication; prescription medication; non-medical products

1. Introduction

Pharmacy technicians (in Denmark called pharmaconomists), with a three-year degree, are the largest group of staff at Danish community pharmacies. Their roles are expansive and bear some resemblance to those of pharmacists in some countries. They play a vital role in counselling customers on prescription medication, over-the-counter (OTC) medication and non-medical products. In general, pharmacy technicians perform a broad array of tasks in community pharmacies, except for the more complex pharmacotherapeutic ones. In Denmark, pharmacy technicians can deliver services, such as Inhaler Technique Assessment Service, teaching and quality assurance. Some community pharmacy services, such as medication review and New Medicine Service, are restricted to be delivered by pharmacists. In Denmark, all pharmacy technicians are educated at the Danish College of Pharmacy Practice, Department of Education.

Denmark has a population of 5.7 million people; they are served by 237 community pharmacies, 254 branch pharmacies and two online pharmacies that offer prescription medication, OTC medication and a restricted selection of non-medical products [1]. This means that there is a community pharmacy or a branch pharmacy for every 11,600 inhabitants. Furthermore, there are 29 medicine distribution units that offer OTC medication, a restricted selection of non-medical products and pre-ordered prescription medication. Normally, counselling at these units is provided by pharmacy technicians [1]. Finally, there are 750 medicine distribution units, where only pre-ordered medicine is provided. No counselling is offered here as there are no pharmacists or pharmacy technicians, and unskilled staff are not allowed to give information on medicines [1]. Having all these different units ensures easy access to medicines in all regions of Denmark.

Community pharmacies and the appurtenant branch pharmacies in Denmark provide medical supplies, information, counselling and preventive health services by pharmacy technicians, along with pharmacists, to ensure the safe use of drugs [2].

Drug-related problems (DRPs) are common and associated with economic and patient-related costs [3,4]. A drug-related problem is defined by Hepler and Strand as: "an event or a circumstance involving drug treatment that actually or potentially interferes with the patient's experiencing an optimum outcome of medical care" [5]. Examples of DRPs are inappropriate drug use, adverse reactions and non-adherence.

Previous research shows that pharmacists play a role in identifying DRPs for customers at community pharmacies and that they contribute to solving them [6–13]. Research on DRPs focuses on evaluating community pharmacist-driven programmes, mostly at community pharmacies, but also, for example, in care facilities for the elderly [10,11,14,15]. Previous and ongoing research also focus on evaluating counselling, including identification and solving of DRPs in daily practice in community pharmacies. Some of this research also included counselling provided by pharmacy technicians along with pharmacists [13,16,17].

Pharmacy technicians, in general, are being accorded greater scopes of practice in community pharmacies, and, in particular, Danish pharmacy technicians are playing a vital role in counselling customers [18–20]. A previous Danish study on DRPs in self-medication showed that pharmacists and pharmacy technicians identified DRPs for 21% of pharmacy customers presenting a symptom or requesting OTC medication [13]. However, it has, so far, not been documented how pharmacy technicians, in particular, contribute to counselling in general, and handling of DRPs at community pharmacies. It is crucial to document their contribution in order to feed the discussion of their future roles at community pharmacies.

The objective of this study is to map the pharmacy technicians' counselling activities regarding prescription medication, OTC medication and non-medical products at community pharmacies in Denmark and to describe how pharmacy technicians identify and handle DRPs.

This is the first study carried out to specifically analyse how pharmacy technicians contribute to counselling and DRP identification at Danish community pharmacies. The study was carried out in collaboration with the Danish Association of Pharmacy Technicians, the Association of Danish Pharmacies and Pharmakon–Danish College of Pharmacy Practice.

2. Materials and Methods

The design of the study is quantitative, comprising a descriptive approach.

All community pharmacies were invited to participate in the study through different media, including professional groups on LinkedIn and Facebook, newsletters from the Danish Association of Pharmacy Technicians, the Association of Danish Pharmacies and Pharmakon–Danish College of Pharmacy Practice.

To ensure the representativity of community pharmacies in Denmark, a list of Danish community pharmacies was used, and every fourth community pharmacy on the list was called. The community pharmacies were selected so that the number of recruited community pharmacies in each region reflected the number of pharmacies as much as possible. Seventy-six pharmacy technicians from 38 community pharmacies (two pharmacy technicians from each pharmacy) from all Danish regions were recruited after responding to a nationwide invitation. Fourteen community pharmacies were recruited by phone by the research group.

The geographic distribution of the included pharmacies is illustrated in Figure 1.

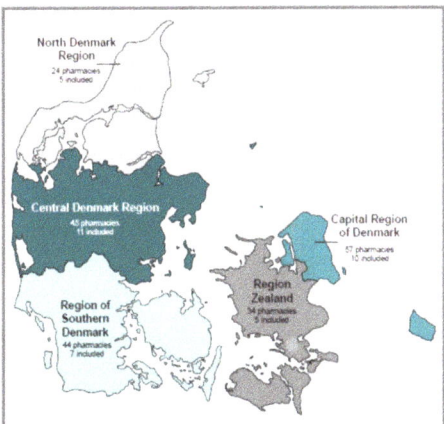

Figure 1. Number of community pharmacies included in each region.

The participating pharmacy technicians registered data on all their customer visits to the community pharmacies for five days over a four-week period between January and March 2019. They registered on different days of the week to cover the normal opening hours of most community pharmacies in Denmark.

At the beginning of the study period, the pharmacy technicians were introduced to the study through a webinar and self-study. They received training on registration consisting of an instruction and eight cases, which they were requested to solve before starting the registration process. During the study period, the research group held two question and answer (Q&A) webinars and could furthermore be contacted for support on registration.

The registration was carried out in an electronic survey developed by researchers and representatives from the Danish Association of Pharmacy Technicians and the Association of Danish Pharmacies. It was also pilot-tested by two pharmacy technicians and adjusted afterwards prior to being used in the study. The registration had the following questions: gender and age of the customer, type of errand(s), type of identified DRP(s), counselling subject(s), solving of DRP(s) and whether the counselling saved a visit to the general practitioner (GP). Most of the questions could be answered by clicking on a drop-down menu to save time. All types of DRPs and the counselling subjects were defined by the research group and adjusted after the pilot study. All questions in the registration were answered by the pharmacy technicians and, therefore, the data is self-reported.

In order to document the proportion of customers registered, the pharmacy technicians registered the total amount of customer visits received on the days chosen for registration.

Data was analysed in SPSS version 24 (IBM Corp., Armonk, NY, USA).

3. Results

Information about a total of 17,692 customers was registered. Of these, 61.0% (n = 10,785) requested prescription medication, 15.7% (n = 2773) requested OTC medication or presented a symptom, 10.9% (n = 1937) requested non-medical products and 12.4% (n = 2197) inquired about a mix of the three categories (Figure 2).

The results are presented for the total study population and for these subgroups:

- customers requesting prescription medication,

- customers requesting OTC medication or presenting a symptom,
- customers requesting non-medical products.

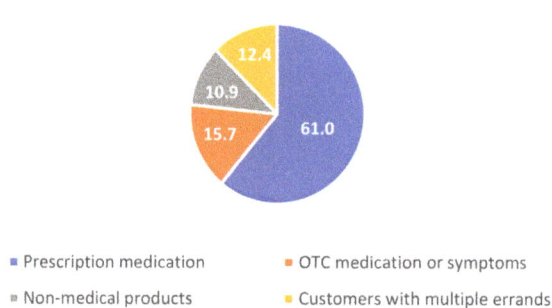

Figure 2. The categories of the customers in the study.

3.1. Description of the Study Population

3.1.1. Proportion of Customers Registered

According to the participating pharmacies check-out systems, they had a total of 21,621 customer visits on the days they registered. The total amount of customers registered was 17,692. That means that 82% of customer visits were registered.

3.1.2. Gender and Age of the Total Study Population

Gender and age were registered for all 17,692 registered customer visits; 58.7% (n = 10,377) were women, 41.3% (n = 7315) were men. Moreover, 52.0% (n = 9199) were between 21 and 64 years old; 38.6% (n = 6835) were 65 years or older; 5.1% of the visits (n = 909) were about children (0–15 years).

3.2. Counselling

3.2.1. Extent of Counselling in the Subgroups

56.1% of customers requesting prescription medication (n = 6050) received counselling on one or more subjects. This was also the case for 68.0% of customers requesting OTC medication or presenting a symptom (n = 1885) and 46.7% of customers requesting non-medical products (n = 905). The reasons why customers did not receive counselling were: the drug/product was for someone else, the customer was familiar with the drug/product, the customer had received counselling at the general practitioner (GP)/hospital, the customer had a language barrier or the customer was a doctor/nurse.

3.2.2. Counselling Subjects

Table 1 presents an overview of the subjects covered by the counselling.

"Drug/product use" was the most frequent subject in counselling for the total study population and in all subgroups. It accounted for 58.4% of all customers who received counselling; 56.4% of customers who requested prescription medication received counselling; 48.8% of customers who requested OTC medication or who presented a symptom received counselling and 67.6% of customers who requested non-medical products received counselling.

In counselling of customers who requested prescription medication, the second and third most frequent subjects were "adverse reactions" and "effect of the drug" (30.9% and 29.0% of customers received counselling).

In counselling costumers who requested OTC medication/presenting a symptom, the second and third most frequent subjects were "effect of the drug" and "personal care" (32.9% and 24.6% of customers received counselling).

In counselling costumers who requested non-medical products, the second and third most frequent subjects were "personal care" and "effect of the drug" (34.0% and 27.6% of customers received counselling).

Table 1. Subjects covered in counselling for the total study population and the three subgroups. The most frequent counselling subjects are highlighted * (threshold value 15.0%).

Subject	All Customers Who Received Counselling (N = 10,417) % (n)	Customers Requesting Prescription Medication Who Received Counselling (N = 6050) % (n)	Customers Requesting OTC Medication or Presenting a Symptom Who Received Counselling (N = 2773) % (n)	Customers Requesting Only Non-Medical Products Who Received Counselling (N = 905) % (n)
Personal care	28.7% (2987) *	23.4% (1414) *	24.6% (683) *	34.0% (308) *
Adverse reactions	26.3% (2743) *	30.9% (1870) *	15.1% (419) *	3.6% (33)
Effect of the drug/product	34.6% (3604) *	29.0% (1754) *	32.9% (913) *	27.6% (250) *
Interactions	4.3% (448)	3.5% (214)	4.5% (126)	2.2% (20)
Drug/product use	58.4% (6079) *	56.4% (3410) *	48.8% (1352) *	67.6% (612) *
Adherence	17.6% (1830) *	19.2% (1162) *	9.2% (256)	7.8% (71)
Recommendation for a drug/product	7.4% (771)	3.6% (218)	9.2% (256)	12.9% (117)
Recommendation for another drug/product than the one requested	4.5% (467)	1.7% (104)	5.9% (164)	8.4% (76)
Recommendation for automated dose dispensing	0.1% (14)	0.2% (13)	0% (0)	0% (0)
Drug/product substitution	18.2% (1901)	25.2% (1525) *	3.5% (96)	1.8% (16)
Reimbursement	6.5% (680)	9.0% (542)	1.3% (36)	0.9% (8)
Medication waste	0.7% (69)	0.9% (57)	0.3% (7)	0.1% (1)
The pharmacy technician contacted the GP	1.2% (121)	1.7% (103)	0.1% (4)	0.1% (1)
The pharmacy technician recommended the customer to contact a GP	12.8% (1336)	13.9% (841)	8.4% (233)	5.6% (51)
Total	221.3% (23,050) **	218.6% (13,227) **	163.9% (4545) **	172.8% (1564) **

** The percentage is over 100% due to the fact that some customers received counselling on more than one subject. GP = general practitioner; OTC = over-the-counter.

The pharmacy technicians estimated that their counselling saved 25.2% of the customers (n = 2621) a visit to the GP, broken down by 22.9% of customers requesting prescription medication (n = 1383), 30.7% of customers requesting OTC medication or presenting a symptom (n = 578) and 17.7% of customers requesting non-medical products (n = 160).

3.3. Occurrence and Types of DRPs

One or more DRPs were identified for 15.8% of the total study population (n = 2800), 17.8% of customers requesting only prescription medication (n = 1917), 12.7% of customers requesting only OTC medication or presenting a symptom (n = 352), and 6.9% of customers requesting only non-medical products (n = 133).

Table 2 shows the types of DRPs identified in the study. The types of DRPs are divided into two categories: (1) treatment effectiveness and safety problems and (2) logistical problems.

Table 2. Drug-related problems (DRPs) in the total study population and in the three categories of customers. The most frequent DRPs are highlighted * (threshold value 8.0%).

DRP	All Customers with DRPs, (N = 2800) % (n)	Customers with DRPs Requesting Only Prescription Medication, (N = 1917) % (n)	Customers with DRPs Requesting Only OTC Medication or Presenting a Symptom, (N = 352) % (n)	Customers with DRPs Requesting Only Non-Medical Products, (N = 133) % (n)
Treatment effectiveness and treatment safety problems				
Inappropriate drug/product	5.8% (163)	1.5% (28)	17.6% (62) *	27.1% (36) *
Contraindication	1.1% (30)	0.4% (7)	3.1% (11)	1.5% (2)
Double dose	2.2% (62)	1.4% (27)	4.5% (16)	1.5% (2)
Interaction	1.8% (51)	1.0% (19)	3.4% (12)	2.3% (3)
Drug dose too high	2.9% (81)	2.3% (45)	5.1% (18)	2.3% (3)
Drug dose too low	3.4% (96)	2.3% (44)	7.4% (26)	5.3% (7)
Duration of treatment too long	2.9% (81)	1.4% (26)	8.8% (31) *	0.8% (1)
Duration of treatment too short	1.8% (50)	1.3% (25)	3.7% (13)	0.8% (1)
Adverse reaction	9.2% (257) *	8.1% (156) *	9.4% (33) *	6.0% (8)
Symptom that requires a visit to a GP	6.4% (179)	3.3% (64)	17.3% (61) *	8.3% (11) *
Problem with practical use of drug/product	4.1% (116)	3.9% (75)	5.7% (20)	6.0% (8)
Non-adherence	7.6% (214)	8.0% (153) *	5.1% (18)	5.3% (7)
Logistical problems				
Prescription is incomplete or inaccurate	6.4% (179)	8.7% (166) *	-	-
Product or prescribed drug not available	20.6% (578) *	22.7% (436) *	12.5% (44) *	21.1% (28) *
Prescription not available	24.0% (673) *	30.6% (586) *	-	-
Other problems				
Other problems	9.5% (265) *	3.1% (60)	-	12.0% (16)
Total	104.0% (3075) **	100.0% (1917)	103.6% (365) **	100.0% (133)

** The percentage is over 100% due to the fact that some customers had more than one DRP.

3.3.1. Types of DRP—Treatment Effectiveness and Safety Problems

The most frequent DRPs related to treatment effectiveness and safety vary between the subgroups (Table 2). "Adverse reactions" and "non-adherence" were the most common DRPs for customers requesting prescription medication (8.1% and 8.0% of customers with DRPs).

The most common DRPs relating to OTC medication or a symptom were "inappropriate drug/product", "symptom that requires a visit to the GP" (17.6% and 17.3% of customers with DRPs).

Regarding customers requesting non-medical products, the most frequent DRPs were "inappropriate drug/product" and "symptom that requires a visit to the GP" (27.1% and 8.3% of customers with DRPs).

3.3.2. Types of DRP—Logistical Problems

The most frequent logistical problems identified for customers requesting prescription medication were that the prescription was not available, the drug/product requested was not available and the prescription was incomplete or inaccurate (30.6%, 22.7% and 8.7% of customers with DRPs).

A frequent DRP for customers requesting OTC medication, or presenting a symptom, was that the drug/product they requested was not available (12.5% of customers with DRPs). This was also a frequent DRP for customers requesting non-medical products (21.1% of customers with DRPs).

3.3.3. Solving of Identified DRPs

The pharmacy technicians estimated that 51.9% of customers with DRPs got their DRP solved, 18.5% of customers with DRPs got their problems partially solved and 20.5% of customers with DRPs did not get their problems solved (n = 1452; n = 517; n = 575). For 9.1% of customers with DRPs, the pharmacy technicians answered "don't know" or gave no answer (n = 256).

4. Discussion

4.1. Discussion of the Results

4.1.1. Proportion of Customers Receiving Counselling

A study mapping Norwegian community pharmacy counselling shows that 60% of the customers receive counselling [17]. Although 80% of the participants in the Norwegian study are community pharmacists, and all of the participants in this study are pharmacy technicians, the proportion of customers receiving counselling in the two studies is comparable.

4.1.2. Counselling Customers Requesting OTC Medication or Presenting a Symptom

In an earlier Danish study mapping DRPs in OTC medication customers, identified by pharmacy technicians and community pharmacists, the most frequent counselling subjects were "counselling on self-medication", "personal care" and "recommendation of a drug/product" [13]. There are similarities between the findings in the two Danish studies because "counselling on self-medication" can cover both of the following subjects: "drug/product use" and "effect of the drug", which were the two most frequent counselling subjects for customers requesting OTC medication or presenting a symptom in this study. In a German study mapping DRPs in OTC medication customers, identified by community pharmacists, the most frequent subjects were "referral to a physician" and "switching to a more appropriate drug" [21]. Pharmacy technicians in this study referred customers to their GP, and they recommended more appropriate drugs/products to some of the customers. However, these two categories were not the most frequent ones. These results show that pharmacy technician counselling is comparable to counselling delivered by community pharmacists, especially in a Danish setting.

4.1.3. Types of DRPs in the Total Study Population

In a German study mapping the DRPs encountered in community pharmacies, identified by pharmacists, the most frequent types of DRPs were "evidence of drug-drug interaction in the literature", "incomplete or unreadable prescription" and "drug not on the market" [7]. It is remarkable that drug-drug interaction is the most frequent DRP in the German study. There are two evidence-based electronic databases in Denmark in which health professionals and patients, respectively, can check for drug-drug interactions. It must be checked if the interactions are clinically relevant; most often only a few of them are. Drug-drug interactions are identified in this study, but are not among the most frequently registered DRPs; but of course, it can be crucial when it is clinically relevant. Otherwise, the next two frequently registered types of DRPs in the German study are similar to the two most frequently registered types of DRPs in this study. Thus, the types of DRPs identified by pharmacy technicians are comparable to those found by pharmacists.

Drug shortage is an international problem and a known and increasing problem in Danish community pharmacies [22,23]. The Association of Danish Pharmacies was contacted by the research group, and they had not detected any extraordinary fluctuation in the frequency of drug shortages in the study period.

A high rate of unavailable prescriptions was shown in this study. A newly published study shows that unavailable prescriptions occur in 1% of all dispensing in Danish community pharmacies. Miscommunication between the patient and GP seems to be the primary source of unavailable prescriptions [24].

4.1.4. Occurrence of DRPs for OTC Medication Customers

DRPs were identified for 15.8% of the total study population and for 12.7% of customers requesting OTC medication or presenting a symptom. The earlier German study documented DRPs in 17.6% of all cases [21]. The earlier Danish study documented DRPs in 21.0% of OTC medication customers [13]. Both studies showed a higher occurrence of identified DRPs in OTC medication customers than this study. It is important to mention that the percentages in the Danish studies are calculated as percentage (%) per customer. The percentages in the German study are calculated as percentage (%) per case or request. So, the Danish results are not comparable with the results from the German study. The percentage in the German study may be lower than 17.6%, as it can be assumed that some of the customers had multiple DRPs. The high occurrence of DRPs identified in the earlier Danish study may be due to extra focus on OTC medication customers during the study period, as it was the aim of the study.

4.1.5. Types of DRPs in Customers Requesting OTC Medication or Presenting a Symptom

The most frequent types of DRPs identified for customers requesting OTC medication or presenting a symptom were "inappropriate drug/product", "symptom that requires a visit to the GP", "adverse reaction" and "duration of treatment too long" (17.6%, 17.3%, 9.4% and 8.8% of customers with DRPs). There are similarities to the German study, which reported that the most frequent DRPs were "self-medication inappropriate", requested drug inappropriate" and "intended duration of drug use too high". In the earlier Danish study, the most frequent types of DRPs were: "the choice of medication is not appropriate/optimal for the condition" (44.8%), "too little of the drug is being taken" (17.0%), "the drug is taken for too long" (15.0%) and "adverse reactions" (13.8%) [13]. The types of identified DRPs are also similar in the two Danish studies. It is remarkable that pharmacy technicians in this study identify symptoms that require a visit to the GP, which probably leads to early diagnosis and treatment, and in this manner, promotes patient safety.

4.1.6. Pharmacy Technicians' Contribution to Counselling and Handling of DRPs

This study documents that pharmacy technicians contribute to counselling in Danish community pharmacies. The subgroup with the highest proportion of customers receiving counselling represents those who request OTC medication or present a symptom (68.0% compared to 58.9% in the total study population). This is probably because most of these customers have not received any prior counselling from a healthcare professional on their OTC medication or their symptom, so they seek counselling at the community pharmacy, and this counselling could be very important for these customers.

Pharmacy technicians have shown that they can identify DRPs for all subgroups. The prevalence of DRPs identified by pharmacy technicians for customers requesting only prescription medication is comparable with the prevalence of DRPs identified by community pharmacists. A Belgian study on the identification and handling of DRPs by community pharmacists in the dispensing process documents that at least one DRP is found in 9869 on a total of 64,962 prescriptions (15%) [25]. The pharmacy technicians in this study solved, or partially solved, DRPs for 70.4% of customers with DRPs. This is also comparable with the Belgian study, where the community pharmacists solved almost 75% of the identified DRPs [25]. Pharmacy technicians contribute to patient safety. In particular, this is documented by the high extent of counselling provided to customers requesting OTC medication or presenting a symptom, and identification and solving of DRPs for customers requesting non-medical products. These customers would probably not have been counselled on DRPs if they had chosen to buy their products from other outlets than the community pharmacy.

4.2. Method Discussion

In order to ensure representativity, a couple of initiatives were carried out.

First, the community pharmacies were selected to reflect the number of pharmacies in each region.

Second, the participants were instructed to choose five days over a four-week period to register all visits and to choose different days of the week to avoid bias. The collected data do not indicate on which days of the week the registration took place, and we therefore cannot tell if the participants followed this instruction. If we look at the proportion of customers registered, which was 82% on average, it can be assumed that the proportion is high enough to conclude that the collected data is representative.

Third, the participants received training on the registration consisting of an instruction and eight cases, which they were requested to solve before starting the registration process. The participants had access to the correct answers, but it might have been better if they had received feedback on their answers from the researchers before starting their registration.

Due to the study design, the pharmacy technicians collected data on their own counselling activities—self-reported data. Questions, such as whether the counselling saved visits to the GP, were answered by the pharmacy technicians by self-estimation. They were asked to estimate whether the customer would have contacted the GP if they had not received counselling from the community pharmacy, and then, whether the counselling had saved the customer a visit to the GP. There might be a bias here. The wording of the question makes it difficult to give an answer as the pharmacy technicians are asked to estimate two scenarios at the same time.

5. Conclusions

Pharmacy technicians contribute to medication safety by counselling and identification and handling of DRPs for customers requesting prescription medication, OTC medication (including those presenting a symptom) and non-medical products.

Moreover, 58.9% of all registered customers (n = 10,417) received counselling.

Pharmacy technicians identified DRPs for 15.8% of all registered customers (n = 2800). Counselling by the pharmacy technicians solved, or partially solved, problems for 70.4% of customers with DRPs. The pharmacy technicians estimated that 25.2% of customers receiving counselling (n = 2621) were saved a visit to the GP.

As community pharmacists get more involved in complex services, it would be necessary to expand the roles of pharmacy technicians. This study maps and documents the important role of pharmacy technicians in counselling at Danish community pharmacies. It provides evidence to researchers and policy makers to support the discussion of the future role of pharmacy technicians in community pharmacies.

Author Contributions: Conceptualization, M.E.-S., R.N.H., B.S., C.R.; methodology, M.E.-S., R.N.H., A.M.R., B.S., C.R.; software, M.E.-S.; validation, R.N.H.; formal analysis, M.E.-S., R.N.H., A.M.R., B.S., C.R.; investigation, M.E.-S.; writing—original draft preparation, M.E.-S.; writing—review and editing, R.N.H., A.M.R., B.S., C.R.; visualization, M.E.-S., C.R.; project administration, M.E.-S., R.N.H., C.R.; funding acquisition, A.M.R., B.S., C.R. All authors have read and agreed to the published version of the manuscript.

Funding: This research was funded by the Danish Association of Pharmacy Technicians, the Association of Danish Pharmacies and Pharmakon–Danish College of Pharmacy Practice.

Acknowledgments: We acknowledge all who contributed to this research, especially the participating pharmacy technicians who registered their customer visits and the community pharmacy owners who gave their permission to include their community pharmacies in the study.

Conflicts of Interest: The funders were included in the recruitment of community pharmacies, analysis and interpretation of data. The design of the study, writing of the manuscript and the decision to publish the results rely on Pharmakon–Danish College of Pharmacy Practice.

References

1. Danish Medicines Agency. Pharmacies in Denmark. Available online: https://laegemiddelstyrelsen.dk/en/pharmacies/pharmacies/ (accessed on 12 September 2019).
2. Abrahamsen, B.; Burgle, H.A.; Rossing, C. Pharmaceutical Care services available in Danish Community Pharmacies. *Int. J. Clin. Pharm.* **2020**, 1–6. [CrossRef] [PubMed]
3. Thomsen, L.A.; Winterstein, A.G.; Sondergaard, B.; Haugbolle, L.S.; Melander, A. Systematic review of the incidence and characteristics of preventable adverse drug events in ambulatory care. *Ann. Pharmacother.* **2007**, *41*, 1411–1426. [CrossRef] [PubMed]
4. Jodar-Sanchez, F.; Malet-Larrea, A.; Martin, J.J.; Garcia-Mochon, L.; Lopez Del Amo, M.P.; Martinez-Martinez, F.; Gastelurrutia-Garralda, M.A.; Garcia-Cardenas, V.; Sabater-Hernandez, D.; Saez-Benito, L.; et al. Cost-utility analysis of a medication review with follow-up service for older adults with polypharmacy in community pharmacies in Spain: The conSIGUE program. *Pharmacoeconomics* **2015**, *33*, 599–610. [CrossRef] [PubMed]
5. Hepler, C.D.; Strand, L.M. Opportunities and responsibilities in pharmaceutical care. *Am. J. Hosp. Pharm.* **1990**, *47*, 533–543. [CrossRef] [PubMed]
6. Herborg, H.; Sørensen, E.W.; Frøkjær, B. Pharmaceutical care in community pharmacies: Practice and research in Denmark. *Ann. Pharmacother.* **2007**, *41*, 681–689. [CrossRef] [PubMed]
7. Hammerlein, A.; Griese, N.; Schulz, M. Survey of drug-related problems identified by community pharmacies. *Ann. Pharmacother.* **2007**, *41*, 1825–1832. [CrossRef]
8. Hämmerlein, A.; Müller, U.; Schulz, M. Pharmacist-led intervention study to improve inhalation technique in asthma and COPD patients. *J. Eval. Clin. Pract.* **2011**, *17*, 61–70. [CrossRef]
9. van Mil, J.W.; Dudok van Heel, M.C.; Boersma, M.; Tromp, T.F. Interventions and documentation for drug-related problems in Dutch community pharmacies. *Am. J. Health Syst. Pharm.* **2001**, *58*, 1428–1431. [CrossRef]
10. Dam, P.; El-Souri, M.; Herborg, H.; Nørgaard, L.S.; Rossing, C.; Sodemann, M.; Thomsen, L.A. Safe and effective use of medicines for ethnic minorities—A pharmacist-delivered counseling program that improves adherence. *J. Pharm. Care Health Syst.* **2015**, 2. [CrossRef]
11. Kjeldsen, L.J.; Bjerrum, L.; Dam, P.; Larsen, B.O.; Rossing, C.; Sondergaard, B.; Herborg, H. Safe and effective use of medicines for patients with type 2 diabetes—A randomized controlled trial of two interventions delivered by local pharmacies. *Res. Soc. Adm. Pharm. RSAP* **2015**, *11*, 47–62. [CrossRef]
12. Rossing, C. *The Practice of Pharmaceutical Care in Denmark—A Quantitative Approach*; University of Copenhagen: København, Denmark, 2003.
13. Frøkjær, B.; Bolvig, T.; Griese, N.; Herborg, H.; Rossing, C. Prevalence of drug-related problems in self-medication in Danish community pharmacies. *INNOVATIONS Pharm.* **2012**, 3. [CrossRef]
14. Kaae, S.; Dam, P.; Rossing, C. Evaluation of a pharmacy service helping patients to get a good start in taking their new medications for chronic diseases. *Res. Soc. Adm. Pharm.* **2016**, *12*, 486–495. [CrossRef] [PubMed]
15. Thomsen, L.A.; Rossing, C.; Trier, H.; Faber, M.; Herborg, H. Improving Safety in the Medicines Use Process for Disabled Persons in Residential Facilities. Results from a Pilot Study. *J. Clin. Toxicol.* **2014**, 4. [CrossRef]
16. Westerlund, L.T.; Marklund, B.R.; Handl, W.H.; Thunberg, M.E.; Allebeck, P. Nonprescription drug-related problems and pharmacy interventions. *Ann. Pharmacother.* **2001**, *35*, 1343–1349. [CrossRef]
17. Brock Nilsen, L. Mapping community pharmacy services: Important information of what is being done [Kartlegging av apotekstjenester: Viktig dokumentasjon av jobben som gjøres]. *Norsk Farmaceutisk Tidsskrift Norwegian* **2017**, *3*, 13–15.
18. Desselle, S.P.; Hoh, R.; Rossing, C.; Holmes, E.R.; Gill, A.; Zamora, L. The caring behaviours of Danish pharmaconomists: Insight for pharmacy technician practice around the world. *Int. J. Pharm. Pract.* **2019**, *27*, 157–165. [CrossRef]

19. Koehler, T.; Brown, A. Documenting the evolution of the relationship between the pharmacy support workforce and pharmacists to support patient care. *Res. Soc. Adm. Pharm. RSAP* **2017**, *13*, 280–285. [CrossRef]
20. Desselle, S.P.; Hoh, R.; Rossing, C.; Holmes, E.R.; Gill, A.; Zamora, L. Work Preferences and General Abilities Among US Pharmacy Technicians and Danish Pharmaconomists. *J. Pharm. Pract.* **2018**. [CrossRef]
21. Eickhoff, C.; Hammerlein, A.; Griese, N.; Schulz, M. Nature and frequency of drug-related problems in self-medication (over-the-counter drugs) in daily community pharmacy practice in Germany. *Pharmacoepidemiol. Drug Saf.* **2012**, *21*, 254–260. [CrossRef]
22. FDA. *Drug Shortages: Root Causes and Potential Solutions*; FDA: Silver Spring, MD, USA, 2019.
23. Lægemiddelstyrelsen. Drug Shortages [Medicinmangel]. Available online: https://laegemiddelstyrelsen.dk/da/godkendelse/kontrol-og-inspektion/mangel-paa-medicin/ (accessed on 20 September 2019).
24. Lundby, C.; Nielsen, A.V.; Bendixen, S.; Almarsdottir, A.B.; Pottegard, A. Unavailable prescriptions at Danish community pharmacies: A descriptive study. *Int. J. Clin. Pharm.* **2019**, *41*, 672–676. [CrossRef]
25. Huysmans, K.; De Wulf, I.; Foulon, V.; De Loof, H.; Steurbaut, S.; Boussery, K.; De Vriese, C.; Lacour, V.; Van Hees, T.; De Meyer, G.R. [Drug related problems in Belgian community pharmacies]. *J. Pharm. Belg.* **2014**, *1*, 4–15.

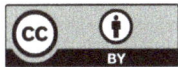

© 2020 by the authors. Licensee MDPI, Basel, Switzerland. This article is an open access article distributed under the terms and conditions of the Creative Commons Attribution (CC BY) license (http://creativecommons.org/licenses/by/4.0/).

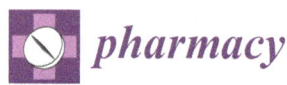

Article

Pharmacy Technicians' Roles and Responsibilities in the Community Pharmacy Sector: A Welsh Perspective

Rebecca Chamberlain [1,2,3,*], Jan Huyton [1] and Delyth James [2]

1. Cardiff School of Education and Social Policy, Cardiff Metropolitan University, Cardiff CF5 2YB, UK; jhuyton@cardiffmet.ac.uk
2. Cardiff School of Sport and Health Sciences, Cardiff Metropolitan University, Cardiff CF5 2YB, UK; dhjames@cardiffmet.ac.uk
3. Health Education Improvement Wales, Ty Dysgu, Cefn Coed, Nantgarw CF15 7QQ, UK
* Correspondence: rebecca.chamberlain2@wales.nhs.uk

Received: 5 March 2020; Accepted: 31 May 2020; Published: 4 June 2020

Abstract: Background: Healthcare delivery models in Wales are changing in response to unprecedented pressure on the National Health Service UK (NHS). Community pharmacies will be prioritised to address public health and clinical needs at a local level. To support the delivery of the new model, pharmacy technicians must be enabled and developed to optimize their roles. The aim of the study was to establish existing roles of pharmacy technicians working in the community pharmacy sector in Wales and to explore barriers and enablers to development. **Methods:** A combination of quantitative and qualitative methodologies was used, with the main focus on quantitative methods. A total of 83 participants completed an online questionnaire and additional qualitative data were obtained from four semi-structured telephone interviews. **Results:** The dispensing and final accuracy checking of medicines were reported as core functions of the community pharmacy technician role, with an average of 43% and 57% of time being spent on these roles, respectively. There was some evidence of engagement in leadership and management roles (average of 19%) and limited evidence of delivery of services (average of 6%). **Conclusions:** There is scope to enable community pharmacy technicians to optimize and further develop their roles. Enablers include the effective use of delegation, workplace support, improved staffing levels and the prioritisation of extended pharmacy technician roles.

Keywords: pharmacy technician; community pharmacy; roles; responsibilities; barriers; enablers; dispenser; pharmacy services; workforce development; wales

---

1. Introduction

The National Health Service (NHS) in the United Kingdom (UK) is under immense pressure to deliver quality healthcare with restricted resources [1]. The devolution of healthcare in the UK has led to significant differences in the commissioning of community pharmacy services across the four nations. In Wales, community pharmacies have been identified as a strategic priority for enabling the local delivery of public health and clinical services, with less focus on the supply of medicines [1–3]. These proposed changes have the potential to impact on the future roles and responsibilities of the community pharmacy workforce in Wales. In order to achieve the Government's strategic objectives, it is crucial that the skill mix of the pharmacy team is utilised to its optimum effectiveness [4]. The General Pharmaceutical Council (GPhC) (2018) reported that there were 23,318 pharmacy technicians (PTs) registered in the UK on 31 March 2017, with 53,967 registered pharmacists and 14,403 registered pharmacy premises [5].

PTs made the transition from an occupation to a profession in 2011, following introduction of professional registration—the title 'Pharmacy Technician' is protected in UK law [6]. Pharmacy technicians must renew their registration every year, by declaring that they remain fit to practice, in accordance with the GPhC's professional standards. The registration requirements are mandated by the GPhC and are the same regardless of sector. These are Level 3 National Vocational Qualification (NVQ) Diploma Pharmacy Services Skills (or equivalent), plus a Level 3 Diploma Pharmaceutical Science (or equivalent) and a minimum of 2 years' relevant work-based experience under the supervision of a pharmacist. Level 3 qualifications are equivalent to A-levels in the UK, a prerequisite to accessing a higher education diploma or degree. Pharmacists in the UK study to reach level 7 (Master's degree) qualifications in higher education institutions (i.e., universities). Pharmacy technicians in the UK are therefore not qualified at degree level.

PTs play an important role within the delivery of pharmacy services in the UK [7]. Defining the role is inherently difficult as there is no agreed definition or clear demarcation of the boundaries with the other members of the pharmacy team [8,9]. As a general overview, PTs are specialists in the technical aspects of medicines supply, e.g., procurement, stock management, sale, dispensing and final accuracy checking of dispensed medicines. PTs may provide guidance on the use of prescribed medicines and public health advice. PTs may manage technical staff and/or the provision of technical pharmacy services. For comparison, pharmacists are considered specialists in the clinical aspects of medicines supply, e.g., ensuring prescribed medicines are safe and appropriate for patients in terms of dose, form, interactions and contra-indications. Pharmacists are legally accountable for the safe and effective provision and delegation of pharmacy services. Current UK pharmacy legislation requires PTs to work under 'supervision' of a pharmacist. The law also recognises that pharmacists have scope to delegate tasks to appropriately trained and competent members of the pharmacy team. Despite the law and professional registration (specifically professional accountability) having been put in place to enable delegation, there appears to have been limited impact on the development of the pharmacy technician role.

The PT role differs significantly across the pharmacy sectors, particularly between community and hospital, which are the two sectors in which most PTs are employed [9]. Anecdotally, PTs working in the community pharmacy sector have traditionally focused on the sale and supply of medicines and related administrative functions. In recent years, accuracy checking of prescriptions has become a more established part of this role [9]. However, there has been limited scope for further development, which could, in part, be due to the lack of career structure and/or progression opportunities [10,11].

Evidence suggests that the PT role in community has remained similar to a 'dispenser' or 'pharmacy assistant' role [12], which is often limited to dispensing medicines and stock related activities. In general, dispensers or pharmacy assistants do not undertake the final accuracy checking of dispensed medicines, provide advice on prescribed medicines or manage pharmacy services. The terms 'dispenser' and 'pharmacy assistant' are used interchangeably (the term 'dispenser' will be used in this paper), to describe non-registered support staff who are trained to NVQ Level 2 or equivalent. Level 2 qualifications are equivalent to GCSE level education in the UK, which is typically completed in Grade 10 and 11 of high school.

1.1. Roles of Pharmacy Technicians

A recent systematic review concluded that PTs who are capable of performing more patient care activities are being underutilised [13]. In 2018, Desselle et al. surveyed 5000 pharmacy technicians across eight states of the United States of America (USA), to establish their involvement with specified practice activities [14]. They reported significant differences between community and hospital roles and a significant involvement with prescription receipt and dispensing. Less involvement was reported for roles such as supervising and checking the work of other technicians, despite participants expressing confidence to undertake such roles. Lower levels of confidence and involvement were reported for clinical roles, e.g., discussing effectiveness of treatment plans and providing medicines related advice.

This is consistent with Koehler and Brown's global online survey of pharmaceutical services in 2017 across 67 countries, where procurement and stock ordering were the most autonomous functions of the PT [15]. John and Brown (2017) also found that the sale and supply of medicines remains the core function of the PT's role in the UK [9].

A 2016 UK study by Boughen et al. [11] explored PT roles across all sectors, including community pharmacy. Survey responses from 71 community pharmacy technicians (CPTs) described a comprehensive list of roles that were undertaken, which mainly related to sale and supply, with some reference made to extended roles. There was no indication of the proportion of time spent on each of the tasks described, in order to provide an accurate picture of the current role. These findings are useful to inform further research, however, they cannot be generalised, due to limitations in the way the sample was recruited. Boughen et al. concluded that community pharmacy technician roles are less expansive and less clinically oriented than hospital pharmacy technician roles.

In 2016, Bradley et al. [7] surveyed a random sample of 1500 pharmacists and pharmacy technicians in England, to explore perceptions of risk associated with the delegation of duties to support staff carrying out roles without direct pharmacist supervision. Participants categorised twenty-two activities as 'safe' (e.g., dispensing), 'borderline' (e.g., issuing prescriptions and sales of medicines) or 'unsafe' (e.g., clinical activities). When compared with PTs and hospital pharmacists, community pharmacists were found to have a significantly higher perception of risk for the delegation of borderline tasks to support staff and were the least ready for change. This may be a barrier to the full realization of changes in practice and development of the PTs role in a community setting.

To date, there has not been any research to explore CPT roles within Wales, where the Welsh Government is prioritising and investing in the community pharmacy sector, as a mechanism to address localised health needs [16].

1.2. Aim

The aim of this study was to establish the existing roles and responsibilities of PTs working in the community pharmacy sector in Wales and to explore potential barriers and enablers to optimal role utilization within the pharmacy team.

2. Materials and Methods

2.1. Overview of Study

A combination of quantitative and qualitative methodologies was used to address the aim of the study. Whilst the focus of the study was predominantly a quantitative approach, an opportunity was provided for participants to add any comments to the survey and to take part in an in-depth telephone interview, to gather supportive and explanatory qualitative data [17]. See Figure 1. An online questionnaire was sent to PTs across Wales. The questionnaire design was based on the existing literature and extensive professional knowledge of the researcher (RC) and one of the study supervisors (DJ). The questionnaire included mainly closed questions, with the opportunity to provide free text comments. At the end of the questionnaire, participants were offered the opportunity to take part in a short telephone interview, if they wished. PTs were not incentivized to complete the questionnaire or participate in an interview.

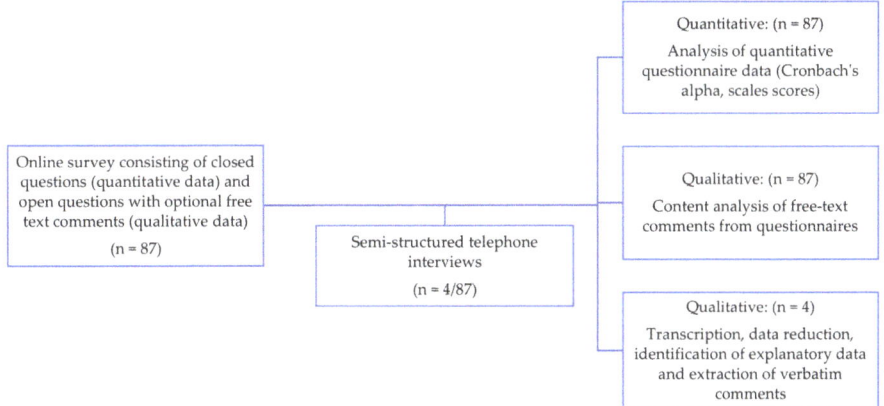

Figure 1. Overview of methodology.

2.2. Approvals and Ethical Considerations

Ethical approval for this study was obtained from the Research Ethics Committee at Cardiff Metropolitan University's School of Education and Social Policy (ethic approval code RC0118JH). Attention was paid to informed consent, anonymity, confidentiality, right to withdraw and data protection [18]. The Research and Insight Manager at GPhC approved the questionnaire, before distribution to all registered PTs who were resident in Wales.

2.3. Questionnaire

An online questionnaire was developed to gather demographic data, data relating to roles and responsibilities and pre- and post-registration training. Specific data were obtained for workplace support, professional identity and delegation, to ascertain whether or not these were barriers and/or enablers to current practice and future role development.

Standardised descriptors were used to categorise the type and size of pharmacy [11,12] —independent pharmacy; small chain (2–4 pharmacies); medium sized multiple (5–25 pharmacies); large multiple (over 25 pharmacies); supermarket pharmacy and other. A five-point Likert scale was used to rate agreement with statements relating to perceived barriers and enablers. (SD = strongly disagree; D = disagree; N = neither agree nor disagree; A = agree; SA = strongly agree. NA = not applicable was added where appropriate).

The wording of some Likert scale statements was reversed to reduce the risk of response bias [19]. Free text boxes were included at the end of each set of questions to enable participants to provide further comment and context [20]. The online questionnaire was piloted using three volunteers within the researcher's [RC] professional network and one of the supervisors (DJ), with expertise in questionnaire design. Revisions were made to improve the clarity of supporting information, the accuracy of rating scales and to resolve technical issues with how the survey was displayed (e.g., when responses to question 7 were filtered through to questions 8 and 9).

2.4. Interviews

Semi-structured, one-to-one telephone interviews were undertaken to obtain further insight into community PT roles and the barriers and enablers experienced. Participants were sent a participant information sheet and provided written consent for the interview to be recorded. A semi-structured interview schedule was developed, based on the existing literature and in-depth knowledge of two authors (RC and DJ) of the pharmacy technician workforce. This was used to identify the main topics for discussion and ensure consistency. Open-ended questions and prompts based on potential responses were prepared in advance to provide structure, whilst retaining some flexibility and allowing participants to determine the level of detail provided [21] (see Supplementary Materials). Interviewees were asked about their current roles, use of knowledge and skills in the workplace, efficacy of initial education and training and any further training undertaken. The interview also explored workplace support, delegation and potential enablers and barriers to conducting their role. Interviews were audio recorded and transcribed verbatim.

2.5. Sampling, Recruitment and Study Procedures

The GPhC register data do not differentiate registrants by sector of pharmacy, so a specific sampling framework could not be identified. The number of CPTs in Wales was estimated based on data indicating that 6.8% of all PTs in the UK live in Wales [22], equivalent to 1586. Of those, it has been estimated that 53% of PTs work in the community pharmacy sector [23], which is equivalent to 841.

The online questionnaire was disseminated to all registered pharmacy technicians in Wales by the GPhC in January 2018 via e-mail. The launch of the questionnaire was advertised via multiple pharmacy related social media platforms, clearly stating that the questionnaire was intended for community pharmacy technicians only. An initial filter question was added to the questionnaire to avoid completion by non-community-based PTs (32 responders who were not CPTs were redirected to the end of the questionnaire). The GPhC sent two follow up e-mails in February and March, both of which increased response rates.

The questionnaire was hosted on Qualtrics © software. An open access web link was added to the e-mail message and social media posts. Responses were captured over a 2-month period between January and March 2018. Interview audio data were transcribed by Sterling Transcription©, using Intelligent Verbatim (Standard Style).

2.6. Data Analysis

Quantitative analysis was undertaken using the report function within Qualtrics software (Version 2018 of Qualtrics, Copyright© 2018 Qualtrics, Provo, UT, USA); e.g., to calculate frequency distribution of demographic and categorical data. Data were extracted from Qualtrics into Microsoft Excel (Excel 97–2004, Microsoft Corporation, Redmond, WA, USA) to calculate central tendencies for interval data; e.g., percentage time spent dispensing per week. Data were also extracted from Qualtrics to the Statistical Package for the Social Sciences (SPSS Version 25.0 2018, IBM Corp, Armonk, NY, USA). Cronbach's alpha analysis was undertaken to estimate the internal consistency (reliability) of the scales. Negatively worded items were reversed scored and items which contributed to a poor alpha score were excluded from the respective scale (i.e., Q31R etc.) Scales with Cronbach's alpha scores > 0.7 were deemed to have good internal reliability [23] and therefore total scale scores were calculated for the following scales: efficacy of initial education (5 items), colleagues' understanding of training (2 items), workplace support (3 items), professional identity (3 items) and delegation (2 items). A Kruskal–Wallis test was used to compare responses from PTs across different categories of pharmacy, for questions relating to workplace support, professional support, recognition of professional identity and use of delegation.

Qualitative content analysis was undertaken by manually coding free-text written comments from questionnaires into categories, e.g., specific job roles, with one exception where quantitative content analysis was undertaken to measure the number of participants who reported a change in role since qualifying as a pharmacy technician. Categories were then grouped together to identify key themes, e.g., areas of pharmacy practice. Interview data were transcribed and simplified using a process known as data reduction [24], to produce a chart summarizing responses to each of the research topics and to identify further explanatory or supporting data. Verbatim quotes were extracted from the interview data for illustrative purposes. Quotes include the participant number, category of pharmacy and year of qualification for context.

3. Results

3.1. Participant Characteristics

A total of 83 questionnaires were fully completed, which represented approximately 10% of the PT population in Wales. Participant characteristics are presented in Table 1.

Table 1. Participant Characteristics (n = 83).

Characteristic	Frequencies
Number of years qualified	Range 1 to 38; Mean = 13 (SD = 8.2)
Qualified pre mandatory registration in 2011	n = 60 (69%)
Worked as a Dispenser prior to becoming a PT	n = 74 (89%)
Number of hours worked a week	Range 12 to 45; Mean 31.7 (SD = 7.84)

The number of years which participants had been qualified varied considerably from 1 year to 38 years, with an average of 13 years. The majority of participants (69%) qualified prior to the introduction of professional registration in 2011. The majority of participants (89%) had worked as a dispenser prior to becoming a PT.

All four participants who indicated their consent for a follow-up interview were contacted by telephone. Two male and two female participants were interviewed. Interviews lasted 29 to 52 min, with an average of 37 min. As the purpose of the interviews was to provide further explanation, relevant summaries of the interview data and verbatim quotes are presented alongside the questionnaire results.

Figure 2 displays the type of community pharmacy in which the participants worked. The majority of participants worked in a large multiple pharmacy (60%).

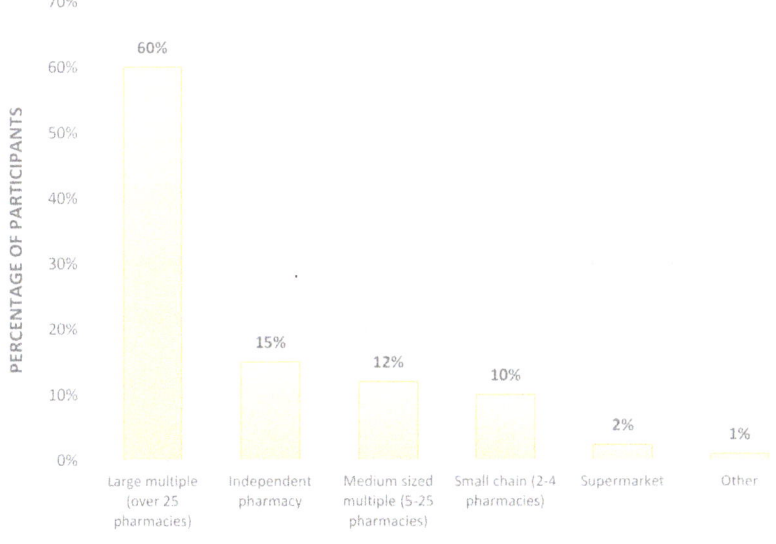

Figure 2. Category of pharmacy in which participants worked.

Figure 3 illustrates the delivery method of initial education and training (IET). The majority of participants studied via distance learning for BTEC and NVQ qualifications. A quarter (25.3%) of participants selected 'other'—where there were multiple references to studying via distance learning.

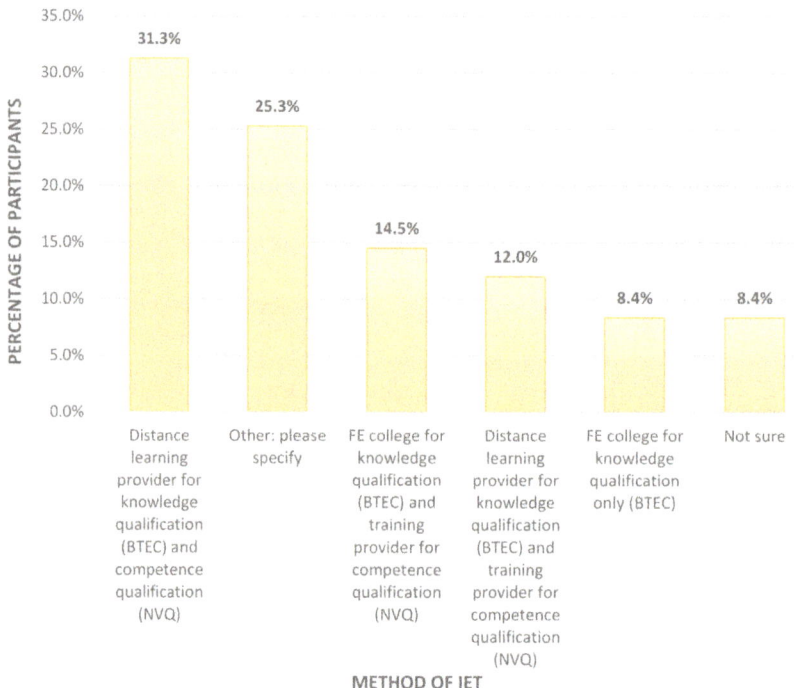

Figure 3. Delivery methods for Initial Education and Training (IET). Key: BTEC = Business and Technology Education Council; NVQ = National Vocational Qualification; FE = Further Education.

Figure 4 presents the post-registration training undertaken by participants. The total number of responses exceeds 83, as participants were able to select as many options as applied. Two thirds (n = 54) of CPTs were trained as accuracy checkers and a third (n = 27) had undergone stop smoking training. A fifth of participants (n = 15) had received advanced inhaler technique (AIT) training.

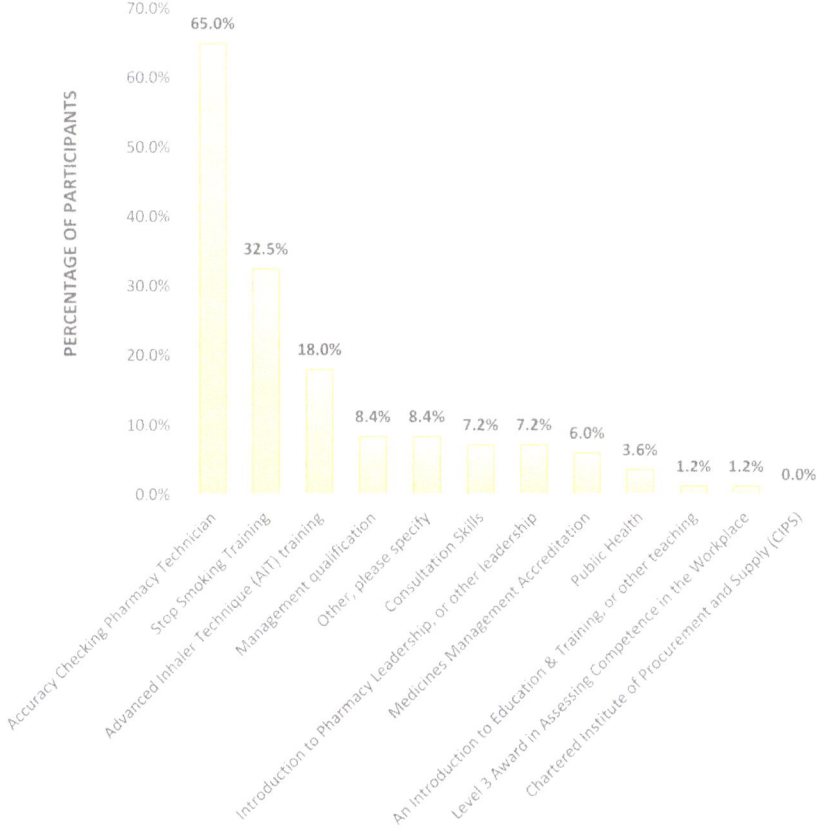

Figure 4. Post Registration training undertaken by participants.

Of the 54 trained accuracy checking pharmacy technicians (ACPTs), 26 reported that it had enabled them to final accuracy check prescriptions. Of the 27 stop smoking trained participants, 4 reported that they were enabled to deliver smoking cessation services. Of the 15 AIT trained participants, four reported that they were enabled to deliver smoking cessation services. Two of these took part in the semi-structured interviews. Interviewee B (independent pharmacy) reported,

> The smoking [training] certainly did [enable me to undertake the role effectively], because we've got a lot of patients on the program, so we do a lot of that in our area, which is good. I—it was just myself and the two pharmacists that—in our two stores and my—the pharmacist here is usually quite busy with other things. So, I tend to take the smoking cessation patients, which is fine with me, because I quite like the—being able to do that service, so—and the training was quite extensive and really in-depth. So, I was able to take that up from day one.

In contrast, Interviewee A (large multiple) stated,

> "Well with the independent [previous employer] I did the smoking with him, did that extra training, so I was certified for that".

Interviewee A wasn't involved in the smoking cessation service at that time of the interview and went on to explain,

> It's lapsed. It's lapsed, I just haven't used it for so long working with the company I work for now, they just—you know most of the pharmacists kind of deal with that, so there are technicians that do do it in the company, but as for me it just never happened.

3.2. PT Roles

Qualitative free text comments describing current roles were categorized to identify core roles. Participants were asked to assign a percentage of time to each role they described—only 40 responses were correctly recorded (i.e., percentages were recorded and totalled 100%). Figure 5 is based on 40 (48%) responders, which shows that the dispensing of medicines remains a core role for CPTs. The data further highlight that CPTs who final accuracy check and spend over half their time engaged in the checking role. The data shows that few CPTs are working in leadership, management and/or training roles, and those who are, spend less than 20% of their time engaged in the role.

The interview data further support the above findings. Interviewee A, C and D's roles related mainly to the sale and supply of medicines, e.g., dispensing and stock management. Interviewee A also described a limited supervisory role, e.g., training new staff and overseeing workload when locum pharmacists are present, and Interviewee C undertook blood pressure checks periodically. In contrast, Interviewee B's role was split between final accuracy checking and supporting delivery of enhanced services, e.g., targeting appropriate patients and administration of the Medicines Use Review (MUR) service. Interviewee B also reported that they were accredited to deliver the Level 3 Smoking Cessation and appeared more involved in the professional aspects of this service.

Participants were asked whether they had previously worked as a dispenser, where 74 (89%) reported that they had. Of those, 64 participants provided further comments, where 13 (20%) reported little or no difference between the two roles, 3 (5%) reported no difference other than the final accuracy checking role and 48 (75%) described important differences. Differences mainly related to a change in level of responsibility, final accuracy checking role, greater knowledge to provide advice and deal with queries, involvement in training, leadership and management and more respect and value for the role.

> More responsibility and more respected as a team leader.
>
> (P83, large multiple, 2017)

> As a PT have the knowledge to answer questions / queries from customers with confidence.
>
> (P75, large multiple, 2005)

> The pharmacist starting delegating more responsible roles to me. The knowledge I gained was used more effectively and I was allowed to demonstrate how my competence had improved. I felt I was trusted with more responsibility, because I worked in a more professional manner.
>
> (P53, medium sized multiple, 2003)

> More responsibility—more involvement in problem solving.
>
> (P40, small chain, 2004)

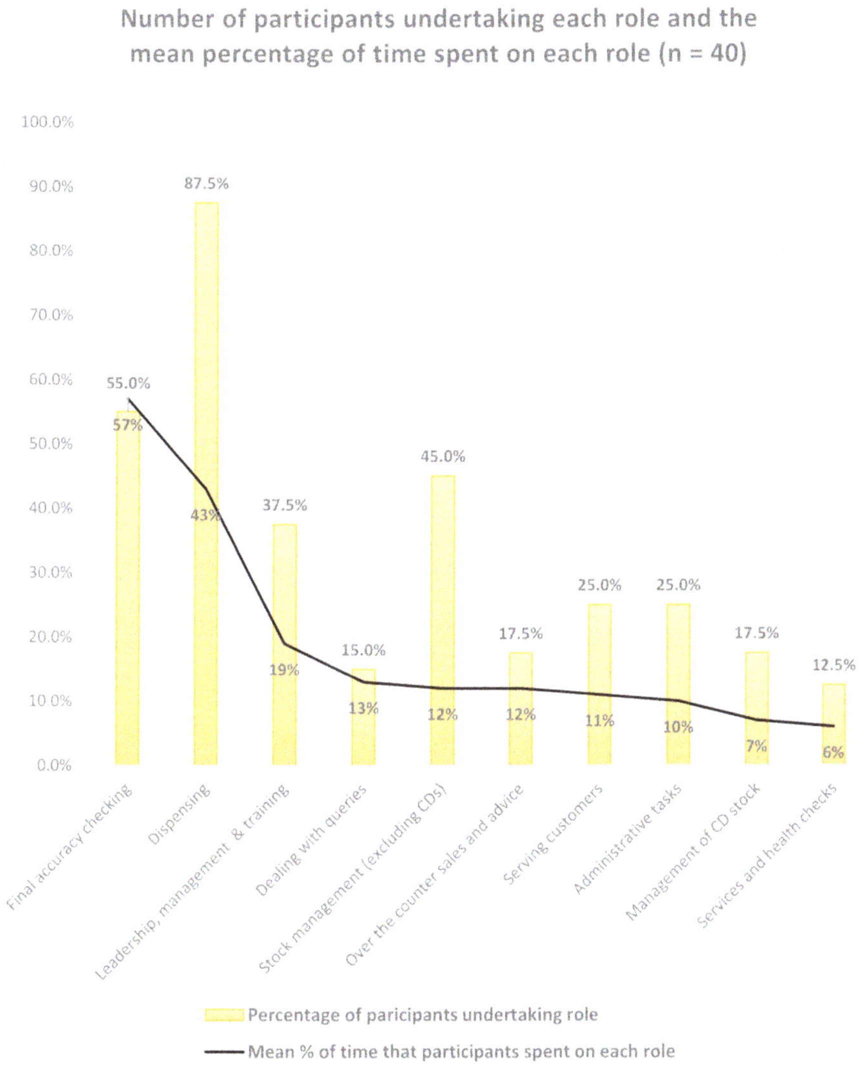

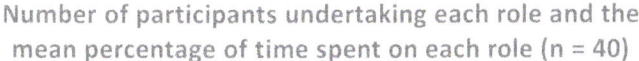

Figure 5. Number of participants and % of time spent undertaking each role.

3.3. Perceived Barriers and Enablers

Table 2 summarises the number of items, Cronbach Alpha, ranges, mid-points and scores for each of the five scales within the questionnaire. Each scale is illustrated and discussed further below.

Table 2. Summary of scale scores.

Scale	Number of Items	Cronbach's Alpha	Scale Range	Scale Mid-Point	% above Scale Mid-Point
Efficacy of Initial Training (scale 5 to 25)	5	0.775	7–25	15	68.7%
Colleagues Understanding of IET (scale 2–10)	2	0.703	2–10	6	43.4%
Workplace Support (scale 3–15)	3	0.663	3–15	9	72.7%
Professional Identity (scale 3–15)	3	0.700	5–15	9	88.0%
Delegation (scale 2–10)	2	0.666	2–10	6	68.7.%

Figure 6 presents participants' views about the efficacy of their initial education and training (Q27, 28, 29, 30 and 32R). The Cronbach alpha for the 'Efficacy of Initial Education and Training' scale was 0.775, with scores ranging from a minimum of 7 to a maximum of 25. The results indicate that two thirds of participants felt their initial training had enabled sufficient development of the knowledge and skills required of the pharmacy technician role, with 68.7% scoring above the mid-point scale score of 15.

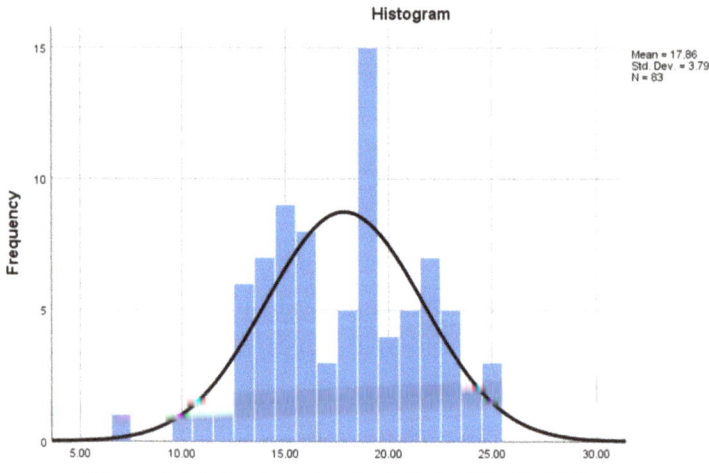

Figure 6. 'Efficacy of Initial Education and Training' scale scores.

Figure 7 presents participants' views on their colleagues' understanding of IET (Q33 and Q34). The Cronbach alpha for the 'Colleague Understanding of IET' scale was 0.703, with scores ranging from a minimum of 2 to a maximum of 10. The results show a wide range in scores, which suggests that there may be a lack of understanding around the IET curriculum and the role of a pre-registration pharmacy technician, with 43.4% scoring at or above the midpoint scale of 6.

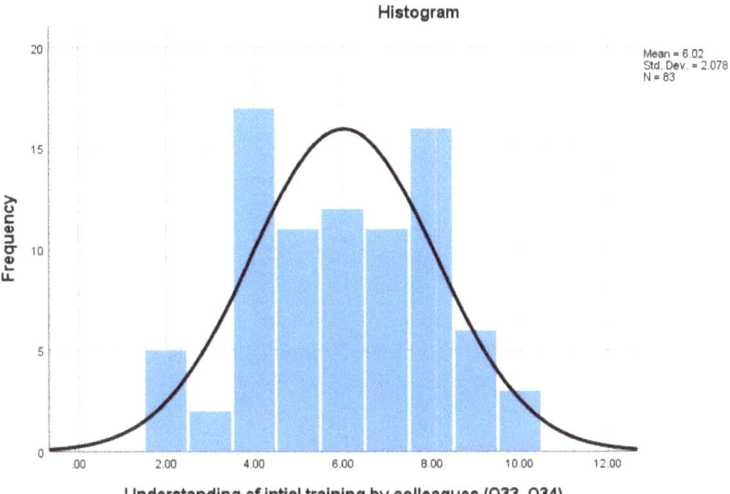

Figure 7. 'Colleague Understanding of IET' scale scores.

Participants were invited to make additional comments about their IET. Twenty-three participants provided qualitative comments and four themes were identified; the need to improve the relevance of IET and opportunities to apply it; the importance of experiential learning to develop skills; the need for workplace support and the challenges of learning in the workplace.

"Whilst interesting most of what I learnt for the NVQ 3 has never been used in my current position".

(P15, large multiple, 2002)

"The training was a base for a pharmacy tech, the skills needed are learnt through experience, it's not an easy job to do and definitely needs in depth training to fully cover all aspects of the job role".

(P49, large multiple, 2011)

"Would have liked an on-site visit to assess my work, found the assessment was not portraying my work, instead of paperwork through my course".

(P46, independent pharmacy, 2012)

Figure 8 presents participants' views about workplace support (Q11, Q12 and Q13). The Cronbach alpha for the 'Workplace Support' scale was 0.663, with scores ranging from a minimum of 3 to a maximum of 17. The results suggest that two thirds of participants felt supported in the workplace, with 72.7% scoring above the mid-point of 9. The results also indicated that CPTs receive most support from pharmacist colleagues and that a quarter ($n = 23$) of CPTs do not have PT colleagues in their workplace.

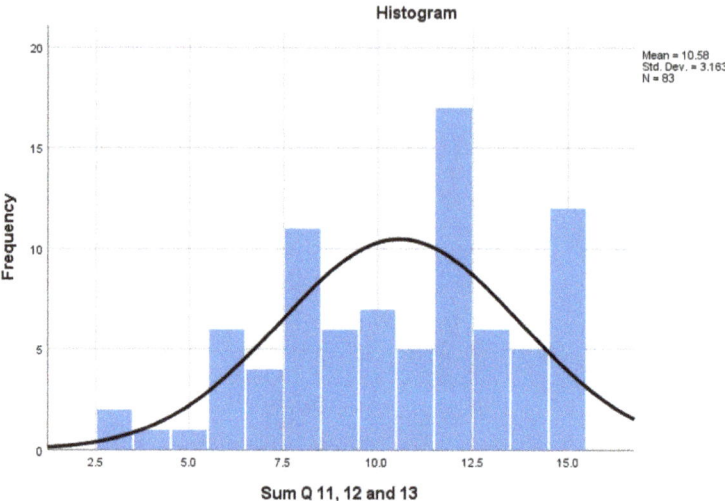

Figure 8. 'Workplace Support' scale scores.

Figure 9 reports participants' views on professional identity (Q15, Q16 and Q18). The Cronbach alpha for 'Professional Identity' was 0.700, with scores ranging from a minimum of 5 to a maximum of 15. The results suggest that the majority of CPTs have adopted a professional identity, with 88% scoring above the mid-point score of 9.

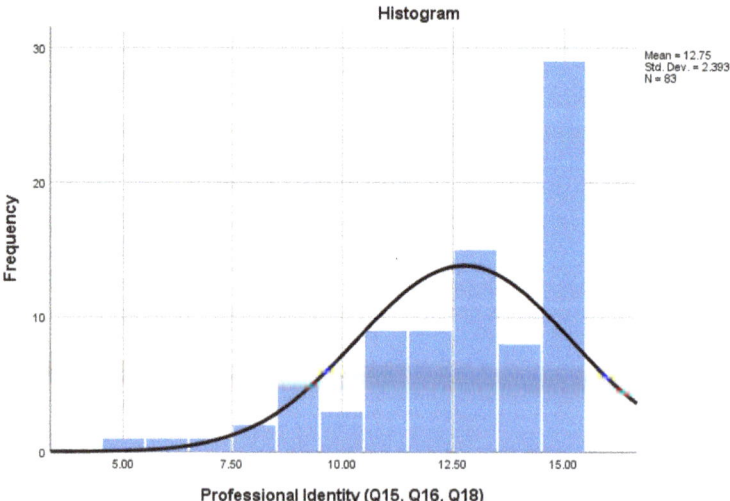

Figure 9. 'Professional Identity' scale scores.

Figure 10 illustrates participants' views on delegation in their workplace (Q20 and Q21). The Cronbach alpha for 'Delegation' was 0.666, with scores ranging from a minimum of 2 to a maximum of 10. The results suggest that although delegation is utilised there, there could be scope to utilise it more effectively, with 68.7% scoring at or above the mid-point score of 6. This is consistent with interview data, in which Interviewees A and D reported that only pharmacists or management staff delegate work, whereas Interviewees B and C reported that they could delegate unscheduled tasks. Interviewees C and D reported that Dispensers and PTs undertook similar tasks, though Interviewee C stated that the dispenser refers any issues to a PT. Interviewee A reported that the PT role was intended to focus on running the pharmacy, but in practice, they often ended up covering dispensers' role, e.g., retail sales. Interviewee B (independent pharmacy) stated,

> So the ACT dispense a lot less that what they used to, because we have people who dispense and then the ACTs do the checking. We—there's a lot more of a defined role now. I mean, I think we could still be better and there's still a lot we could do, but I think we're definitely moving in the right direction.

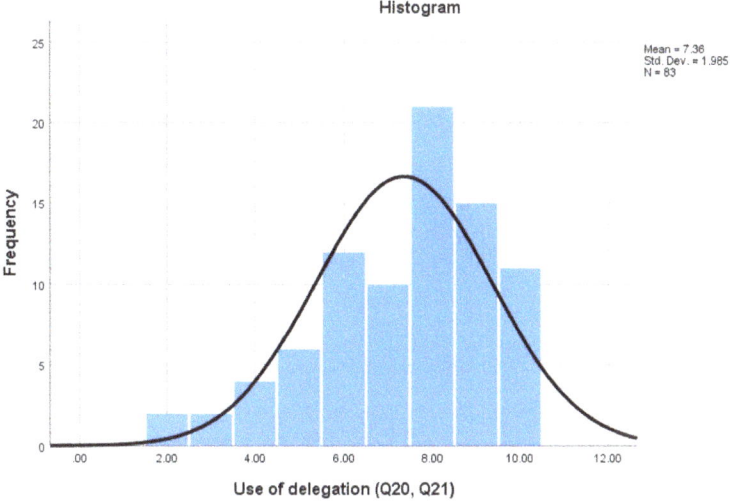

Figure 10. 'Delegation' scale data.

Participants were asked to describe factors which enabled them to undertake their role effectively. Fifty-three (64%) of participants provided qualitative responses and the main theme which emerged was support, i.e., team working, pharmacist support and managerial support. Adequate and on-going training was also highlighted.

> Support of the superintendent pharmacist which enables me to lead and develop my team.
>
> (P6, independent pharmacy, 2009)

> A strong supportive non-pharmacy manager plays a huge role in my pharmacy. Colleagues who work together in a very busy pharmacy.
>
> (P10, medium sized multiple, 2015)

> My pharmacy manager gives me the encouragement and confidence for me to undertake my role effectively.
>
> (P38, large multiple, 2016)

> Quality of training. The right person in the right task. Clean and efficient working environment. Good managerial team.
>
> (P66, large multiple, 2006)

> I have continual trading [training] from my pharmacist to ensure I'm up to date with what I'm checking.
>
> (P73, medium size multiple, 2001)

The interview data provided a contrasting picture, with all four interviewees reporting limited workplace support. Interviewees C and D suggested they accessed support from specific pharmacist colleagues with whom they had a good relationship, whereas Interviewees A and B suggested that the only guidance or support received was from SOPs and annual performance reviews, respectively.

Participants were also asked to describe factors which were barriers to them undertaking their roles effectively. Fifty-nine (71%) participants provided qualitative responses and two key themes were identified. The first was staffing issues, i.e., inadequate staffing and lack of qualified or competent staff. The second was business pressures, i.e., busy environment, insufficient time and the prioritisation of targets.

> We don't have enough staff for me to do my job role. I am the only qualified technician in our dispensary.
>
> (P7, large multiple, 2016)

> Enough staff to have more time to take on the roles I would like to do.
>
> (P36, large multiple, 2003)

> The pressure of a very busy pharmacy sometimes means you don't have enough time to interact with patients.
>
> (P9, large multiple, 1993)

> Pharmacists having to take on too many services. Not enough time for them to do any prescription checking.
>
> (P58, large multiple, 2002)

Finally, participants were asked to identify any roles which they felt confident to do but did not currently undertake. From the thirty-one qualitative responses, four key themes emerged; enhanced services (e.g., weight loss, stop smoking and medicines usage review); extended roles (e.g., final accuracy checking); training and development and counselling and advice. The reasons given for non-engagement in these roles included; lack of relevant training, lack of time, staff shortages, minimal pay increase, domain of the pharmacist, demands of repeat dispensing, automation of dispensing process, lapsed accreditation and health board restrictions.

> Offering weight loss service and stop smoking device [service] in pharmacy, unable to at present as not undertaken relevant training yet.
>
> (P77, independent pharmacy, 2013)

> More enhanced services, specifically DMR (discharge) and flu jabs. I see no reason why fully qualified technicians can't learn and provide the service. Also we should be carrying out MURs in the home to the patients who need more assistance. Technicians should somehow be able to assist with that and be able to do the home visits and the medicines management.
>
> (P60, independent pharmacy, 2008)

> There are lots of service roles that are aimed at pharmacists—no smoking, weight control etc. that both technicians or pharmacists could do but both are hampered by the continuous and increasing demands or repeat dispensing.
>
> (P56, independent pharmacy, 2009)

> Checking prescriptions which I can no longer do due to the introduction on [of] advance dispensing and robot dispensing.
>
> (P55, large multiple, 2002)

> Mentor staff when doing courses. I do this but only in a casual way. The pharmacist does this officially.
>
> (P45, independent pharmacy, 2001)

3.4. Relationship between Type of Pharmacy and Barriers and Enablers

There were no statistically significant differences between the category of pharmacy and the median responses to the sets of questions relating to efficacy of IET (H (df = 5) = 4.249, p = 0.514), colleague understanding of IET (H (df = 5) = 6.645, p = 0.248), workplace support (H (df = 5) = 6.751, p = 0.240), professional identity (H (df = 5) = 7.514, p = 0.185) and delegation (H (df = 5) = 4.410, p = 0.492).

4. Discussion

Survey responses provided data from across all categories of pharmacy and from CPTs, with varying educational backgrounds. The GPhC 'Survey of registered pharmacy professionals 2019' [25] provides data to suggest that the sample within this research could be considered representative of CPTs in Wales. The GPhC reported that 6% of the 23,506 registered PTs were resident in Wales (1410) and that 56% of PTs in Wales work in community pharmacy. This suggests there were 789 CPTs in Wales in 2019, which is consistent with the estimated sample size of 841 in 2018. The 2019 survey showed that 64% of CPTs in Wales accessed the register via the grandparent route, i.e., prior to 2011, which is comparable with the research sample in which over two-thirds of CPTs qualified prior to 2011. The average number of hours worked per week by CPTs in Wales in 2019 was reported as 32.4, which is broadly equivalent to the average reported in this study. The 2019 survey showed that 55% of CPTs in Wales worked in a large multiple and 20% in a small to medium chain; again, this is consistent with our findings, where over half worked in a large community pharmacy and a fifth worked in a small or medium sized chain. Finally, 57% of PTs across all sectors in Wales reported that they held an ACPT qualification—which was slightly higher (two-thirds) in our study sample. It is therefore reasonable to conclude that the research sample is representative of CPTs in Wales and therefore the results can be generalised to the wider population of CPTs in Wales.

The aim of this study was to explore the roles and responsibilities of CPTs in Wales and identify potential barriers and enablers to role development. In summary, the dispensing of medicines remains a core role for CPTs in Wales, despite there being opportunity to delegate the role to appropriately trained, non-registered support staff, which make up 64% full time equivalent (FTE) roles in community pharmacies in Wales [26]. This finding is consistent with Salameh et al.'s (2018) [27] exploratory study, in which all 16 PT participants reported dispensing as a day-to-day responsibility, and the recent 2019 GPhC survey [25], in which 85% of CPTs in Wales reported supplying medicines and medical devices as a main role. Failure to enable delegation of the dispensing process and fully utilise the skill mix within the pharmacy team, is a barrier to CPTs in Wales fulfilling their potential, even within their existing roles.

The results also suggest that final accuracy checking is becoming a core role and that ACPTs spend approximately half their time final accuracy checking. However, the data also suggest that not all trained ACPTs are being enabled to final accuracy check, often due to capacity issues. This finding is consistent with a recent workforce survey [26], which concluded that "the required opportunities and infrastructure should be made available to increase the percentage of community pharmacy technicians accredited to accuracy check prescriptions to match hospital levels over the next 3 years". Similarly, the data suggest that there is limited engagement in service-based roles, e.g., smoking cessation and inhaler techniques counselling, even when CPTs have completed the required training and there are data suggesting CPTs are willing to undertake these roles. These findings are consistent with Doucette and Schommer's [28] survey research, which found that insufficient staffing levels, insufficient time and lack of employer recognition for specialized skills, were barriers to PTs engaging in emerging tasks. These findings support the need for the community pharmacy sector in Wales to urgently address the capacity issues which are a current barrier to CPTs engaging in roles which they are trained and/or are willing to be trained to undertake. Taking these measures would support the Welsh Government's vision of localised delivery of public health and clinical services.

There is evidence of an explicit career pathway, from Dispenser to PT in the community pharmacy sector in Wales. In 2018, the Welsh Government announced a commitment to support the education of up to two hundred PRPTs over three years and community pharmacy contractors were invited to nominate suitable candidates—it is likely that this funding will continue to support the development of dispensers to PTs [29]. The data suggest that many PTs recognise important differences between the two roles in terms of responsibility, knowledge required and respect or value for the PT role—this is a marked divergence from existing research [12,27]. The majority of participants previously worked as dispensers, and despite this, they appear to have transitioned and adopted a professional identity. Salameh et al. (2018) [27] found that professional identity formation was one of four key areas required to optimise the PT role in the community sector, hence these results are encouraging in terms of laying the foundations for future role development.

The existing IET appears to be sufficient to support the foundation PT role, with the majority of PTs reporting that their initial training enabled them to undertake their role on day one. IET could be further improved by ensuring the curriculum accurately reflects the PT role, placing a greater emphasis on experiential learning and improving workplace support for PRPTs. What appears to be more of a barrier is the lack of understanding of the IET and/or the role of a pre-registration pharmacy technician (PRPT) by colleagues. This could be related to the use of distance learning courses, where PRPT training is often facilitated by a single pharmacist who may review work and/or act as an expert witness, but where summative assessment decisions are made by external assessors employed by the education provider [12]. The new combined qualification which is currently being introduced [30], must meet the GPhC (2017) revised standards for IET [31], which state that systems must enable PRPTs to meet regularly with colleagues to review and document their progress. Similarly, the GPhC 'Guidance on tutoring and supervising pharmacy professionals in training' [32] explicitly states that a designated educational supervisor must have oversight of training and assessment in the workplace, overall responsibility for supervision and sign the final supervisory declaration. The new qualification standards allow PRPT training to be supervised by a PT, not just a pharmacist, as was previously the case. It is hoped that the new standards will improve colleague engagement and understanding of the IET curriculum and the PRPT role, which could lead to increased confidence in PT competencies and facilitate more informed decision making around the use of delegation and potential PT roles.

Despite some conflicts within the data, it does appear that workplace support is an important enabler for CPTs, particularly support from pharmacists and managers. The support provided appears to be informal in nature, e.g., encouragement and confidence building, and often provided by colleagues with whom the CPT has a good working relationship. Whilst this could be sufficient to support CPTs within their existing roles, CPTs would benefit from access to more formal support in the workplace, such as mentoring or peer support, to enable them to further develop their roles with confidence.

This study has several limitations. The questionnaire data did not include the participants' age or gender. The authors acknowledge that gender could be considered a relevant factor, as 90% of the PT profession are female [22], whilst noting that the gender of the interviewees was balanced. The quality of data could have been affected by recall bias, when participants were asked to report on their practice as a 'day one' pharmacy technician and their career since. It may also have been affected by the willingness of participants to report on some topics, e.g., being open about the barriers experienced [33]. The validity of the survey data could have been affected by non-response bias, though the authors note that the 2019 GPhC study [25] yielded a 25% response rate for PTs in Wales across all sectors (not just community sector), and this highlights the difficulty in reaching this population. Although the response rate is low, this is consistent with those of similar studies with PTs. However, the authors acknowledge that care should be taken when generalising these findings. Due to the limited volume of research into PT roles in Wales, or indeed the UK, there was little opportunity to use previously validated questions. The wording of one question, 'Which role/s did your further training enable you to undertake' was potentially ambiguous. The word 'enable' could have been interpreted as competence and/or confidence to undertake the role, or as opportunities to undertake the role within the workplace. The limitations of Likert scales include the assumption that subjective data can be quantified and that intervals on a Likert scale are equally spaced. The issue of quantifying subjective data was addressed to some degree, by the inclusion of free text boxes, to enable participants to provide further context [20]. The questionnaire was purposely designed to enable participants to describe their role in their own words, rather than compelling participants to select roles from a pre-determined list. However, the use of open-ended questions is a known factor in survey fatigue [34] and may have affected completion rates. The questionnaire was also designed to quantify the amount of time participants spent undertaking each role, to identify core roles and responsibilities. Unfortunately, under half of respondents completed this section correctly. Some participants simply did not assign a percentage to each role, whereas other participants assigned percentages which did not add up to 100%. The erroneous responses had to be omitted from the analysis of this section, which reduced the reliability of the data.

The authors recognise that the validity of the interview data may be compromised by the low response rate and note that time constraints did not allow for further recruitment of participants. Telephone interviews present specific challenges for researchers; e.g., the sample of participants who are accessible via telephone may not be representative, it may be more challenging to develop a rapport with participants over the telephone [35], participant responses may be affected by the perceived anonymity that distance provides, researchers cannot use visual aids and neither party has access to non-verbal language and cues [36].

The lead author and interviewer (RC) is a PT and acknowledged that their experiential knowledge of the profession shaped their approach to the research, e.g., the barriers and enablers explored. RC also considered the potential impact of 'role power' and was careful to differentiate the research from other employed roles. To avoid a one-way discourse during the interviews, a semi-structured interview format was favoured.

An alternative approach to undertaking this research may have been to observe CPTs in the workplace, or to conduct more in-depth interviews to establish core roles. This approach would also have enabled further exploration of how professional identities are developed, which was beyond the scope of this study, but could highlight another important area for further qualitative research. The scope of this study was limited by time and resources; however, it is recognised that future research would benefit from the inclusion of pharmacist perspectives, particularly around the issues of delegation and efficacy of IET.

This study has been circulated internally at the General Pharmaceutical Council (GPhC) to individuals working in education, policy, revalidation, communications and insight, intelligence and inspection. At the time of writing, the outcomes of this are as yet unknown. The study has also been shared with the Pharmacy Dean at Health Education and Improvement Wales (HEIW) and the Chief Pharmaceutical Officer for Wales. The study has been referenced within HEIW's Wales Community Pharmacy Workforce Survey 2019 [26].

5. Recommendations and Conclusions

The findings of this study indicate that CPTs' knowledge and skills are not being utilised to the full extent even within existing roles. There is also evidence to suggest that CPTs are willing and able to undertake extended roles such as smoking cessation services, if they are enabled to do so. If the Welsh Government's vision for community pharmacy services is to be fully realised, the existing potential of the PT workforce within Wales must be recognised and the further development of PT roles must be prioritised. Whilst the ability to make firm conclusions is limited by the small response rate, there are a number of recommendations that could be taken forward, based on these findings. These are:

1. Community pharmacy employers and stakeholders should recognise the potential of the CPT workforce and address the barriers to optimisation of the current CPT role in Wales.

2. Community pharmacy employers and stakeholders should prioritise the training and development of CPTs and enable them to undertake extended roles, which will support the future delivery of pharmacy services in Wales.
3. Following the introduction of the new IET standards and guidance on tutoring, the GPhC should explore the impact of the standards and guidance on the training experiences of PRPTs and the understanding of the IET requirements by the wider pharmacy team.
4. Further qualitative research into the CPT workforce in Wales should include further exploration of time spent on specific roles, and the exploration of how professional identities are developed, as well as the views of pharmacists on issues such as the delegation and efficacy of IET.

Supplementary Materials: The following are available online at http://www.mdpi.com/2226-4787/8/2/97/s1, Participant Interview Schedule.

Author Contributions: Conceptualization, R.C. and J.H; Methodology, R.C., J.H. and D.J.; Validation; D.J.; Data curation, R.C. and D.J.; Formal analysis, R.C. and D.J.; Investigation, R.C.; Supervision, J.H. and D.J.; Writing—original draft, R.C. and D.J.; Writing—review and editing, R.C., J.H. and D.J. All authors have read and agreed to the published version of the manuscript.

Funding: This research received no external funding. Funding for the academic Master's fees was received from the Wales Centre for Professional Pharmacy Education, Cardiff University (prior to transfer to Health Education and Improvement Wales).

Acknowledgments: The authors would like to acknowledge the contributions of the pharmacy technicians who participated in this study.

Conflicts of Interest: The authors declare no conflict of interest.

References

1. Welsh Government. A Healthier Wales: Our Plan for Health and Social Care. 2018. Available online: https://www.basw.co.uk/system/files/resources/180608healthier-wales-mainen.pdf (accessed on 4 March 2020).
2. Welsh Government. Written Statement Community Pharmacy Funding 2017-18 and beyond. 2017. Available online: https://gov.wales/written-statement-community-pharmacy-funding-2017-18-and-beyond (accessed on 4 March 2020).
3. Robinson, J. Diverging community pharmacy practice across the four UK nations. *Pharm J.* **2017**, *299*. [CrossRef]
4. Welsh Government. Written Statement Delivering Prudent Healthcare within Wales. 2014. Available online: https://gov.wales/written-statement-delivering-prudent-healthcare-wales (accessed on 4 March 2020).
5. General Pharmaceutical Council. Annual Report 2016-2017. 2018. Available online: https://www.pharmacyregulation.org/sites/default/files/gphc_annual_report_2016-17.pdf (accessed on 1 October 2018).
6. General Pharmaceutical Council. Criteria for Registration as a Pharmacy Technician. 2013. Available online: https://www.pharmacyregulation.org/sites/default/files/Registration%20criteria%20for%20pharmacy%20technicians%20May%202013.pdf (accessed on 28 November 2019).
7. Bradley, F.; Willia, S.C.; Noyce, P.R.; Schafheutle, E.I. Restructuring supervision and reconfiguration of skill mix in community pharmacy: Classification of perceived safety and risk. *Res. Soc. Admin. Pharm.* **2016**, *12*, 733–746. [CrossRef] [PubMed]
8. General Pharmaceutical Council. Tomorrow's Pharmacy Team, Future Standards for the Initial Education and Training of Pharmacists, Pharmacy Technicians and Pharmacy Support Staff. 2015. Available online: https://www.pharmacyregulation.org/sites/default/files/tomorrows_pharmacy_team_june_2015.pdf (accessed on 1 October 2018).
9. John, C.; Brown, A. Technicians and other pharmacy support workforce cadres working with pharmacists: United Kingdom Case Study. *Res. Soc. Admin. Pharm.* **2017**, *13*, 297–299. [CrossRef] [PubMed]

10. Howe, H.; Wilson, K. (2012) Modernising Pharmacy Careers Programme. Review of Post-Registration Career Development of Pharmacists and Pharmacy Technicians, Background Pape. 2012. Available online: http://docplayer.net/3056835-%C2%AD%E2%80%90Modernising-%C2%AD%E2%80%90pharmacy-%C2%AD%E2%80%90careers-%C2%AD%E2%80%90programme-%C2%AD%E2%80%90review-%C2%AD%E2%80%90of-%C2%AD%E2%80%90post-%C2%AD%E2%80%90registration-%C2%AD%E2%80%90career-%C2%AD%E2%80%90development-%C2%AD%E2%80%90of-%C2%AD%E2%80%90pharmacists-%C2%AD%E2%80%90and-%C2%AD%E2%80%90pharmacy-%C2%AD%E2%80%90technicians.html (accessed on 11 September 2018).
11. Boughen, M.; Fenn, T.; Croot, J.; Frost, K.; Family, H.; Wright, D.; Sutton, J. Identifying the Roles of Pharmacy Technicians in the UK, Final Report, September 2016. Available online: https://www.uea.ac.uk/documents/899297/15294873/Identifying+The+Role+Of+Pharmacy+Technicians+In+The+UK/d6d60e7b-f527-481a-8f16-9f3f04037b6c (accessed on 1 October 2018).
12. Schafheutle, E.I.; Jee, S.D.; Willis, S.C. The influence of learning environments on trainee pharmacy technicians' education and training experiences. *Res. Soc. Admin. Pharm.* **2018**, *14*, 1020–1026. [CrossRef] [PubMed]
13. Mattingly, A.N.; Mattingly, T.J. Advancing the role of the pharmacy technician: A systematic review. *JAPhA* **2018**, *58*, 94–108. [CrossRef] [PubMed]
14. Desselle, S.P.; Hoh, R.; Holmes, E.R.; Gill, A.; Zamora, L. Pharmacy Technician self-efficacies: Insight to aid future education, staff development, and workforce planning. *Res. Soc. Admin. Pharm.* **2018**, *14*, 581–588. [CrossRef] [PubMed]
15. Koehler, T.; Brown, A. A global picture of pharmacy technician and other pharmacy support workforce cadres. *Res. Soc. Admin. Pharm.* **2017**, *13*, 271–279. [CrossRef] [PubMed]
16. Welsh Government. A Healthier Wales: Our Plan for Health and Social Care. 2019. Available online: https://gov.wales/sites/default/files/publications/2019-10/a-healthier-wales-action-plan.pdf (accessed on 2 March 2020).
17. Bryman, A. *Soc. Research Methods*, 5th ed.; Oxford University Press: Oxford, UK, 2016.
18. British Educational Research Association Ethical Guidelines for Educational Research. Available online: https://www.bera.ac.uk/wp-content/uploads/2014/02/BERA-Ethical-Guidelines-2011.pdf?noredirect=1 (accessed on 22 September 2018).
19. Bowling, A. Quantitative Social Science: The survey. In *Handbook of Health Research Methods*; Bowling, A., Ebrahim, S., Eds.; Open University Press: Berkshire, UK, 2005.
20. Rattray, J.; Jones, M.C. Essential elements of questionnaire design and development. *J. Clin. Nurse* **2007**, *16*, 234–243. [CrossRef] [PubMed]
21. Miller, R.L.; Brewer, J.D. *The A-Z of Soc. Research*; SAGE Publications Ltd.: London, UK, 2007.
22. Seston, L.; Hassell, K. Briefing Paper: GPhC Pharmacy Technician Register Analysis 2012. Available online: https://www.pharmacyregulation.org/sites/default/files/document/gphc-pharmacy-technician-register-analysis-2012.pdf (accessed on 1 October 2018).
23. General Pharmaceutical Council. Registrant Survey 2013, Initial Analysis. 2014. Available online: https://www.pharmacyregulation.org/sites/default/files/gphc_registrant_survey_2013_initial_analysis.pdf (accessed on 4 July 2018).
24. Cohen, L.; Manion, L.; Morrison, K. *Research Methods in Education*; Routledge: Abingdon, UK, 2011.
25. General Pharmaceutical Council. Survey of Registered Pharmacy Professionals 2019. Available online: https://www.pharmacyregulation.org/sites/default/files/document/gphc-2019-survey-pharmacy-professionals-main-report-2019.pdf (accessed on 16 February 2018).
26. Health Education and Improvement Wales (HEIW). *(2020) Wales Community Workforce Survey Report 2019*; Health Education and Improvement Wales (HEIW): Nantgarw, Wales; p. 50, (Unpublished report).
27. Salameh, L.; Yeung, D.; Surkic, N.; Gregory, P.; Austin, Z. Facilitating integration of regulated pharmacy technicians into community pharmacy practice in Ontario: Results of an exploratory study. *CPJ* **2018**, *151*, 189–196. [CrossRef] [PubMed]
28. Doucette, W.R.; Schommer, J.C. Pharmacy Technicians' Willingness to Perform Emerging Tasks in Community Practice. *Pharmacy* **2018**, *6*. [CrossRef] [PubMed]

29. Allan, M.; (Director, Wales Centre for Pharmacy Professional Education). Letter to: Community Pharmacy Wales. 1 leaf. Available online: http://www.cpwales.org.uk/getattachment/Services-and-commissioning/Workforce-Development/Pharmacy-Technician-training/PRPT-Letter-to-CPW-Aug18.pdf.aspx?lang=en-GB (accessed on 31 August 2018).
30. General Pharmaceutical Council. Approved Pharmacy Technician Courses 2019. Available online: https://www.pharmacyregulation.org/education/pharmacy-technician/accredited-courses (accessed on 27 April 2020).
31. General Pharmaceutical Council. Standards for the Initial Education and Training of Pharmacy Technicians. 2017. Available online: https://www.pharmacyregulation.org/sites/default/files/standards_for_the_initial_education_and_training_of_pharmacy_technicians_october_2017.pdf (accessed on 1 March 2020).
32. General Pharmaceutical Council. Guidance on Tutoring and Supervising Pharmacy Professionals in Training. 2018. Available online: https://www.pharmacyregulation.org/sites/default/files/document/guidance_on_supervising_pharmacy_professionals_in_training_august_2018.pdf (accessed on 3 March 2020).
33. Alderman, A.K.; Salem, B. Survey Research. *Plast. Reconstr. Surg.* **2010**, *126*. [CrossRef] [PubMed]
34. O'Reilly-Shah, V.N. Factors influencing healthcare provider respondent fatigue answering a globally administered in-app survey. *Peer J.* **2017**, *5*, e3785. [CrossRef] [PubMed]
35. Hughes, M. Interviewing. In *Research Methods for Postgraduate*; Greenfield, T., Ed.; Arnold: London, UK, 2002; pp. 209–217.
36. Block, E.S.; Erskine, L. Interviewing by Telephone: Specific Considerations, Opportunities and Challenges. *Int. J. Qual. Methods* **2012**, *11*. [CrossRef]

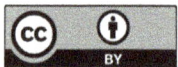

© 2020 by the authors. Licensee MDPI, Basel, Switzerland. This article is an open access article distributed under the terms and conditions of the Creative Commons Attribution (CC BY) license (http://creativecommons.org/licenses/by/4.0/).

MDPI
St. Alban-Anlage 66
4052 Basel
Switzerland
Tel. +41 61 683 77 34
Fax +41 61 302 89 18
www.mdpi.com

Pharmacy Editorial Office
E-mail: pharmacy@mdpi.com
www.mdpi.com/journal/pharmacy

www.ingramcontent.com/pod-product-compliance
Lightning Source LLC
Chambersburg PA
CBHW051618020226
39067CB00061B/125